Essentials of Nursing Leadership and Management

Fourth Edition

Essentials of Nursing Leadership and Management

Fourth Edition

DIANE K. WHITEHEAD, EdD, RN
Department Chair and Professor
Nova Southeastern University Nursing Department
Fort Lauderdale, Florida

SALLY A. WEISS, RN, EdD
Program Coordinator and Professor
Nova Southeastern University Nursing Department
Fort Lauderdale, Florida

RUTH M. TAPPEN, EdD, RN, FAAN
Christine E. Lynn Eminent Scholar and Professor
Florida Atlantic University College of Nursing
Boca Raton, Florida

 F. A. DAVIS COMPANY • Philadelphia

F. A. Davis Company
1915 Arch Street
Philadelphia, PA 19103
www.fadavis.com

Printed in the United States of America.

Last digit indicates print number: 10 9 8 7 6 5 4 3 2

Publisher: Joanne P. DaCunha, RN, MSN
Developmental Editor: Kristin L. Kern
Manager of Art & Design: Carolyn O'Brien

As new scientific information becomes available through basic and clinical research, recommended treatments and drug therapies undergo changes. The author(s) and publisher have done everything possible to make this book accurate, up to date, and in accord with accepted standards at the time of publication. The author(s), editors, and publisher are not responsible for errors or omissions or for consequences from application of the book, and make no warranty, expressed or implied, in regard to the contents of the book. Any practice described in this book should be applied by the reader in accordance with professional standards of care used in regard to the unique circumstances that may apply in each situation. The reader is advised always to check product information (package inserts) for changes and new information regarding dose and contraindications before administering any drug. Caution is especially urged when using new or infrequently ordered drugs.

Library of Congress Cataloging-in-Publication Data

Whitehead, Diane K., 1945-
Essentials of nursing leadership and management / Diane K. Whitehead,
Sally A. Weiss, Ruth M. Tappen. — 4th ed.
p. ; cm.
Tappen's name appears first on the previous edition.
Includes bibliographical references and index.
ISBN-10: 0-8036-1568-X (alk. paper)
ISBN-13: 978-0-8036-1568-7
1. Nursing services—Administration. 2. Leadership. I. Weiss, Sally A.,
1950-. II. Tappen, Ruth M. III. Title.
[DNLM: 1. Nursing—United States. 2. Leadership—United States.
3. Nursing Services—organization & administration—United States.
WY 16 T175e 2006]
RT89.T357 2006
362.1′73068—dc22
2006012801

Dedication

To our students, colleagues, and mentors who continue to enrich our lives.

To our families for the joy they bring to our lives.

preface

We are delighted to bring our readers this Fourth Edition of *Essentials of Nursing Leadership and Management*. The Fourth Edition has been updated to reflect the current health-care environment. The content, examples, and diagrams were designed with the goal of assisting the new graduate to make the transition to professional nursing practice.

This textbook focuses on the staff nurse as a vital member of the health-care team and manager of patient care. As a manager of care, the staff nurse must have the knowledge and skills necessary to make decisions on setting priorities, delegation, quality improvement, legal parameters of nursing practice, and ethical issues confronting nursing today. These issues are presented with up-to-date information and relevant examples.

We continue to bring you comprehensive, practical information on developing a nursing career. Based on input from our students, faculty, and reviewers, we have separated the leader and manager chapters and emphasized the understanding of followership. Workplace issues such as change, conflict management, client and workplace safety, stress, burnout, and cultural diversity are addressed in an easy-to-understand style. We have included many of the issues surrounding compliance and regulation facing health-care institutions today. It is our hope that this textbook will assist new graduates in developing their professional roles in the ever-changing health-care environment.

We realize that the demand for new graduates to have a basic understanding of health-care finance is increasing. Included in this edition is an optional chapter on the financial environment of health care. Topics included in this chapter include financial trends, legal and ethical issues that impact costs, financial viability of health-care organizations, basic budgeting and financial skills for nurses, and personnel cost issues and calculation of FTEs. This chapter is available on the FA Davis Web site.

We would like to thank the people at F.A. Davis for their assistance and our colleagues, reviewers, and students for their helpful suggestions.

Diane K. Whitehead
Sally A. Weiss
Ruth Tappen

Gerri Althenn-LaBonte, RN, MN
CCRN
Nursing Division Faculty
Greenville Technical College
Greenville, South Carolina

Edna M. Berg, RN, BScN, Med
Faculty/Coordinator of Theory Courses
Grant McEwan College
Edmonton, Alberta, Canada

Rosalinda Haddon, RN, BSN, MA
Assistant Clinical Professor
Northern Arizona University
Flagstaff, Arizona

Pamela Harrison, TN, MS, EdD,
APRN-BC
Associate Professor
Indiana Wesleyan University
Marion, Indiana

Beth Hickey, RN, MSN, CCRN
Assistant Professor
Northern Kentucky University
Highland Heights, Kentucky

Joan C. Martin, RN, MN
Assistant Professor of Nursing
Central Missouri State University
North Kansas City, Missouri

Kathleen Stroh, RN, MSN
Assistant Professor
Edinboro University of Pennsylvania
Edinboro, Pennsylvania

Jean Ternus, RN, MS
Nursing Professor
Kansas City Community College
Kansas City, Kansas

Sonia Ann Udod, RN, MN, PhD(c)
Lecturer
University of Manitoba
Winnipeg, Manitoba, Canada

Michelle Willihnganz, RN, MS
Nursing Instructor
Rochester Community and Technical College
Rochester, Minnesota

contents

Professional Considerations

Leadership and Followership

OBJECTIVES

After reading this chapter, the student should be able to:

◆ Define the terms *leadership* and *followership*.

◆ Discuss the importance of effective leadership and followership for the new nurse.

◆ Discuss the qualities and behaviors that contribute to effective followership.

◆ Discuss the qualities and behaviors that contribute to effective leadership.

OUTLINE

CHAPTER 1 SELF-ASSESSMENT
Are You Ready to Be a Leader?

Before you read this chapter, evaluate your current Leadership Quotient. How often do you...

1. Critically analyze new information or opinions you encounter:
   Never _____ Every once in a while _____ Sometimes _____ Often _____

2. Provide positive feedback to classmates, colleagues, coworkers:
   Never _____ Every once in a while _____ Sometimes _____ Often _____

3. Provide negative feedback to classmates, colleagues, coworkers:
   Never _____ Every once in a while _____ Sometimes _____ Often _____

4. Talk about your vision for the future:
   Never _____ Every once in a while _____ Sometimes _____ Often _____

5. Initiate discussion of a problem or misunderstanding:
   Never _____ Every once in a while _____ Sometimes _____ Often _____

6. Pursue new learning opportunities:
   Never _____ Every once in a while _____ Sometimes _____ Often _____

You will read about each of the above leadership actions and more in this chapter.

Nurses work with an extraordinary variety of people: doctors, respiratory therapists, physical therapists, social workers, psychologists, technicians, aides, unit managers, housekeepers, clients, and clients' families.

The reason why we study leadership is to learn how to work well, or *effectively*, with other people. In this chapter, we define *leadership* and *followership* and the relationships between them. We also discuss the characteristics and behaviors that can make you an effective leader and follower.

LEADERSHIP

Are You Ready to Be a Leader?

You may be thinking, "I'm just beginning my career in nursing. How can you expect me to be a leader now?" This is an important question. You will need time to refine your clinical skills and learn how to function in a new environment. But you can begin to assume some leadership right away within your new nursing roles. Consider the following example:

Billie Blair Thomas is a new staff nurse at Green Valley Nursing Care Center. After orientation, she was assigned to a rehabilitation unit with high admission and discharge rates. Billie noticed that admissions and discharges were assigned rather haphazardly. Anyone who was "free" at the moment was directed to handle them. Sometimes, unlicensed assistant personnel were directed to admit or discharge residents. Billie believed that using them was inappropriate because their assessment skills were limited and they had no training in discharge planning.

Billie thought there was a better way to do this but was not sure that she should say so because she was so new. "Maybe they've already thought of this," she said to a former classmate. "It's such an obvious solution." They began to talk about what they had learned in their leadership course before graduation. "I just keep hearing our instructor saying, 'There's only one manager, but anyone can be a leader of our group.'"

"If you want to be a leader, you have to act on your idea," her friend said.

"Maybe I will," Billie replied.

Billie decided to speak with her nurse manager, an experienced rehabilitation nurse who seemed not only approachable but also open to new ideas. "I have been so busy getting our new record system on line before the surveyors come that I wasn't paying attention to that," the nurse manager told her. "I'm so glad you brought it to my attention."

Billie's nurse manager raised the issue at the next executive meeting, giving credit to Billie for having brought it to her attention. The other nurse managers had the same response. "We were so focused on the new record system that we overlooked that. We need to take care of this situation as soon as possible. Billie Blair Thomas has leadership potential."

Leadership Defined

The essence of leadership is the *ability to influence other people*. Effective leaders enable people to move "in the same direction, toward the same destination, at the same speed, not because they have been forced to, but because they want to" (Lansdale, 2002, p. 63). The three primary tasks of a leader in health care are to help people:

◆ Develop a sense of direction and purpose.
◆ Build the group's commitment to its goals.
◆ Face the numerous challenges that arise in a health care setting (Drath, 2001). See Table 1-1.

Effective nurse leaders are those who engage others to work together effectively in pursuit of a shared goal. Examples of shared goals are providing excellent client care, designing a cost-saving procedure, and challenging the ethics of a new policy.

▚ FOLLOWERSHIP

Followership and leadership are separate but reciprocal roles. Without followers, one cannot be a leader; conversely, one cannot be a follower without a leader (Lyons, 2002).

TABLE 1-1
Three Primary Tasks of a Leader in Health Care
1. Set direction: Mission, goals, vision, purpose
2. Build commitment: Motivation, spirit, teamwork
3. Confront challenges: Innovation, change, turbulence

Adapted from Drath, W. (2001). *The Deep Blue Sea.* San Francisco: Jossey-Bass.

Being an effective follower is as important to the new nurse as is being an effective leader. In fact, most of the time most of us are followers: members of a team, attendees at a meeting, staff of a care nursing care unit, and so forth.

Followership Defined

Followership is not a passive role. On the contrary, the most valuable follower (team member, staff nurse, etc.) is a skilled, self-directed employee, one who participates actively in setting the group's direction, invests his or her time and energy in the work of the group, thinks critically, and advocates for new ideas (Grossman & Valiga, 2000). Imagine working on a client care unit where all staff members, from the unit secretary to the assistant nurse manager, willingly take on extra tasks without being asked (Spreitzer & Quinn, 2001), come back early from coffee breaks, complete their charting on time, suggest ways to improve client care, and are proud of the high quality care they provide. Wouldn't it be wonderful to be a part of that team?

Becoming a Better Follower

There are a number of things you can do to become a better follower:

◆ If you discover a problem, inform your team leader or manager right away. Even better, include a suggestion for solving the problem in your report.
◆ Freely invest your interest and energy in your work.
◆ Be supportive of new ideas and new directions suggested by others.
◆ When you disagree, explain why you do not support an idea or suggestion.
◆ Listen carefully, and reflect on what your leader or manager says.
◆ Continue to learn as much as you can about your specialty area.
◆ Share what you learn with others.

Being an effective follower will not only make you a more valuable employee but also increase the meaning and satisfaction you can get from your work.

Most, but not all, team leaders and nurse managers will respond very positively to having staff who are good followers. Occasionally, you will encounter a poor leader or manager who can confuse, frustrate, and even distress you. Here are a few suggestions for handling this:

◆ Continue to do your best work and to provide leadership for the rest of the group.

◆ Avoid adopting the ineffective behaviors of this individual.

◆ If the situation worsens, enlist the support of others on your team to seek a remedy; do not try to do this alone as a new graduate.

◆ If the situation becomes intolerable, consider the option of transferring to another unit or seeking another position (Deutschman, 2005; Korn, 2004).

WHAT MAKES A PERSON A LEADER?

Leadership Theories

There are many different ideas about how a person becomes a good leader. Despite years of research on this subject, none has emerged as the clear winner. The reason for this may be that different qualities and behaviors are most important in different situations. In nursing, for example, some situations require quick thinking and fast action. Others require some time to figure out the best solution to a complicated problem. Different leadership qualities and behaviors are needed in these two instances. The result is that there is not yet a single best answer to the question: "What makes a person a leader?"

Let's look now at some of the best-known leadership theories and the many qualities and behaviors that have been identified as those of the effective nurse leader (Pavitt, 1999; Tappen, 2001).

Trait Theories

At one time or another, you have probably heard someone say, "Leaders are born, not made." In other words, some of us are natural leaders but others of us are not. In reality, leadership may come more easily to some of us than to others, but every one of us can be a leader, given the necessary knowledge and skill.

Many of the early research studies on leadership attempted to identify the qualities, or *traits*, that distinguish a leader from a nonleader. The traits most often identified are:

◆ Intelligence.

◆ Initiative.

Other qualities that were found to be associated with leadership are:

◆ Excellent interpersonal skills.

◆ High self-esteem.

◆ Creativity.

◆ Willingness to take risks.

◆ Ability to tolerate the consequences of taking risks.

Although these theories were focused on characteristics of a leader, they do hint at common behaviors of good leaders.

Behavioral Theories

The behavioral theories are concerned with what the leader does. One of the most influential theories is concerned with leadership style (White & Lippitt, 1960) (Table 1-2).

The three styles are:

◆ **Autocratic leadership** (also called *directive, controlling,* or *authoritarian*). The autocratic leader gives orders and makes decisions for the group as a whole. For example, when a decision needs to be made, an autocratic leader says, "I've given this a great deal of thought and decided that this is the way we're going to solve our problem." Although this is an efficient way to run things, it usually dampens creativity and may inhibit motivation.

◆ **Democratic leadership** (also called *participative*). Democratic leaders share leadership. Important plans and decisions are made jointly with the rest of the team (Chrispeels, 2004). Although this is often a less efficient way to run things, it is more

	Autocratic	Democratic	Laissez-Faire
TABLE 1-2 **Comparison of Autocratic, Democratic, and Laissez-Faire Leadership Styles**			
Degree of freedom	Little freedom	Moderate freedom	Much freedom
Degree of control	High control	Moderate control	Little control
Decision making	By the leader	Leader and group together	By the group or by no one
Leader activity level	High	High	Minimal
Assumption of responsibility	Leader	Shared	Abdicated
Output of the group	High quantity, good quality	Creative, high quality	Variable, may be poor quality
Efficiency	Very efficient	Less efficient than auto-cratic style	Inefficient

Adapted from White, R.K., & Lippitt, R. (1960). *Autocracy and Democracy: An Experimental Inquiry.* New York: Harper & Row.

flexible and usually increases motivation and creativity. Democratic leadership is characterized by guidance from the leader rather than control by the leader.

◆ **Laissez-faire leadership** (also called *permissive* or *nondirective*). The laissez-faire ("let it alone") leader does very little planning or decision making and fails to encourage others to do so. It is really a lack of leadership. For example, when a decision needs to be made, a laissez-faire leader may postpone making the decision or never make the decision at all. In most instances, the laissez-faire leader leaves people feeling confused and frustrated because there is no goal, no guidance, and no direction. Some very mature individuals thrive under laissez-faire leadership because they need little guidance. Most people, however, flounder under this kind of leadership.

Pavitt summed up the difference among these three styles nicely: a democratic leader tries to move the group toward its goals; an autocratic leader tries to move the group toward the leader's goals; and a laissez-faire leader makes no attempt to move the group (1999, pp. 330ff).

Task vs. Relationship

Another important distinction in leadership style is between a task focus and a relationship focus (Blake, Mouton, & Tapper, 1981). Some nurses emphasize the tasks (e.g., reducing medication errors, completing patient records) and fail to realize that interpersonal relationships

(e.g., attitude of physicians toward nursing staff, treatment of housekeeping staff by nurses) affect the morale and productivity of employees. Other nurses focus on the interpersonal aspects and ignore the quality of the job being done as long as people get along with each other. The most effective leader is able to balance the two, attending to both the task and the relationship aspects of working together.

Emotional Intelligence

The relationship aspects of leadership are again brought to our attention in the work on emotional intelligence (Goleman, Boyatzes, & McKee, 2002). Part of what distinguishes ordinary leaders from leadership "stars" is consciously addressing the effect of people's feelings on the team's emotional reality. How is this done?

First, learn how to recognize and understand your own emotions, and learn how to manage them, channel them, and stay calm and clear-headed and suspend judgment until all the facts are in when a crisis occurs (Baggett & Baggett, 2005). The emotionally intelligent leader welcomes constructive criticism, asks for help when needed, can juggle multiple demands without losing focus, and can turn problems into opportunities.

Second, the emotionally intelligent leader listens attentively to others, picks up unspoken concerns, acknowledges others' perspectives, and brings people together in an atmosphere of respect, cooperation, collegiality, and helpfulness so that they can direct their energies toward achieving the team's goals. "The enthusiastic, caring, and supportive leader generates those same feelings throughout the team," wrote Porter-O'Grady of the emotionally intelligent leader (2003, p. 109).

Situational Theories

People and leadership situations are far more complex than the early theories recognized. In addition, situations can change rapidly, requiring more complex theories to explain leadership (Bennis, Spreitzer, & Cummings, 2001).

Adaptability is the key to the situational approach (McNichol, 2000). Instead of assuming that one particular approach works in all situations, situational theories recognize the complexity of work situations and encourage the leader to consider many factors when deciding what action to take.

The following is an illustration of how just one factor in a situation can affect people's response to change.

Two nurse managers were talking before the council meeting began. "How did your staff react to the new 6 a.m. to 2 p.m. hours for the day tour?" Jennifer Chinn asked her friend Esther Cabriollo.

"They love it," said Esther.

"Really?" said Jennifer. "My staff is so upset. They said it was an inhumane schedule and that they have to be at work before the birds get up in the morning. You should hear their complaints."

"Most of my staff thinks it's just the opposite," said Esther. "Many have young children. With this new schedule, their spouses can take the children to school in the morning, and they can be home in time to meet the school bus. They said it's the most humane change the administration has ever made."

"That explains it," said Jennifer. "Most of my staff have older children who have a lot of activities in the evening, and they're all having trouble getting up an hour earlier in the morning. Their situation is entirely different."

Every situation is different. A change that is welcomed by one group of people may be hated by another group. Similarly, the type of leadership approach that is being used may affect people's responses. Another important situational factor is the type of organization in which the leader works (see Chapter 5). Situational theories emphasize the importance of understanding all the factors that affect a particular group of people in a particular environment.

Transformational Leadership

Although the situational theories were an improvement over earlier theories, there was still something missing. Meaning, inspiration, and vision were still not given enough attention (Tappen, 2001). These are the distinguishing features of transformational leadership.

The transformational theory of leadership emphasizes that people need a sense of mission that goes beyond good interpersonal relationships or the appropriate reward for a job well done (Bass & Avolio, 1993). This is especially true in nursing. Caring for people, sick or well, is the goal of our profession. Most of us chose nursing to do something for the good of humankind: this is our vision. One responsibility of nursing leadership is to help us achieve our vision.

Transformational leaders can communicate their vision in a manner that is so meaningful and exciting that it reduces negativity (Leach, 2005) and inspires commitment in the people with whom they work (Trofino, 1995). If successful, the goals of the leader and staff will "become fused, creating unity, wholeness, and a collective purpose" (Barker, 1992, p. 42).

Moral Leadership

The corporate scandals of recent years have redirected our attention to the values and ethics that underlie our practice of leadership as well as client care (Dantley, 2005). Caring about the people who work for you as people as well as employees (Spears & Lawrence, 2004) is part of moral leadership. This can be a great challenge in times of limited financial resources.

Molly Benedict was a team leader on the acute geriatric unit (AGU) when a question of moral leadership arose. Faced with large budget cuts in the middle of the year and feeling a little desparate to figure out how to run the AGU with fewer staff, her nurse manager suggested that reducing the time that unlicensed assistive personnel (UAP) spent ambulating the clients wiould enable them to increase UAP workload from 10 to 15 clients. "George," responded Molly, "you know that inactivity has many harmful effects, from emboli to disorientation in our very elderly population. Instead, let's try to figure out how to encourage more self-care or even family involvement in care so the UAP can still walk clients and prevent their becoming nonambulatory." Molly based her response on important values, particularly those of prevention.

Qualities of an Effective Leader

Effective leadership is defined as the accomplishment of the goals shared by leader and followers. Integrity, courage, initiative, energy, optimism, perseverance, balance, ability to handle stress, and self-awareness are qualities of effective leaders in nursing (Fig. 1-1):

◆ **Integrity.** Integrity is expected of healthcare professionals. Clients, colleagues, and employers all expect nurses to be honest, law-abiding, and trustworthy. Adherence to both a code of personal ethics and a code of professional ethics (Appendix 1, American Nurses Association Code for Nurses) is expected of every nurse. Would-be leaders who do not exhibit these characteristics cannot expect them of their followers. This is an essential component of moral leadership.

◆ **Courage.** Sometimes, being a leader means taking some risks. In the story of Billie Blair Thomas, for example, Billie needed some courage to speak to her nurse manager about a problem she had observed.

◆ **Initiative.** Good ideas are not enough. To be a leader, you must act on those good ideas. This requires initiative on your part.

◆ **Energy.** Leadership also requires energy. Both leadership and followership are hard but satisfying endeavors that require effort.

It is also important that you use your energy wisely.

◆ **Optimism.** When the work is difficult and one crisis seems to follow another in rapid succession, it is easy to become discouraged. It is important not to let discouragement keep you and your coworkers from seeking ways to resolve these problems. In fact, the ability to see a problem as an opportunity is part of the optimism that makes a person an effective leader. Like energy, optimism is "catching." Holman (1995) called this being a *winner* instead of a *whiner* (Table 1-3).

◆ **Perseverance.** Effective leaders do not give up easily. Instead, they persist, continuing their efforts when others are tempted to stop trying. This persistence often pays off.

◆ **Balance.** In our effort to become the best nurses we can be, we may forget that other aspects of life are equally important. As important as our clients and colleagues are to us, family and friends are important too. Although school and work are meaningful activities, cultural, social, recreational, and spiritual activities also have meaning. We need to find a balance between work and play.

◆ **Ability to handle stress.** There is some stress in almost every job. Coping with stress in as positive and healthy a manner as possible helps you conserve your energy and be a model for others. Maintaining balance and handling stress are reviewed in Chapter 10.

◆ **Self-awareness.** How is your emotional intelligence? People who do not understand themselves are limited in their ability to

Qualities

Integrity	Perseverance
Courage	Balance
Initiative	Ability to handle stress
Energy	Self-awareness
Optimism	

Behaviors

Think critically	Set goals, share vision
Solve problems	Develop self and others
Communicate skillfully	

FIGURE 1-1 ◆ Keys to effective leadership.

TABLE 1-3
Winner or Whiner—Which Are You?

A winner says ...	A whiner says ...
We have a real challenge here.	This is really a problem.
I'll give it my best.	Do I have to?
That's great!	That's nice, I guess.
We can do it!	Will never succeed.
Yes!	Maybe...

Adapted from Holman, L. (1995). *Eleven Lessons in Self-leadership: Insights for Personal and Professional Success.* Lexington, KY: A Lessons in Leadership Book.

understand the motivations of others. They are far more likely to fool themselves than are self-aware people. For example, it is much easier to be fair with a coworker you like than with one you do not like. Recognizing that you like some people more than others is the first step in avoiding unfair treatment based on personal likes and dislikes.

Behaviors of an Effective Leader

Leadership requires action. The effective leader chooses the action carefully. Important leadership behaviors include thinking critically, solving problems, respecting people, communicating skillfully, setting specific goals, communicating a vision for the future, and developing oneself and others:

◆ **Thinking critically.** Critical thinking is the careful, deliberate use of reasoned analysis to reach a decision about what to believe or what to do (Feldman, 2002). The essence of critical thinking is a willingness to ask questions and to be open to new ideas, new ways to do things. To avoid falling prey to assumptions and biases of your own and those of others, ask yourself frequently, "Do I have the information I need? Is it accurate? Am I prejudging a situation?" (Jackson, Ignatavicius, & Case, 2004).

◆ **Solving problems.** Client problems, paperwork problems, staff problems: these and others occur frequently and need to be solved. The effective leader helps people identify problems and to work through the problem-solving process to find a reasonable solution.

◆ **Respecting the individual.** Although people have much in common, each individual has different wants and needs and has had different life experiences. For example, some people really value the psychological rewards of helping others; other people are more concerned about earning a decent salary. There is nothing wrong with either of these points of view; they are simply different. The effective leader recognizes these differences in people and helps them find the rewards in their work that mean the most to them.

◆ **Skillful communication.** This includes listening to others, encouraging exchange of information, and providing feedback:

Listening to others. We have separated listening from talking with other people to emphasize that communication involves both giving and receiving information. The only way to find out people's individual wants and needs is to watch what they do and to listen to what they tell you. It is amazing how often leaders fail simply because they did not listen to what other people were trying to tell them.

Encouraging the exchange of information. Many misunderstandings and mistakes occur because people fail to share enough information with each other. The leader's role is to make sure that the channels of communication remain open and that people use them.

Providing feedback. Everyone needs some information about the effectiveness of his or her performance. Frequent feedback, both positive and negative, is needed so that people can continually improve their performance.

Some nurse leaders find it difficult to give negative feedback because they fear that they will upset the other person. How else can a person know where improvement is needed? Negative feedback can be given in a manner that is neither hurtful nor resented by the individual receiving it. In fact, it is often appreciated.

Other nurse leaders fail to give positive feedback, assuming that coworkers will know when they are doing a good job. This is also a mistake because everyone appreciates positive feedback. In fact, for some people, it is the most important reward they get from their jobs.

◆ **Setting specific goals.** Just as each one of us is unique in terms of our experiences, needs, and wants, we are also likely to have unique goals for ourselves. An important leadership task is to find the common thread in all of those goals and to help the group reach a consensus about its goals. This may require considerable discussion before it is achieved.

◆ **Communicating a vision for the future.** The effective leader has a vision for the future. Communicating this vision to the group and involving everyone in working toward that vision create the inspiration that keeps people going when things become difficult. Even better, involving people in creating the vision is not only more satisfying for employees but also has the potential for the most creative and innovative outcomes (Kerfott, 2000). It is this vision that helps make work meaningful.

◆ **Developing oneself and others.** Learning does not end on leaving school. In fact, experienced nurses will tell you that school is just the beginning, that it only prepares you to continue learning throughout your career. As new and better ways to care for clients are discovered, it is your responsibility as a professional to critically analyze these new approaches and decide whether they would be better for your clients than current approaches to care.

Effective leaders not only continue to learn but also encourage others to do the same. Sometimes, leaders function as teachers. At other times, their role is primarily to encourage and guide others to seek more knowledge. Observant, reflective, analytical practitioners know that learning takes place every day if people are open to it (Kagan, 1999).

CONCLUSION

The key elements of leadership and followership have been discussed in this chapter. Every registered nurse needs leadership and followership skills to be effective as a practitioner and employee. Many of the leadership qualities and behaviors mentioned here are discussed in more detail in later chapters.

STUDY QUESTIONS

1   Why is it important for nurses to be good leaders?

2   Why are effective followers as important as effective leaders?

3   Compare and contrast the autocratic, democratic, and laissez-faire styles of leadership. List alternative names for each of these styles. What effect does each of these leadership styles have on followers?

4   Select an individual whose leadership skills you particularly admire. What are some qualities and behaviors that this individual displays? How do these relate to the leadership theories discussed in this chapter? In what ways could you emulate this person?

CRITICAL THINKING EXERCISE

Two new associate degree graduates were hired for the pediatric unit. Both worked three 12-hour shifts a week, Jan in the day-to-evening shift and Ronnie at night. Whenever their shifts connected, they would compare notes on their experience. Jan felt she was learning rapidly, gaining clinical skills and beginning to feel at ease with her colleagues.

(Continued on following page)

Ronnie, however, still felt unsure of herself and often isolated. "There have been times," she told Jan, "that I am the only registered nurse on the unit all night. The aides and LPNs are really experienced, but that's not enough. I wish I could work with an experienced nurse as you are doing."

"Ronnie, you are not even finished with your 3-month orientation program," said Jan. "You should never be left alone with all these sick children. Neither of us is ready for that kind of responsibility yet. And how will you get the experience you need with no experienced nurses to help you? You must speak to our nurse manager about this."

"I know I should, but she's so hard to reach. I've called several times and she's never available. She leaves all the shift assignments to her assistant. I'm not sure she even reviews the schedule before it's posted."

"You will have to try harder to reach her. Maybe you could stay past the end of your shift one morning and meet with her," suggested Jan. "If something happens when you are the only nurse on the unit, you will be held responsible."

1. In your own words, summarize the problem that Jan and Ronnie are discussing. To what extent is this problem due to a failure to lead? Who has failed to act?

2. What style of leadership was displayed by Ronnie and the nurse manager? How effective was their leadership? Did Jan's leadership differ from that of Ronnie and the nurse manager? In what way?

3. In what ways has Ronnie been an effective follower? In what ways has Ronnie not been so effective as a follower?

4. If an emergency occurred and was not handled well while Ronnie was the only nurse on the unit, who would be responsible? Explain why this person or persons would be responsible.

5. If you found yourself in Ronnie's situation, what steps would you take to resolve the problem? Show how the leader characteristics and behaviors found in this chapter support your solution to the problem.

REFERENCES

Baggett, M.M., & Baggett, F.B. (2005). Move from management to high-level leadership. *Nursing Management,* 36(7), 12.

Barker, A.M. (1992). *Transformational Nursing Leadership: A Vision for the Future.* New York: National League for Nursing Press.

Bass, B.M., & Avolio, B.J. (1993). Transformational leadership: A response to critiques. In Chemers, M.M., & Ayman, R. (eds.). *Leadership Theory and Research: Perspectives and Direction.* San Diego: Academic Press.

Bennis, W., Spreitzer, G.M., & Cummings, T.G. (2001). *The Future of Leadership.* San Francisco: Jossey-Bass.

Blake, R.R., Mouton, J.S., & Tapper, M., et al. (1981). *Grid Approaches for Managerial Leadership in Nursing.* St. Louis: C.V. Mosby.

Chrispeels, J.H. (2004). *Learning to Lead Together.* Thousand Oaks, CA: Sage Publications.

Dantley, M.E. (2005). Moral leadership: Shifting the management paradigm. In English, F.W. *The Sage Handbook of Educational Leadership* (pp. 34–46). Thousand Oaks, CA: Sage Publications.

Deutschman, A. (2005). Is your boss a psychopath? *Making Change.* Fast Company, 96, 43–51.

Drath, W. (2001). *The Deep Blue Sea.* San Francisco: Jossey-Bass.

Feldman, D.A. (2002). *Critical Thinking: Strategies for Decision Making.* Menlo Park, CA: Crisp Publications.

Goleman, D., Boyatzes, R., & McKee, A. (2002). *Primal*

Leadership: Realizing the Power of Emotional Intelligence. Boston: Harvard Business School Press.

Grossman, S., & Valiga, T.M. (2000). *The New Leadership Challenge: Creating the Future of Nursing.* Philadelphia: FA Davis.

Holman, L. (1995). *Eleven Lessons in Self-Leadership: Insights for Personal and Professional Success.* Lexington, KY: A Lessons in Leadership Book.

Jackson, M., Ignatavicius, D., & Case, B. (eds.). (2004). *Conversations in Critical Thinking and Clinical Judgement.* Pensacola, FL: Pohl.

Kagan, S.S. (1999). *Leadership Games: Experiential Learning for Organizational Development.* Thousand Oaks, CA: Sage Publications.

Kerfott, K. (2000). Leadership: Creating a shared destiny. *Dermatological Nursing,* 12(5), 363–364.

Korn, M. (2004). *Toxic Cleanup: How to Deal With a Dangerous Leader.* Fast Company, 88, 17.

Lansdale, B.M. (2002). *Cultivating Inspired Leaders.* West Hartford, CN: Kumarian Press.

Leach, L.S. (2005). Nurse Executive Transformational Leadership and Organizational Commitment. *Journal of Nursing Administration,* 35(5), 228–237.

Lyons, M.F. (2002). Leadership and followership. *The Physician Executive,* Jan/Feb, 91–93.

McNichol, E. (2000). How to be a model leader. *Nursing Standard,* 14(45), 24.

Pavitt, C. (1999). Theorizing about the group communication-leadership relationship. In Frey, L.R. (ed.). *The Handbook of Group Communication Theory and Research.* Thousand Oaks, CA: Sage Publications.

Porter-O'Grady, T. (2003). A different age for leadership, Part II. *Journal of Nursing Administration,* 33(2), 105–110.

Spears, L.C., & Lawrence, M. (2004). *Practicing Servant-Leadership.* New York: Jossey-Bass.

Spreitzer, G.M., & Quinn, R.E. (2001). *A Company of Leaders: Five Disciplines for Unleashing the Power in Your Workforce.* San Francisco: Jossey-Bass.

Tappen, R.M. (2001). *Nursing Leadership and Management: Concepts and Practice.* Philadelphia: FA Davis.

Trofino, J. (1995). Transformational leadership in health care. *Nursing Management,* 26(8), 42–47.

White, R.K., & Lippitt, R. (1960). *Autocracy and Democracy: An Experimental Inquiry.* New York: Harper & Row.

chapter 2

Manager

CHAPTER 2 SELF-ASSESSMENT
Do You Know How to Provide Feedback?

Indicate whether you think each of the following recommendations for providing feedback is correct. Then check your answers.

1. It is more important to correct people than to praise them.
   True _____ False _____

2. Always allow yourself to "cool off" before correcting someone.
   True _____ False _____

3. It is preferable to correct someone in private rather than in front of others.
   True _____ False _____

4. General statements are preferable to descriptions of specific incidents when providing feedback.
   True _____ False _____

5. Seek feedback on your performance from others, including your patients.
   True _____ False _____

6. Include suggestions for improvement when giving negative feedback.
   True _____ False _____

7. Save your corrective comments for the annual formal evaluation sessions.
   True _____ False _____

Answers: 1. F, 2. F, 3. T, 4. F, 5. T, 6. T, 7. F

Every nurse should be a good leader and a good follower. Not everyone can or should be a manager, however. In fact, new graduates simply are not ready to take on management responsibilities. Once you have had time to develop your clinical and leadership skills, you can begin to think about taking on management responsibilities (Table 2-1).

MANAGEMENT

Are You Ready to Be a Manager?

For most new nurses, the answer is *no,* you should not accept managerial responsibility. The breadth and depth of your experience are still undeveloped. You need to direct your

energies to building your own skills before you begin supervising other people.

What Is Management?

The essence of management is getting work done through others. The classic definition of management is Henri Fayol's 1916 list of managerial tasks: planning, organizing, commanding, coordinating, and controlling the work of a group of employees (Wren, 1972). But Mintzberg (1989) argued that managers really do whatever is needed to make sure that employees do their work and do it well. Lombardi (2001) points out that two-thirds of a manager's time is spent on people problems. The rest is taken up by budget work, going

TABLE 2-1
Differences Between Leadership and Management

Leadership	Management
Based on influence and shared meaning	Based on authority
An informal role	A formally designated role
An achieved position	An assigned position
Part of every nurse's responsibility	Usually responsible for budgets, hiring and firing people
Requires initiative and independent thinking	Improved by the use of effective leadership skills

to meetings, preparing reports, and other "administration."

THE DIFFERENCE BETWEEN LEADERSHIP AND MANAGEMENT

Management Theories

There are two major but opposing schools of thought in management: scientific management and the human relations–based approach. The latter emphasizes the interpersonal aspects of managing people, and the former emphasizes the task aspects of management.

Scientific Management

Almost 100 years ago, Frederick Taylor argued that most jobs could be done more efficiently if they were thoroughly analyzed (Lee, 1980; Locke, 1982). With a well-designed task and enough incentive to get the work done, workers could be more productive. For example, he encouraged paying people by the piece instead of by the hour. In health care, the equivalent would be by the number of clients bathed or visited at home rather than by the number of hours worked. This would create an incentive to get the most work done in the least amount of time, Taylor theorized. Taylorism stresses that there is a best way to do a job. Usually, this is also the fastest way to do the job (Dantley, 2005).

The work itself is analyzed to improve efficiency. In health care, for example, there has been a lot of discussion about the time it takes to bring clients to radiology or to physical therapy versus bringing the technician or therapist to the client. Emphasis on eliminating excess staff or increasing the productivity of remaining employees is also based on this kind of thinking.

Nurse managers who use the principles of scientific management will pay particular attention to the type of assessments and procedures done on the unit, the equipment needed to do this efficiently, and the strategies that would facilitate efficient accomplishment of these tasks. Typically, these nurse managers keep careful records of the amount of work accomplished and reward those who accomplish the most.

Human Relations–Based Management

McGregor's theories X and Y provide a good example of the difference between scientific management and human relations–based management. Theory X, said McGregor (1960), reflects a common attitude among managers that most people really do not want to work very hard and that the manager's job is to make sure that they do work hard. To accomplish this, according to theory X, a manager needs to employ strict rules, constant supervision, and the threat of punishment (reprimands, withheld raises, and threats of job loss) to create industrious, conscientious workers.

Theory Y, which McGregor preferred, is the opposite viewpoint. Theory Y managers believe that the work itself can be motivating and that people will work hard if their managers provide a supportive environment. A theory Y manager emphasizes guidance rather than control, development rather than close supervision, and reward rather than punishment (Fig. 2-1). A theory Y nurse manager is concerned with keeping employee morale as high as possible, assuming that satisfied, motivated employees will do the best work. Employees' attitudes, opinions, hopes, and fears are important to this type of nurse manager. Considerable effort is expended to work out conflicts and promote mutual understanding to provide

THEORY X

Work is something to be avoided

People want to do as little as possible

Use control-supervision-punishment

THEORY Y

The work itself can be motivating

People really want to do their job well

Use guidance-development-reward

FIGURE 2-1 ◆ Theory X versus theory Y.

an environment in which people can do their best work.

Servant Leadership

The emphasis on people and interpersonal reationships is taken one step further by Greenleaf (2004), who wrote an essay in 1970 that began the servant leadership movement. Like transformational leadership, servant leadership has a special appeal to nurses and other health-care professionals. Despite its name, however, servant leadership applies more to people in supervisory or administrative positions than to people in staff positions.

The servant leadership staff manager believes that people have value as people, not just as workers (Spears & Lawrence, 2004). The manager is committed to improving the way each employee is treated at work. The attitude is employee first, not manager first. So the manager sees himself or himself as being there for the employee. Here is an example:

Hope Marshall is a relatively new staff nurse at Jefferson County Hospital. When she was invited to be the staff nurse representative on the search committee for a new VP for Nursing, she was very excited and a little anxious about being on a committee with so many managerial and administrative people. As the interviews of candidates began,

however, she forgot about her concerns and focused on what the candidates had to say. Each had very impressive resumes and spoke confidently about their accomplishments. Hope was impressed but did not yet prefer one over the other. Then the fifth and last candidate spoke to the committee. "My primary job," he said, "is to make it possible for each nurse to the very best job he or she can do. I am here to make their work easier, to remove barriers and provide them with whatever they need to provide the best client care possible." Hope had not heard the term servant leadership but she knew immediately that this last candidate was the one she would support for this important position.

QUALITIES OF AN EFFECTIVE MANAGER

A Gallup poll found that two-thirds of people who leave their jobs say the main reason was an ineffective or incompetent manager (Hunter, 2004).

The effective nurse manager possesses a combination of qualities: leadership, clinical expertise, and business sense. None of these alone is enough; it is the combination that prepares an individual for the complex task of managing a unit or team of health-care providers. Let's look at each of these briefly:

◆ **Leadership.** All of the people skills of the leader are essential to the effective manager. They are skills needed to function as a manager.

◆ **Clinical expertise.** It is very difficult to help others develop their skills and evaluate how well they have done this without possessing clinical expertise oneself. It is probably not necessary (or even possible) to know everything all other professionals on the team know, but it is important to be able to assess the effectiveness of their work in terms of client outcomes.

◆ **Business sense.** Nurse managers also need to be concerned with the "bottom line"; that is, with the *cost* of providing the care that is given, especially in comparison with the benefit received from that care and the funding available to pay for it, whether from insurance, Medicare, Medicaid, or out of the client's own pocket. This is a complex task that requires knowledge of budgeting, staffing, and measurement of client outcomes, much of which is beyond the scope of this textbook.

There is some controversy over the amount of clinical expertise versus business sense that is needed to be an effective nurse manager. Some argue that a person can be a "generic" manager, that the job of managing people is the same no matter what tasks he or she performs. Others argue that managers must understand the tasks themselves, better than anyone else in the work group. Our position is that equal amounts of clinical skill and business acumen are needed, along with excellent leadership skills.

BEHAVIORS OF AN EFFECTIVE MANAGER

Mintzberg (1989) divided a manager's activities into three categories: interpersonal, decisional,

Informational

Representing employees
Representing the organization
Public relations monitoring

Interpersonal

Networking
Conflict negotiation and resolution
Employee development and coaching
Rewards and punishment

Decisional

Employee evaluation
Resource allocation
Hiring and firing employees
Planning
Job analysis and redesign

FIGURE 2-2 ◆ Keys to effective management.

and informational. We will use these categories but have taken some liberties with them and added some activities suggested by other authors (Dunham-Taylor, 1995; Montebello, 1994) and by our own observations of nurse managers (Fig. 2-2).

Interpersonal Activities

The interpersonal area is one in which leaders and managers have overlapping concerns. However, the manager has some additional responsibilities that are seldom given to leaders. These include the following:

◆ **Networking.** Within their organization's hierarchy, nurse managers have many opportunities to influence the status and treatment of staff nurses. It is important that they are able to clearly articulate nurses' roles and value to the institution.

◆ **Conflict negotiation and resolution.** Managers often find themselves resolving conflicts between employees, clients, and administration.

◆ **Employee development.** Providing for the continuing learning and upgrading of the skills of employees is a managerial responsibility.

◆ **Coaching.** This is one of the ways in which nurse managers can share their experience and expertise with the rest of the staff. The goal is to help the employee (the "coachee") to do a better job through learning (McCauly & Van Velson, 2004).

Some managers use a directive approach:

◆ This is how it's done. Watch me.
◆ Let me show you how to do this.

Others prefer a nondirective approach:

◆ Let's try to figure out what's wrong here (Hart & Waisman, 2005).
◆ How do you think we can improve our outcomes?

You can probably see the parallel with democratic and autocratic leadership styles described in Chapter 1. The decision whether to be directive (e.g., in an emergency) or nondirective (e.g., when developing a long-term plan to improve infection control) will depend on the situation. This overlaps with managers' informational responsibilities.

◆ **Rewards and punishments.** Managers are in a position to provide both specific (e.g., salary increases, time off) and general (e.g., praise, recognition) rewards as well as punishments.

Decisional Activities

Nurse managers are also responsible for making many decisions:

◆ **Employee evaluation.** Managers are responsible for conducting formal performance appraisals of their staff members.

◆ **Resource allocation.** In decentralized organizations, nurse managers are often given a set amount of money for running their units or departments and must allocate these resources wisely. This can be difficult when resources are very limited.

◆ **Hiring and firing employees.** Most nurse managers either decide or participate in employment and termination decisions for their units.

◆ **Planning for the future.** The day-to-day operation of most units is complex and time-consuming, but nurse managers must also look ahead in order to prepare themselves and their units for future changes in budgets, organizational priorities, and client populations.

◆ **Job analysis and redesign.** In a time of extreme cost sensitvity, nurse managers are often called on to analyze and redesign the work of their units to make them as efficient as possible.

Informational Activities

Nurse managers often find themselves in positions within the organizational hierarchy in which they acquire much information that is not available to their staff. They also have much information about their staff that is not readily available to the administration, placing them in a strategic position within the information web of any organization. The effective manager uses this position for the benefit of both the staff and the organization. The following are some examples:

◆ **Spokesperson.** Managers often speak for administration when relaying information to their staff members. Likewise, they often speak for staff members when relaying information to administration.

◆ **Monitoring.** Effective nurse managers purposely spend much of their day out of their offices (Hardesty, 2002). Nurse managers are expected to monitor the activities of their units or departments. This may include the number of clients seen, average length of stay, infection rates, and so forth. They also monitor the staff (e.g., absentee rates, tardiness, unproductive time) and the budget (e.g., money spent, money left to spend in comparison with money needed to operate the unit).

◆ **Public Relations.** Nurse managers share information with their clients, staff members, and employers. This information may be related to the results of their monitoring efforts, new developments in health care, policy changes, and so forth.

◼ CONCLUSION

Nurse managers have complex, responsible positions within health-care organizations. Ineffective managers may do harm to their employees, their clients, and to the organization, but effective managers can help their staff members grow and develop as health-care professionals while providing the highest quality care to their clients.

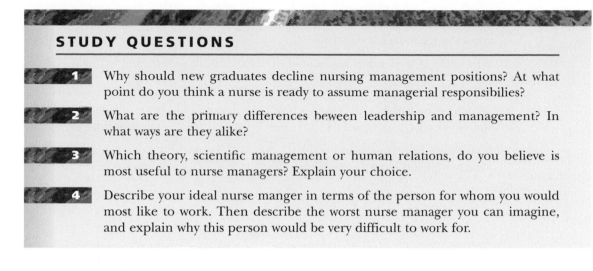

STUDY QUESTIONS

1   Why should new graduates decline nursing management positions? At what point do you think a nurse is ready to assume managerial responsibilies?

2   What are the primary differences beween leadership and management? In what ways are they alike?

3   Which theory, scientific management or human relations, do you believe is most useful to nurse managers? Explain your choice.

4   Describe your ideal nurse manger in terms of the person for whom you would most like to work. Then describe the worst nurse manager you can imagine, and explain why this person would be very difficult to work for.

CRITICAL THINKING EXERCISE

Joe Garcia has been an operating room nurse for 5 years. He was often on call on Saturday and Sunday, but he enjoyed his work and knew that he would not be called unless he was really needed. When a large health-care corporation bought the hospital he worked for, Joe was initially pleased because he thought that this would increase his opportunities for advancement.

A multicar accident on a nearby interstate highway occurred on the second weekend after the hospital had been purchased. Most of the accident victims were taken to the city-owned hospital, but two were brought to the emergency room of the hospital where Joe worked. One was critically injured; the other had minor cuts and bruises. Joe was called in to prepare for emergency surgery. When he arrived, he was told that the client had died.

As usual, Joe requested payment for the time spent traveling to and from the hospital on the emergency call. Joe was not paid for this time on his next paycheck. When he asked about it, his nurse manager told him that he would not be paid because he did not do any work. "That's not fair," he said, "I'm going to speak with the director about this."

"The last person who complained to the director was fired," the nurse manager warned him.

"I can't believe that," said Joe. "The director has always been fair with all of us."

"No more," replied the nurse manager. "The director has been replaced. This is no longer the fair, employee-centered organization we used to work for. With this new management, your protest, however justified it is, will be harshly received and you might regret having raised the issue. The choice is up to you."

Joe decided that he did not want to work in such an institution. With his 4 years of operating room experience, he quickly found another operating room position in an organization that utilized a more humanistically oriented approach to management.

(Continued on following page)

1. What style of leadership and school of management thought seem to be preferred by Joe Garcia's employer?

2. What style of leadership and school of management were preferred by Joe?

3. What effect did the change in approach have on Joe?

4. Which of the listed qualites of leaders and managers did the nurse manager display? Which behaviors? Which ones did the nurse manager not display?

5. If you were Joe, what would you have done? If you were the nurse manager, what would you have done? Why?

REFERENCES

Dantley, M.E. (2005). Moral Leadership: Shifting the Management Paradigm. In English, F.W. *The Sage Handbook of Educational Leadership* (pp. 34–46). Thousand Oaks, CA: Sage Publications.

Dunham-Taylor, J. (1995). Identifying the best in nurse executive leadership. *Journal of Nursing Administration,* 25(7/8), 24–31.

Greenleaf, R.K. (2004). Who is the Servant-Leader? In Spears, L.C., & Lawrence, M. *Practicing Servant-Leadership.* New York: Jossey-Bass.

Hardesty, P. (2002). Full circle. *Nursing-Spectrum,* 12(12), 3.

Hunter, J.C. (2004). *The World's Most Powerful Leadership Principle.* New York: Crown Business.

Lee, J.A. (1980). *The Gold and the Garbage in Management Theories and Prescriptions.* Athens, OH: Ohio University Press.

Locke, E.A. (1982). The Ideas of Frederick Taylor: An Evaluation. *Academy of Management Review,* 7(1), 14.

Lombardi, D.N. (2001). *Handbook for the New Health Care Manager.* San Francisco: Jossey-Bass/AHA Press.

McCauley, C.D, & Van Velson, E. (eds.). (2004). *The Center for Creative Leadership Handbook of Leadership Development.* New York: Jossey-Bass.

McGregor, D. (1960). *The Human Side of Enterprise.* New York: McGraw-Hill.

Mintzberg, H. (1989). *Mintzberg on Managment: Inside Our Strange World of Organizations.* New York: Free Press.

Montebello, A. (1994). *Work Teams That Work.* Minneapolis: Best Sellers Publishing.

Spears, L.C., & Lawrence, M. (2004). *Practicing Servant-Leadership.* New York: Jossey-Bass.

Wren, D.A. (1972). *The Evolution of Management Thought.* New York: Ronald Press.

chapter 3

Nursing Practice and the Law

OBJECTIVES

After reading this chapter, the student should be able to:

◆ Identify three major sources of laws.

◆ Explain the differences between various types of laws.

◆ Differentiate between negligence and malpractice.

◆ Explain the difference between an intentional and an unintentional tort.

◆ Explain how standards of care are used in determining negligence and malpractice.

◆ Describe how nurse practice acts guide nursing practice.

◆ Explain the purpose of licensure.

◆ Discuss issues of licensure.

◆ Explain the difference between internal standards and external standards.

◆ Discuss advance directives and how they pertain to clients' rights.

◆ Discuss the legal implications of the Health Insurance Portability and Accountability Act

OUTLINE

General Principles
Meaning of Law
Sources of Law
  The Constitution
  Statutes
  Administrative Law

Types of Laws
Criminal Law
Civil Law
  Tort
  Quasi-Intentional Tort
  Negligence
  Malpractice

Other Laws Relevant to Nursing Practice
Good Samaritan Laws
Confidentiality
Slander and Libel
False Imprisonment
Assault and Battery

Standards of Practice
Use of Standards in Nursing
  Negligence Malpractice
  Actions
Patient's Bill of Rights
Informed Consent

Staying Out of Court
Prevention
  Appropriate Documentation

Common Actions Leading to
  Malpractice Suits
If a Problem Arises

Professional Liability Insurance

End-of-Life Decisions and the Law
Do Not Resuscitate
  Orders
Advance Directives
  Living Will and Durable Power of Attorney for Health Care (Health-Care Surrogate)
Nursing Implications

Legal Implications of Mandatory Overtime

Licensure
Qualifications for
  Licensure
Licensure by Examination
  NCLEX-RN
  Preparing for the NCLEX-RN
  Licensure Through Endorsement
  Multistate Licensure
Disciplinary Action

Conclusion

The courtroom seemd cold and sterile. Scanning her surroundings with nervous eyes, Germaine decided she knew how Alice must have felt when the Queen of Hearts screamed for her head. The image of the White Rabbit running through the woods, looking at his watch, yelling, "I'm late! I'm late!" flashed before her eyes. For a few moments, she indulged herself in thoughts of being able to turn back the clock and rewrite the past. The future certainly looked grim at that moment. The calling of her name broke her reverie. Mr. Ellison, the attorney for the plaintiff, wanted her undivided attention regarding the fateful day when she committed a fatal medication error. That day, the client died following a cardiac arrest because Germaine failed to check the appropriate dosage and route for the medication. She had administered 40 mEq of potassium chloride by intravenous push. Her 15 years of nursing experience meant little to the court. Because she had not followed hospital protocol and had violated an important standard of practice, Germaine stood alone. She was being sued for malpractice.

As client advocates, nurses have a responsibility to deliver safe care to their clients. This expectation requires that nurses have professional knowledge at their expected level of practice and be proficient in technological skills. A working knowledge of the legal system, client rights, and behaviors that may result in lawsuits helps nurses to act as client advocates. As long as nurses practice according to established standards of care, they will be able to avoid the kind of day in court that Germaine experienced.

GENERAL PRINCIPLES

Meaning of Law

The word *law* has several meanings. For the purposes of this chapter, *law* means those rules that prescribe and control social conduct in a formal and legally binding manner (Bernzweig, 1996). Laws are created in one of three ways:

1. *Statutory laws* are created by various legislative bodies, such as state legislatures or Congress. Some examples of federal statutes include the Patient Self-Determination Act of 1990 and the Americans With Disabilities Act. State statutes include the state nurse practice act, the state board of nursing, and the Good Samaritan Act. Laws that govern nursing practice are statutory laws.

2. *Common law* develops within the court system as judicial decisions are made in various cases and precedents for future cases are set. In this way, a decision made in one case can affect decisions made in later cases of a similar nature. This portion of American law is based on the English tradition of case law. This is "judge-made law" (Black, 2004). Many times a judge in a subsequent case will follow the reasoning of a judge in a previous case. Therefore, one case sets a precedent for another.

3. *Administrative law* is established through the authority given to government agencies, such as state boards of nursing, by a legislative body. It is then the duty of these governing boards to meet the intent of the law or statute.

Sources of Law

The Constitution

The Constitution is the foundation of American law. The Bill of Rights, comprising the first 10 amendments to the U.S. Constitution, is the basis for protection of individual rights. These laws define and limit the power of the government and protect citizens' freedom of speech, freedom of assembly, freedom of religion, freedom of the press, and freedom from unwarranted intrusion by government into personal choices. State constitutions can expand individual rights but cannot deprive people of rights guaranteed by the U.S. Constitution.

Constitutional law evolves. As individuals or groups bring suit to challenge interpretations of the Constitution, decisions are made concerning application of the law to that particular event. An example is the protection of freedom of speech. Are obscenities protected? Can one person threaten or criticize another person? The freedom to criticize is protected; threats are not protected. The definition of what constitutes obscenity is often debated and has not been fully clarified by the courts.

Statutes

Localities, state legislatures, and the U.S. Congress create statutes. These can be found in multivolume sets of books and computerized databases.

At the federal level, conference committees comprising representatives of both houses of Congress negotiate the resolution of any differences on wording of the final bill before it becomes law. If the bill does not meet with the approval of the executive branch of government, the president can veto it. If that occurs, the legislative branch must have enough votes to override the veto or the bill will not become law.

Nurses have an opportunity to influence the development of statutory law both as citizens and as health-care providers. Writing to or meeting with state legislators or members of Congress is a way to demonstrate interest in such issues and their outcomes in terms of the laws passed. Passage of a new law is often a long process that includes compromise of all interested individuals.

Administrative Law

The Department of Health and Human Services, the Department of Labor, and the Department of Education are federal agencies that have been given the responsibility for administering health-care–related laws. At the state level are departments of health and mental health and licensing boards.

Administrative agencies are staffed with professionals who develop the specific rules and regulations that direct the implementation of statutory law. These rules must be reasonable and consistent with existing statutory law and the intent of the legislature. Usually, the rules go into effect only after review and comment by affected persons or groups. For example, the state nursing board receives the authority to issue and revoke licenses from specific statutory laws, which means that each board of nursing has the responsibility to oversee the professional nurse's competence.

TYPES OF LAWS

Another way to look at the legal system is to divide it into two categories: criminal law and civil law.

Criminal Law

Criminal laws were developed to protect society from actions that threaten its existence. Criminal acts, although directed toward individuals, are considered offenses against the state. The perpetrator of the act is punished, and the victim receives no compensation for injury or damages. There are three categories of criminal law:

1. *Felony.* The most serious category, including such acts as homicide, grand larceny, and nurse practice act violation
2. *Misdemeanor.* Includes lesser offenses such as traffic violations or shoplifting of a small dollar amount
3. *Juvenile.* Crimes carried out by individuals younger than 18 years; specific age varies by state and crime

There are occasions when a nurse breaks a law and is tried in criminal court. A nurse who illegally distributes controlled substances, either for personal use or for the use of others, for example, is violating the law. Falsification of records of controlled substances is also a criminal action. In some states, altering a patient record may be a misdemeanor (Northrop & Kelly, 1987). For example:

Nurse V. needed to administer a blood transfusion. Because she was in a hurry, she did not check the paperwork properly and violated the standard of practice established for blood administration. Because the nurse failed to follow the designated protocol, the client was transfused with incompatible blood, suffered from a transfusion reaction, and died. Nurse V. attempted to conceal her conduct and falsified the records. She was found guilty of manslaughter (Northrop & Kelly, 1987).

Civil Law

Civil laws usually involve the violation of one person's rights by another person. Areas of civil law that particularly affect nurses are tort law, contract law, antitrust law, employment discrimination, and labor laws.

Tort

The remainder of this chapter focuses primarily on tort law. A tort is a legal or civil wrong carried out by one person against the person or property of another (Black, 2004). Tort law recognizes that individuals in their relationships with each other have a general duty not to harm others (Cushing, 1999). For example, as drivers of automobiles, everyone has a duty to drive safely so that others will not be harmed. A roofer has a duty to install a roof properly so that it will not collapse and injure individuals within the structure. Nurses have a duty to deliver care in such a manner that the consumers of care are not harmed. These legal duties of care may be violated intentionally or unintentionally.

Quasi-Intentional Tort

A quasi-intentional tort has its basis in speech. These are voluntary acts that directly cause injury or anguish without meaning to harm or to cause distress. The elements of cause and desire are present, but the element of intent is missing. Quasi-intentional torts usually involve problems in communication that result in damage to a person's reputation, violation of personal privacy, or infringement of an individual's civil rights. These include defamation of character, invasion of privacy, and breach of confidentiality (Aiken, 2004, p. 139).

Negligence

Negligence is the unintentional tort of acting or failing to act as an ordinary, reasonable, prudent person, resulting in harm to the person to whom the duty of care is owed (Black, 2004). The legal elements of negligence consist of duty, breach of duty, causation, and harm or injury (Cushing, 1999). All four elements must be present in the determination. For example, if a nurse administers the wrong medication to a client, but the client is not injured, the element of harm has not been met. However, if a nurse administers appropriate pain medication but fails to put up the side rails, and the client falls and breaks a hip, all four elements have been satisfied. The duty of care is the standard of care. The law defines standard of care as that which a reasonable, prudent practitioner with similar education and experience would do or not do in similar circumstances (Prosser & Keeton, 1984).

Malpractice

Malpractice is the term used for professional negligence. When fulfillment of duties requires specialized education, the term malpractice is used. In most malpractice suits, the facilities employing the nurses who cared for a client are named as defendents in the suit. Vicarious liability is the legal principle cited in these cases. *Respondeat superior,* the borrowed servant doctrine, and the captain of the ship doctrine fall under vicarious liability.

An important principle in understanding negligence is *respondeat superior.* Translated literally, this phrase means, "let the master answer" (Aiken, 2004, p. 279). This doctrine holds employers liable for any negligence by their employees when the employees were acting within the realm of employment and when the alleged negligent acts happened during employment (Aiken, 2004).

Consider the following scenario:

A nursing instructor on a clinical unit in a busy metropolitan hospital instructed his students not to administer any medications unless he was present. Marcos, a second-level student, was unable to find his instructor, so he decided to administer digoxin to his client without supervision. The dose was 0.125 mg. The unit dose came as digoxin 0.5 mg/mL. Marcos administered the entire amount without checking the digoxin dose or the client's blood and potassium levels. The client became toxic, developed a dysrhythmia, and was transferred to the intensive care unit. The family sued the hospital and the nursing school for malpractice. The nursing instructor was also sued under the principle of respondeat superior, even though specific instructions to the contrary had been given to the students.

OTHER LAWS RELEVANT TO NURSING PRACTICE

Good Samaritan Laws

In the past, fear of being sued often prevented trained professionals from assisting during an emergency. To encourage physicians and nurses to respond to emergencies, many states developed what are now known as the Good Samaritan laws. When administering emergency care, nurses and physicians are protected from civil liability by Good Samaritan laws as long as they behave in the same manner as an ordinary, reasonable, and prudent professional would have in the same or similar circumstances (Prosser & Keeton, 1984). In other words, when assisting during an emergency, nurses must still observe professional standards of care. However, if a payment is received for the care given, the Good Samaritan laws do not hold.

Confidentiality

It is possible for nurses to be involved in lawsuits other than those involving negligence. For example, clients have the right to confidentiality, and it is the duty of the professional nurse to ensure this right. This assures the client that information obtained by a nurse while providing care will not be communicated to anyone who does not have a need to know. This includes giving information over the telephone to individuals claiming to be related to a client, giving out information without a client's signed release, or removing documents from a health-care provider with a client's name or other information.

The Health Insurance Portability and Accountability Act (HIPAA) of 1996 was passed as an effort to preserve confidentiality and protect the privacy of health information and improve the portability and continuation of health-care coverage. The HIPAA gave Congress until August 1999 to pass this legislation. Congress failed to act, and the Department of Health and Human Services took over developing the appropriate regulations (Charters, 2003). The latest version of this privacy act was published in the Federal Register in 2002 (Charters, 2003).

The increased use of electronic sources of documentation and transfer of client information present many confidentiality issues. It is important for nurses to be aware of the guidelines protecting the sharing and transfer of information through electronic sources. Most health-care institutions have internal procedures to protect client confidentiality.

Take the following example:

Bill was admitted for pneumonia. With Bill's permission, an HIV test was performed, and the result was positive. This information was available on the computerized laboratory result printout. A nurse inadvertently left the laboratory results on the computer screen that was partially facing the hallway. One of Bill's coworkers, who had come to visit him, saw the report on the screen. This individual reported the test results to Bill's supervisor. When Bill returned to work, he was fired for "poor job performance," although he had had superior job evaluations. In the process of filing a discrimination suit against his employer, Bill discovered that the information on his health status had come from this source. A lawsuit was filed against the hospital and the nurse involved based on a breach of confidentiality.

Slander and Libel

Slander and libel fall under the category of quasi-intentional torts. Nurses rarely think of themselves as being guilty of slander or libel. The term *slander* refers to the spoken word and *libel* to the written word. Making a false statement about a client's condition that may result in an injury to that client is considered slander. Putting a false statement into writing is libel. For example, stating that a client who had blood drawn for drug testing has a substance abuse problem, when in fact the client does not carry that diagnosis, could be considered a slanderous statement.

Slander and libel also refer to statements made about coworkers or other individuals whom you may encounter in both your professional and educational life. Think before you speak and write. Sometimes what may appear to be harmless to you, such as a complaint, may contain statements that damage another person's credibility personally and professionally. Consider this example:

Several nurses on a unit were having difficulty with the nurse manager. Rather than approach the manager or follow the chain of command, they decided to send a written statement to the chief executive officer (CEO) of the hospital. In this letter, they embellished some of the incidents that occurred and took out of context statements the nurse manager had made, changing the meanings of the remarks. The nurse manager was called to the CEO's office and reprimanded for these events and statements, which in fact had not occurred. The nurse manager sued the nurses for slander and libel based on the premise that her personal and professional reputation had been tainted.

False Imprisonment

False imprisonment is confining an individual against his or her will by either physical (restraining) or verbal (detaining) means. The following examples fall within the definition of false imprisonment:

◆ Using restraints on individuals without the appropriate written consent.

◆ Restraining mentally handicapped individuals who do not represent a threat to themselves or others.

◆ Detaining unwilling clients in an institution when they desire to leave.

◆ Keeping persons who are medically cleared for discharge for an unreasonable amount of time.

◆ Removing the clothing of clients to prevent them from leaving the institution.

◆ Threatening clients with some form of physical, emotional, or legal action if they insist on leaving.

Sometimes clients are a danger to themselves and to others. Nurses often need to decide on the appropriateness of restraints as a protective measure. Nurses should try to obtain the cooperation of the client before applying any type of restraints. The first step is to attempt to identify a reason for the risky behavior and resolve the problem. If this fails, document the need for restraints, consult with the physician, and carefully follow the institution's policies and standards of practice. Failure to follow these guidelines may result in greater harm to the client and possibly a lawsuit for the staff. Consider the following:

Mr. Harrison, who is 87 years old, was admitted through the emergency department with severe lower abdominal pain of 3 days' duration. Physical assessment revealed severe dehydration in a man in acute distress. A surgeon was called, and an abdominal laparotomy was performed, revealing a ruptured appendix. Surgery was successful, and the client was sent to the intensive care unit for 24 hours. On transfer to the surgical floor the next day, Mr. Harrison was in stable condition. Later that night, he became confused, irritable, and anxious. He attempted to climb out of bed and pulled out his indwelling urinary catheter. The nurse restrained him. The next day, his irritability and confusion continued. Mr. Harrison's nurse placed him in a chair, tying him in and restraining his hands. Three hours later he was found in cardiopulmonary arrest.

A lawsuit of wrongful death and false imprisonment was brought against the nurse manager, the nurses caring for Mr. Harrison, and the institution. During discovery, it was determined that the primary cause of Mr. Harrison's behavior was hypoxemia. A violation of law occurred with the failure of the nursing staff to notify the physician of the client's condition and to follow the institution's standard of practice on the use of restraints.

To protect themselves against charges of negligence or false imprisonment in such cases, nurses should discuss safety needs with clients, their families, or other members of the health-care team. Careful assessment and documentation of client status are also imperative; confusion, irritability, and anxiety often have metabolic causes that need correction, not restraint.

There are statutes and case laws specific to the admission of clients to psychiatric institutions. Most states have guidelines for emergency involuntary hospitalization for a specific period. Involuntary admission is considered necessary when clients are a danger to themselves or others. Specific procedures must be followed. A determination by a judge or administrative agency or certification by a specified number of physicians that a person's mental health justifies detention and treatment may be required. Once admitted, these clients may not be restrained unless the guidelines established by state law and the institution's policies so provide. Clients who voluntarily admit themselves to psychiatric institutions are also protected against false imprisonment. Nurses need to make themselves aware of the policies of their state and employing institution.

Assault and Battery

Assault is a threat to harm. *Battery* is touching another person without his or her consent. Most medical treatments, particularly surgery, would be battery if it were not for informed consent from the client. The significance of an assault is in the threat. "If you don't stop pushing that call bell, I'll give you this injection with the biggest needle I can find" is considered an assaultive statement. Battery would occur if the injection were given when it was refused, even if medical personnel deemed it was for the "client's good." Holding down a violent client against his or her will and injecting a sedative is battery. With few exceptions, clients have a right to refuse treatment.

STANDARDS OF PRACTICE

Concern for the quality of care is a major part of nursing's responsibility to the public. Therefore, the nursing profession is accountable to the consumer for the quality of its services. One of the defining characteristics of a profession is the ability to set its own standards. Nursing standards were established as guidelines for the profession to ensure acceptable quality of care (Beckman, 1995). Standards of practice are also used as criteria to determine whether appropriate care has been delivered. In practice, they represent the minimum acceptable level of care. Nurses are judged on generally accepted standards of practice for their level of education, experience, position, and specialty area. Standards of the profession take many forms. Some are written and may be included in recommendations by professional organizations, job descriptions, agency policies and procedures, and textbooks. Others, which may be intrinsic to the custom of practice, are not found in writing (Beckman, 1995).

State boards of nursing and professional organizations vary by role and responsibility in relation to standards of development and implementation (ANA, 1998; 2004). Statutes, professional organizations, and health-care institutions establish standards of practice. The nurse practice acts of individual states define the boundaries of nursing practice within the state. In Canada, the provincial and territorial associations define practice.

The courts have upheld the authority of boards of nursing to regulate standards. The boards accomplish this through direct or delegated statutory language (ANA, 1998; 2004). The American Nurses Association (ANA) also has specific standards of practice in general and in several clinical areas (see Appendix 2). In Canada, the colleges of registered nurses or the registered nurses associations of the various provinces and territories have developed published practice standards. These may be found at cna-aiic.ca

Internal standards of practice are those that institutions develop. They are usually explained in a specific institutional policy, and the institution includes these standards in policy and procedure manuals. For example, guidelines for the appropriate administration of a specific chemotherapeutic agent or agents are included in an institutional policy and procedure manual. The guidelines are based on the current literature and research. It is the nurse's responsibility to maintain currency with an institution's standards of practice. It is the institution's responsibility to notify the health-care personnel of any changes and instruct the personnel about the changes. Institutions may accomplish this task through written memos or meetings and in-service education.

With the expansion of advanced nursing practice, it has become particularly important to clarify the legal distinction between nursing and medical practice. It is important to be aware of the boundaries between these professional domains because crossing them can result in legal consequences and disciplinary action. The nurse practice act and related regulations developed by most state legislatures and state boards of nursing help to clarify nursing roles at the various levels of practice.

Use of Standards in Nursing Negligence Malpractice Actions

When omission of prudent care or acts committed by a nurse or those under his or her supervision cause harm to a client, standards are used as a guide to determine whether appropriate care was administered. Many nurses assume that the standards of nursing practice are the only ones used to determine whether malpractice or negligence exists. Other standards may be used. These may include, but are not limited to (ANA, 1998):

◆ State, local, or national standards.

◆ Institutional policies that alter or adhere to the nursing standards of care.

◆ Expert opinions on the appropriate standard of care at the time.

◆ Available literature and research that substantiates a standard of care or changes in the standard.

Patient's Bill of Rights

In 1973, the American Hospital Association approved a statement called the Patient's Bill of Rights. These were revised in October 1992. Patient rights were developed with the belief that hospitals and health-care institutions would support these with the goal of delivering effective client care. In 2003, these were replaced by the Patient Care Partnership. These standards were derived from the ethical principle of autonomy. A copy of this document may be found at aha.org/aha/ptcommunication/partnership/index.

Informed Consent

Without consent, many of the procedures performed on clients in a health-care setting may be considered battery or unwarranted touching. When clients consent to treatment, they give health-care personnel the right to deliver care and perform specific treatments without fear of prosecution. Although physicians are responsible for obtaining informed consent, nurses often find themselves involved in the process. It is the physician's responsibility to give information to a client about a specific treatment or medical intervention (*Giese v. Stice*, 1997). The individual institution is not responsible for obtaining the informed consent unless (1) the physician or practitioner is employed by the institution or (2) the institution was aware or should have been aware of the lack of informed consent and did not act on this fact (Guido, 2001). Some institutions require the physician or independent practitioner to obtain his or her own informed consent by obtaining the client's signature at the time the explanation for treatment is given.

The informed consent form should contain all the possible negative outcomes as well as the positive ones. Nurses may be asked to obtain the signatures on this form. The following are some criteria to help ensure that a client has actually given an informed consent (Guido, 2001; Kozier, Erb, Blais, & Wilkinson, 1995):

◆ A mentally competent adult has voluntarily given the consent.

◆ The client understands exactly to what he or she is consenting.

◆ The consent includes the risks involved in the procedure, alternative treatments that may be available, and the possible result if the treatment is refused.

◆ The consent is written.

◆ A minor's parent or guardian usually gives consent for treatment.

Ideally, a nurse should be present when the physician is explaining the treatment to the client. Before obtaining the client's signature, the nurse asks the client to recall exactly what the physician has told him or her about the treatment. If at any point the nurse thinks that the client does not understand the treatment or the expected outcome, the nurse must notify the physician of this fact.

To be able to give informed consent, the client must be fully informed. Clients have the right to refuse treatment, and nurses must respect this right. If a client refuses the recommended treatment, a client must be informed of the possible consequences of this decision.

Implied consent is a form of consent in which the consent is assumed. This may be an issue in an emergency when an individual is unable to give consent, as in the following scenario:

An elderly woman is involved in a car accident on a major highway. The paramedics called to the scene find her unresponsive and in acute respiratory distress; her vital signs are unstable. The paramedics immediately intubate her and begin treating her cardiac dysrhythmias. Because she is unconscious and unable to give verbal consent, there is an implied consent for treatment.

▨ STAYING OUT OF COURT

Prevention

Unfortunately, the public's trust in the medical profession has declined over recent years. Consumers are better informed and more assertive in their approach to health care. They demand good and responsible care. If clients and their families believe that behaviors are uncaring or that attitudes are impersonal, they are more likely to sue for what they view as errors in treatment. The same applies to nurses. If nurses demonstrate an interest in and caring behaviors toward clients, a relationship develops. Individuals do not sue those they view as "caring friends." The potential to change the attitudes of health-care consumers is within the power of health-care personnel. Demonstrating care and concern and making clients and families aware of choices and methods can help decrease liability. Nurses who involve clients and their families in decisions about care reduce the likelihood of a lawsuit. Tips to prevent legal problems are listed in Box 3-1.

All health-care personnel are accountable for their own actions and adherence to the accepted standards of health care. Most negligence and malpractice cases arise from a violation of the accepted standards of practice and the policies of the employing institution. Common causes of negligence are listed in Table 3-1. Expert witnesses on both sides are called to cite the accepted standards and assist attorneys in formulating the legal strategies pertaining to those standards. For example, most medication errors can be traced to a violation of the accepted standard of medication administration, the *five rights* (Kozier et al., 1995), which have been amended to include a sixth right (Iyer & Camp, 2005):

1. Right drug.
2. Right dose.
3. Right route.

TABLE 3-1 Common Causes of Negligence	
Problem	**Prevention**
Client falls	Identify clients at risk. Place notices about fall precautions. Follow institutional policies on the use of restraints. Always be sure beds are in their lowest positions. Use side rails appropriately.
Equipment injuries	Check thermostats and temperature in equipment used for heat or cold application. Check wiring on all electrical equipment.
Failure to monitor	Observe IV infusion sites as directed by institutional policy. Obtain and record vital signs, urinary output, cardiac status, etc. as directed by institutional policy and more often if client condition dictates. Check pertinent laboratory values.
Failure to communicate	Report pertinent changes in client status to appropriate personnel. Document changes accurately. Document communication with appropriate source.
Medication errors	Follow the Six Rights. Monitor client responses. Check client medications for multiple drugs for the same actions.

BOX 3-1

Tips for Avoiding Legal Problems

- Keep yourself informed regarding new research findings related to your area of practice.
- Insist that the health-care institution keep personnel apprised of all changes in policies and procedures and in the management of new technological equipment.
- Always follow the standards of care or practice for the institution.
- Delegate tasks and procedures only to appropriate personnel.
- Identify clients at risk for problems, such as falls or the development of decubiti.
- Establish and maintain a safe environment.
- Document precisely and carefully.
- Write detailed incident reports, and file them with the appropriate personnel or department.
- Recognize certain client behaviors that may indicate the possibility of a lawsuit.

4. Right time.
5. Right client.
6. Right documentation.

Appropriate Documentation

The adage "not documented, not done" holds true in nursing. According to the law, if something is not documented, then the responsible party did not do whatever needed to be done. If a nurse did not "do" something, that leaves the nurse open to negligence or malpractice charges.

Nursing documentation needs to be legally credible. Legally credible documentation is an accurate accounting of the care the client received. It also indicates the competence of the individual who delivered the care.

Charting by exception creates defense difficulties. When this method of documentation is used, investigators need to review the entire patient record in an attempt to reconstruct the care given to the client. Clear, concise, and accurate documentation helps nurses when they are named in lawsuits. Often, this documentation clears the individual of any negligence or malpractice. Documentation is credible when it is:

◆ **Contemporaneous.** Documenting at the time care was provided.

◆ **Accurate.** Documenting exactly what was done.

◆ **Truthful.** Documenting only what was actually done or observed.

◆ **Appropriate.** Documenting only what could be discussed comfortably in a public setting.

Box 3-2 lists some documentation tips.

In the case of Luis, the nursing student violated the *right dose* principle and therefore made a medication error. By signing off on medications for all clients for a shift before the medications are administered, a nurse is leaving himself or herself open to charges of medication error.

In the case of Mr. Harrison, the institutional personnel were found negligent because of a direct violation of the institution's standards regarding the application of restraints.

Nursing units are busy and often understaffed. These realities exist but should not be allowed to interfere with the safe delivery of health care. Clients have a right to safe and effective health care, and nurses have an obligation to deliver this care.

Common Actions Leading to Malpractice Suits

◆ Failure to appropriately assess a client.

◆ Failure to report changes in client status to the appropriate personnel.

◆ Failure to document in the patient record.

◆ Altering or falsifying a patient record.

◆ Failure to obtain informed consent.

◆ Failure to report a coworker's negligence or poor practice.

◆ Failure to provide appropriate education to a client and/or family members.

◆ Violation of internal or external standards of practice.

BOX 3-2

Some Documentation Guidelines

◆ Medications:
  Always chart the time, route, dose, and response.
  Always chart prn medications and the client response.
  Always chart when a medication was not given, the reason (client in radiology, physical therapy, etc.; do not chart that the medication was not on the floor), and the nursing intervention.
  Chart all medication refusals and report them to the appropriate source.
◆ Physician communication:
  Document each time a call is made to a physician, even if he or she is not reached. Include the exact time of the call. If the physician is reached, document the details of the message and the physician's response.
  Read back verbal orders to the physician, and confirm the client's identity as written on the chart. Chart only verbal orders that you have heard from the source, not those told to you by another nurse or unit personnel.
◆ Formal issues in charting:

Before writing on the chart, check to be sure you have the correct patient record.
Check to make sure each page has the client's name and the current date stamped in the appropriate area.
If you forgot to make an entry, chart "late entry" and place the date and time at the entry.
Correct all charting mistakes according to the policy and procedures of your institution.
Chart in an organized fashion, following the nursing process.
Write legibly and concisely, and avoid subjective statements.
Write specific and accurate descriptions.
When charting a symptom or situation, chart the interventions taken and the client response.
Document your own observations, not those that were told to you by another party.
Chart frequently to demonstrate ongoing care, and chart routine activities.
Chart client and family teaching and the response.

In the case *Tovar v. Methodist Healthcare* (2005), a 75-year-old female client came to the emergency department complaining of a headache and weakness in the right arm. Although an order for admission to the neurological care unit was written, the client was not transported until 3 hours later. Once in the unit, the nurses called one physician regarding the client's status. Another physician returned the call 90 minutes later. Three hours later, the nurses called to report a change in neurological status. A STAT computed tomography scan was ordered, which revealed a massive brain hemorrhage. The nurses were cited for the following:

1. Delay in transferring the client to the neurological unit.
2. Failure to advocate for the client.

The client presented with an acute neurological problem requiring admission to an intensive care unit where appropriate observation and interventions were available. A delay in transfer may lead to delay in appropriate treatment. According to the ANA standards of care for neuroscience nurses (2002), nurses need to correctly assess the client's changing neurological status and advocate for the client. In this instance, the court stated that the nurses should have been more assertive in attempting to reach the physician and request a prompt medical evaluation. The Court sided with the family, agreeing with the plantiff's medical expert's conclusion that the client's death was related to improper management by the nursing staff.

If a Problem Arises

When served with a summons or complaint, people often panic, allowing fear to overcome reason and sanity. First, simply answer the complaint. Failure to do this may result in a default judgment, causing greater distress and difficulties.

Second, many things can be done to protect oneself if named in a lawsuit. Legal representation can be obtained to protect personal property. Never sign any documents without consulting the malpractice insurance carrier or a legal representative. If you are personally covered by malpractice insurance, notify the company immediately, and follow their instructions carefully.

Institutions usually have lawyers to defend themselves and their employees. Whether or not you are personally insured, contact the legal department of the institution where the act took place. Maintain a file of all papers, proceedings, meetings, and telephone conversations about the case. Do not withhold any information from your attorneys, even if that information can be harmful to you. A pending or ongoing legal case should not be discussed with coworkers or friends.

Let the attorneys and the insurance company help decide how to handle the difficult situation. They are in charge of damage control. Concealing information usually causes more damage than disclosing it.

Sometimes, nurses believe they are not being adequately protected or represented by the attorneys from their employing institution. If this happens, consider hiring a personal attorney who is experienced in malpractice. This information can be obtained through either the state bar association or the local trial lawyer's association.

Anyone has the right to sue; however, that does not mean that there is a case. Many negligence and malpractice courses find in favor of the health-care providers, not the client or the client's family. The following case demonstrates this situation:

The Supreme Court of Arkansas heard a case that originated from the Court of Appeals in Arkansas. A client died in a single car motor vehicle accident shortly after undergoing an outpatient colonoscopy performed under conscious sedation. The family sued the center for performing the procedure and permitting the client to drive home. The Court agreed that sedation should not be admininstered without the confirmation of a designated driver for later. It also agreed that an outpatient facility needs to have directives stating that nurses and physicians may not admininster sedation unless transportation is available for later. However, the Court ruled physicians and nurses may rely on information from the client. If the client states that someone will be available for transportation after the procedure, sedation may be administered.

The second aspect of the case revolved around the client's insistence on leaving the facility and driving himself. When a client leaves against medical advice, the health-care personnel have a legal duty to warn and strongly advise the client against the highly dangerous action. However, nurses and physicians do not have a legal right to restrain the client physically, keep his clothes, or take away car keys. The nurses are not obligated to call a taxi, call the police, admit the client to the hospital, or personally escort the client home if the client insists on leaving. Clients have some responsibility for their own safety (*Young v. GastroIntestinal Center, Inc.*, 2005). In this case, the nurses acted appropriately. They adhered to the standard of practice, documented that the client stated that someone would be available to transport him home, and filled the duty to warn.

PROFESSIONAL LIABILITY INSURANCE

We live in a litigious society. Although there are a variety of opinions on the issue, in today's world nurses need to consider obtaining professional liability insurance (Aiken, 2004). Various forms of professional liability insurance are available. These policies have been developed to protect nurses against personal financial losses if they are involved in a medical malpractice suit. If a nurse is charged with malpractice and found guilty, the employing institution has the right to sue the nurse to reclaim damages. Professional malpractice insurance protects the nurse in these situations.

END-OF-LIFE DECISIONS AND THE LAW

When a heart ceases to beat, a client is in a state of cardiac arrest. In health-care institutions and in the community, it is common to begin cardiopulmonary resuscitation (CPR) when cardiac arrest occurs. In health-care institutions, an elaborate mechanism is put into action when a client "codes." Much controversy exists concerning when these mechanisms should be used and whether individuals who have no chance of regaining full viability should be resuscitated.

Do Not Resuscitate Orders

A do not resuscitate (DNR) order is a specific directive to health-care personnel not to initiate CPR measures. Only a physician can write a DNR order, usually after consulting with the client or family. Other members of the health-care team are expected to comply with the order. Clients have the right to request a DNR order. However, they may make this request without a full understanding of what it really means. Consider the following example:

When Mrs. Vincent, 58 years old, was admitted to the hospital for a hysterectomy, she explicitly stated, "I want to be made a DNR." The nurse, rather concerned by the statement, questioned Mrs. Vincent's understanding of a DNR order. The nurse asked her, "Do you mean that if you are walking down the hall after your surgery and your heart stops beating, you do not want the nurses or physicians to do anything? You want us to just let you die?" Mrs. Vincent responded with a resounding, "No, that is not what I mean. I mean if something happens to me and I won't be able to be the way I am now, I want to be a DNR!" The nurse then explained the concept of a DNR order.

New York state has one of the most complete laws regarding DNR orders for acute and long-term care facilities. The New York law sets up a hierarchy of surrogates who may ask for a DNR status for incompetent clients. The state has also ordered that all health-care facilities ask clients their wishes regarding resuscitation (Guido, 2001). The American Nurses Association advocates that every facility have a written policy regarding the initiation of such orders (ANA, 1992). The client or, if the client is unable to speak for himself or herself, a family member or guardian should make clear the client's preference for either having as much as possible done or withholding treatment (see the next section, Advance Directives). Elements to include in a DNR order are listed in Box 3-3.

Advance Directives

The legal dilemmas that may arise in relation to DNR orders often require court decisions. For this reason, in 1990 Senator John Danforth of Missouri and Senator Daniel Moynihan of New York introduced the Patient Self-

---

BOX 3-3

Elements to Include in a Do Not Resuscitate (DNR) Order

◆ Statement of the institution's policy that resuscitation will be initiated unless there is a specific order to withhold resuscitative measures.
◆ Statement from the client regarding specific desires.
◆ Description of the client's medical condition to justify a DNR order.
◆ Statement about the role of family members or significant others.
◆ Definition of the scope of the DNR order.
◆ Delineation of the roles of various caregivers.

American Nurses Association. (1992). Position statement on nursing care and do not resuscitate decisions. Washington, DC: ANA.

Determination Act to address questions regarding life-sustaining treatment. The act was created to allow people the opportunity to make decisions about treatment in advance of a time when they might become unable to participate in the decision-making process. Through this mechanism, families can be spared the burden of having to decide what the family member would have wanted.

Federal law requires that health-care institutions that receive federal money (from Medicare, for example) inform clients of their right to create advance directives. The Patient Self-Determination Act (S.R. 13566) provides guidelines for developing advance directives concerning what will be done for individuals if they are no longer able to participate actively in making decisions about care options. The Patient Self-Determination Act states that institutions must do several things:

◆ **Provide information to every client.** On admission, all clients must be informed in writing of their rights under state law to accept or refuse medical treatment while they are competent to make decisions about their care. This includes the right to execute advance directives.

◆ **Document.** All clients must be asked whether they have a living will or have chosen a durable power of attorney for health care (also known as a health-care surrogate). The response must be indicated on the medical record, and a copy of the documents, if available, should be placed on the client's chart.

◆ **Educate.** Nurses, other health-care personnel, and the community need to understand what the Patient Self-Determination Act as well as state laws regarding advance directives require.

◆ **Be respectful of clients' rights.** All clients are to be treated with respectful care regardless of their decision regarding life-prolonging treatments.

Living Will and Durable Power of Attorney for Health Care (Health-Care Surrogate)

The two most common forms of advance directives are living wills and durable power of attorney for health care (health-care surrogate).

A living will is a legally executed document that states an individual's wishes regarding the use of life-prolonging medical treatment in the event that he or she is no longer competent to make informed treatment decisions on his or her own behalf and is suffering from a terminal condition (Catalano, 2000; Flarey, 1991).

A condition is considered terminal when, to a reasonable degree of medical certainty, there is little likelihood of recovery or the condition is expected to cause death. A terminal condition may also refer to a persistent vegetative state characterized by a permanent and irreversible condition of unconsciousness in which there is (1) absence of voluntary action or cognitive behavior of any kind and (2) an inability to communicate or interact purposefully with the environment (Hickey, 2002).

Another form of advance directive is the appointment of a health-care surrogate. Chosen by the client, the health-care surrogate is usually a family member or close personal friend. The role of the health-care surrogate is to make the client's wishes known to medical and nursing personnel. Imperative in the designation of a health-care surrogate is a clear understanding of the client's wishes should the need arise to know them.

In some situations, clients are unable to express themselves adequately or competently, although they are not terminally ill. For example, clients with advanced Alzheimer's disease or other forms of dementia cannot communicate their wishes; clients under anesthesia are temporarily unable to communicate; and the condition of comatose clients does not allow for expression of health-care wishes. In these situations, the health-care surrogate can make treatment decisions on the behalf of the client. However, when a client regains the ability to make his or her own decisions and is capable of expressing them effectively, he or she resumes control of all decision making pertaining to medical treatment (Reigle, 1992). Nurses and physicians may be held accountable when they go against a client's wishes regarding DNR orders and advance directives.

In the case *Wendland v. Sparks* (1998), the physician and nurses were sued for "not initiating CPR." In this particular case, the client had been in the hospital for more than 2 months for lung disease and multiple myeloma. Although improving at the time, during the hospitalization she had experienced three cardiac arrests. Even after this, the client had not requested a DNR order. Her family had not discussed this either. After one of the arrests, the client's husband had told the physician that he wanted his wife placed on artificial life support if it was necessary (Guido, 2001). The client had a fourth cardiac arrest. One nurse went to obtain the crash cart, and another went to get the physician who happened to be in the area. The physician checked the heart rate, pupils, and respirations and stated, "I just cannot do it to her." (Guido, 2001, p. 158). She ordered the nurses to stop the resuscitation and the physician pronounced the death of the client. The nurses stated that if they had not been given a direct order they would have continued their attempts at resuscitation. "The court ruled that the physician's judgment was faulty and that the family had the right to sue the physician for wrongful death" (Guido, 2001, p. 158). The nurses were cleared in this case because they were following a physician's order.

Nursing Implications

The Patient Self-Determination Act does not specify who should discuss treatment decisions or advance directives with clients. Because directives are often implemented on nursing units, however, nurses need to be knowledgeable about living wills and health-care surrogates and be prepared to answer questions that clients may have about directives and the forms used by the health-care institution.

As client advocates, the responsibility for creating an awareness of individual rights often falls on nurses. It is the responsibility of the health-care institution to educate personnel about the policies of the institution so that nurses and others involved in client care can inform health-care consumers of their choices. Nurses who are unsure of the policies in their health-care institution should contact the appropriate department.

LEGAL IMPLICATIONS OF MANDATORY OVERTIME

Although mostly a workplace and safety issue, there are legal implications to mandatory overtime. Due to the nursing shortages, there has been an increased demand by hospitals forcing nurses to work overtime (ANA, 2000). Overtime causes physical and mental fatigue, increased stress, and decreased concentration. Subsequently, these conditions lead to medical errors such as failure to assess appropriately, report, document, and administer medications safely. This practice of overtime ignores other responsibilities nurses have outside of their professional lives, which affects their mood, motivation, and productivity (Vernarec, 2000).

Forced overtime causes already fatigued nurses to deliver nursing care that may be less than optimum, which in turn may lead to negligence and malpractice. This can result in the nurse losing his or her license and perhaps even facing a wrongful death suit due to an error in judgment.

Nurses practice under state or provincial (Canada) nurse practice acts. These state the nurses are held accountable for the safety of their clients (AACN, 2003; CNA, 2002). Once a nurse accepts an assignment for the client, the nurse becomes liable under his/her license.

Many states are working to create legislation restricting mandatory overtime for nurses.

LICENSURE

Licensure is defined by the National Council of State Boards of Nursing as the "process by which an agency of state government grants permission to an individual to engage in a given profession upon finding that the applicant has attained the essential degree of competency necessary to perform a unique scope of practice" (NCSBN, 2004). Licenses are given by a government agency to allow an individual to engage in a professional practice and use a specific title. State boards of nursing issue nursing licenses, thus limiting practice to a specific jurisdiction (Blais, Hayes, Kozier, & Erb, 2006).

Canadian nurses take the Canadian Registered Nurse Examination (CRNE). The purpose of the CRNE is to protect the public by ensuring that the entry-level registered nurse possesses the competencies required to practise safely and effectively. The level of competence of registered nurses in all provinces and territories except Quebec is measured, in part, by the CRNE. Quebec gives a separate examination for licensure.

Each provincial or territorial nursing regulatory body in Canada is responsible for ensuring that the individuals it registers as nurses meet an acceptable level of competence before beginning to practice. The Canadian Nurses Association (CNA) develops and maintains the CRNE. The provincial and territorial nursing regulatory authorities administer the examination and determine eligibility to write it (cna-aiic.ca).

Licensure can be mandatory or permissive. Permissive licensure is a voluntary arrangement whereby an individual chooses to become licensed to demonstrate competence. However, the license is not required to practice. Mandatory licensure requires a nurse to be licensed in order to practice. In the United States and Canada, licensure is mandatory.

Qualifications for Licensure

The basic qualification for licensure requires graduation from an approved nursing program. In the United States and the Canadian territories with the exception of Quebec, candidates must be proficient in English. To sit for the licensure examination in Quebec, the candidate must demonstrate fluency in French. States may add additional requirements, such as disclosures regarding health or medications that could affect practice. Most states require disclosure of criminal conviction.

The CNA has a similar system for licensure. Candidates must be graduates of an approved school of nursing, apply directly to the nursing regulatory body in the province or territory, and receive a letter of recommendation stating that they are qualified to sit for the examination (cna-aiic.ca).

Licensure by Examination

A major accomplishment in the history of nursing licensure was the creation of the Bureau of State Boards of Nurse Examiners. The formation of this agency led to the development of an identical examination in all states. The original examination, called the State Board Test Pool Examination, was created by the testing department of the National League for Nursing. This was done through a collaborating contract with the state boards. Initially, each state determined its own passing score; however, the states did adopt a common passing score for this examination. The present examination is referred to as the NCLEX-RN and is used in all states and territories of the United States. This test is prepared and administered through a testing company, Pearson Professional Testing of Minnesota (Ellis & Hartley, 2004).

NCLEX-RN

The NCLEX-RN is administered through computerized adaptive testing (CAT). Candidates must register to take the examination at an approved testing center in their area. Because of a large test bank, CAT permits a variety of questions to be administered to a group of candidates. Candidates taking the examination at the same time may not necessarily receive the same questions. Once a candidate answers a question, the computer analyzes the response and then chooses an appropriate question to ask next. If the question was answered correctly, the following question may be more difficult; if the question was answered incorrectly, the next question may be easier.

The minimum number of questions given is 75, and the maximum is 265. Although the maximum amount of time for taking the examination is 5 hours, candidates who do well or those who are not performing well may finish as soon as 1 hour. The test ends once the analysis of the examination clearly determines that the candidate has successfully passed, has undoubtedly failed, the maximum number of questions have been answered, or the time limit has been reached (Ellis & Hartley, 2004, p. 254). The computer scores the test at the time it is taken, however, candidates are not notified of their status at the time of completion. The information first goes to the testing service, which in turn notifies the appropriate state board. The state board notifies the candidate of the examination results.

Nursing practice requires the application of knowledge, skills, and abilities (NCSBN, 2004, p.3). The items are written to reflect the candidates' ability to make nursing decisions regarding client care through application and analysis of the information. The examination is organized into categories and subcategories based on client needs and the nursing process (NCSBN, 2004). Integrated throughout the client needs categories are processes basic to the practice of nursing.

These processes include:

◆ The nursing process.

◆ Caring.

◆ Communication and documentation.

◆ Teaching/learning (NCSBN, 2004, p. 4).

Table 3-2 summarizes the categories and subcategories.

Previously all questions were written in a multiple-choice format. In 2003, alternative item formats were introduced. These alternative format questions include fill-in-the-blank; multiple-response answers; "hot spots" that require the candidate to identify an area on a picture, graph, or chart; and drag and drop (NCSBN, 2005, p. 2). More information on alternative item formats can be found on the NCSBN Web site: ncsbn.org

TABLE 3-2
Major Categories and Subcategories of Client Needs

Category	Subcategories
Safe Effective Care Environment	Management of Care
	Safety and Infection Control
Health Promotion and Maintenance	
Psychosocial Integrity	
Physiological Integrity	Basic Care and Comfort
	Pharmacological and Parental Therapies
	Reduction of Risk Potential
	Physiological Adaptation

Adapted from NCSBN NCLEX-RN test plan (NCSBN, 2004, p. 3).

The CRNE is in the pencil-and-paper format. Candidates may take the examination in either French or English. The examination consists of 240-260 multiple-choice and short-answer questions designed to measure a specific competency expected of entry-level nurses. About 15%–25% of the examination questions are in a short-answer format, and 75%–85% percent are multiple-choice questions.

The examination measures the competencies that Canadian nurses have identified as necessary for safe and effective nursing practice. For the 2005–2010 examination cycle, approximately 190 competencies will be measured. These competencies have been organized into a framework that reflects a primary health-care model (cna-aiic.ca). More information can be found on the CNA Web site cna-aiic.ca

Preparing for the NCLEX-RN

There are several ways to prepare for the NCLEX-RN. Some candidates attend review courses, others view videos and DVDs, while others prefer to review books. These methods assist in reviewing information that was learned during education. Everyone needs to decide what works best for himself or herself. It is helpful to take practice tests, because it familiarizes one with the computer and the examination format. The NCSBN offers an on-line NCLEX-RN study program.

The CNA, which developed and owns the CRNE, offers two official tools to help candidates study for the examination: the Canadian Registered Nurse Exam Prep Guide and the LeaRN CRNE Readiness Test. These are available from the CNA.

Licensure Through Endorsement

Nurses licensed in one state may obtain a license in another state through the process of endorsement. Each application is considered independently and is granted a license based on the rules and regulations of the state. There is commonality among the states regarding licensing laws allowing nurses who have current licenses in one state to receive licensure through endorsement.

States differ in the number of continuing education credits required, legal requirements, and other educational requirements. Some states require that nurses meet the current criteria for licensure at the time of application, whereas others may grant the license based on the criteria in effect at the time of the original licensure (Ellis & Hartley, 2004). When applying for a license through endorsement, a nurse should always contact the board of nursing for the state and find out the exact requirements for licensure. This information can usually be found on the board of nursing Web site for that particular state.

Canada has a similar process as the licensure examination in the Canadian provinces and territories (with the exception of Quebec) is standardized. Licensed nurses in Canada contact the nursing organization of the province or territory to apply for licensure in that particular area (cna-aiic.ca)

Multistate Licensure

The concept of multistate licensure allows a nurse licensed in one state to practice in additional states without obtaining additional licenses. NCSBN created a Multistate Licensure Compact, which permits this practice. States that belong to the compact have passed legislation adopting the terms of this agreement. States that have signed the compact are known as party states. The nurse's home state is the state where he or she lives and received his or her original license. Renewal of the license is completed in the home state.

The nurse can hold only one home state license. If the nurse moves to another state that belongs to the compact, the nurse applies for licensure within that state based on residency. The nurse is expected to follow the guidelines for nursing practice for that new state. The multistate licensure applies only to a basic registered nurse license, not to advanced practice. More information on multistate licensure can be found on the NCSBN Web site.

Disciplinary Action

State boards of nursing and the CNA and its associated provinces maintain the rules and regulations for the practice of nursing. Violation of these regulations results in disciplinary actions delineated by these boards. Issues of primary concern today include, but are not limited to, the following:

◆ Falsifying documents to obtain a license.

◆ Conviction of a felony.

◆ Practicing while under the influence of drugs or alcohol.

◆ Functioning outside the delineated scope of practice.

◆ Child or elder abuse.

Nurses convicted of a felony or found guilty in a malpractice action may find themselves before their state board of nursing or, in Canada, the provincial or territorial regulatory body.

Disciplinary action may include but is not limited to the suspension or revocation of a nursing license, mandatory fines, and mandatory continuing education. For more information regarding the regulations that guide nursing practice, consult the board of nursing in your state or, in Canada, your provincial or territorial regulatory body.

CONCLUSION

Nurses need to understand the legalities involved in the delivery of safe health care. It is important to know the standards of care established within your institution and the rules and regulations in the nurse practice acts of your state, province, or territory because these are the standards to which you will be held accountable. Health-care consumers have a right to quality care and the expectation that all information regarding diagnosis and treatment will remain confidential. Nurses have an obligation to deliver quality care and respect client confidentiality. Caring for clients safely and avoiding legal difficulties require nurses to adhere to the expected standards of care and carefully document changes in client status. Licensure helps to ensure that health-care consumers are receive competent and safe care from their nurses.

STUDY QUESTIONS

1. How do federal laws, court decisions, and state boards of nursing affect nursing practice? Give an example of each.

2. Obtain a copy of the nurse practice act in your state. What are some of the penalties for violation of the rules and regulations delineated in the act?

3. The next time you are on your clinical unit, look at the nursing documentation done by several different staff members. Do you believe it is adequate? Explain your rationale.

4. How does your institution handle medication errors?

5. If a nurse is found to be less than proficient in the delivery of safe care, how should the nurse manager remedy the situation?

6. Describe the areas that should be accessed in determining standards of care. Explain whether each is an example of an internal or external standard of care.

7. Explain the importance of federal agencies in setting standards of care in health-care institutions.

8. What is the difference between consent and informed consent?

9. Look at the forms for advance directives and DNR policies in your institution. Do they follow the guidelines of the Patient Self-Determination Act?

10. What should a practicing nurse do to stay out of court? What should a nurse not do?

11. What impact would a law that prevents mandatory overtime have on nurses, nursing care, and the health-care industry?

CRITICAL THINKING EXERCISE

Mr. Evans, 40 years old, was admitted to the medical-surgical unit from the emergency department with a diagnosis of acute abdomen. He had a 20-year history of Crohn's disease and had been on prednisone, 20 mg, every day for the past year. Three months ago he was started on the new biologic, etanercept, 50 mg. s.c. q weekly. His last dose was 4 days ago. Because he was allowed nothing by mouth (NPO), total parenteral nutrition was started through a triple-lumen central venous catheter line, and his steroids were changed to Solu-Medrol, 60 mg by IV push q6h. He was also receiving several IV antibiotics and medication for pain and nausea.

Over the next 3 days, his condition worsened. He was in severe pain and needed more analgesics. One evening at 9 p.m., it was discovered that his central venous catheter line was out. The registered nurse notified the physician, who stated that a surgeon would come in the morning to replace it. The nurse failed to ask the physician what to do about the IV steroids, antibiotics, and fluid replacement because the client was still NPO. She also failed to ask about the etanercept. At 7 a.m., the night nurse noticed that the client had had no urinary output since 11 p.m. the night before. She failed to report this information to the day shift.

The client's physician made rounds at 9 a.m. The nurse for Mr. Evans did not discuss the fact that the client had not voided since 11 p.m. the previous night, nor did she request orders for alternative delivery of the steroids and antibiotics nor ask about administering the etanercept. At 5 p.m. that evening, while Mr. Evans was having a computed tomography scan, his blood pressure dropped to 70 mm Hg, and because no one was in the scan room with him, he coded. He was transported to the ICU and intubated. He developed severe sepsis and acute respiratory distress syndrome.

1. List all the problems you can find with the nursing care in this case.

2. What were the nursing responsibilities in reporting information?

3. What do you think was the possible cause of the drop in Mr. Evans' blood pressure and his subsequent code?

4. If you worked in risk management, how would you discuss this situation with the nurse manager and the staff?

STUDENT ACTIVITIES

1. Make arrangements to attend a court case regarding negligence or malpractice.

2. Interview the risk manager at your clinical institution.

3. Review three charts on your clinical unit. Identify documentation issues that could possibly lead to legal problems.

(Continued on following page)

4. Develop an in-service program to help the nurses on your clinical unit avoid possible legal issues with documentation.

5. Search the board of nursing Web site in your state. What information is provided on the site? Is your state a member of the NCSBN Multistate Licensure Compact?

REFERENCES

Aiken, T.D. (2004). *Legal, Ethical and Political Issues in Nursing,* 2nd ed. Philadelphia: FA Davis.

American Nurses Association (ANA). (1998). Legal aspects of standards and guidelines for clinical nursing practice. Washington, DC: ANA.

American Nurses Association (ANA). (2004). Nursing: Scope and standards of practice. Pub 03SSNP. Washington, DC: ANA.

American Nurses Association (ANA). (1992). Position statement on nursing care and do not resuscitate decisions. Washington, DC: ANA.

American Nurses Association (ANA). (2002). Scope and standards of neuroscience nursing practice. Pub NNS22. Washington, DC: ANA.

Beckman, J.P. (1995). *Nursing Malpractice: Implications for Clinical Practice and Nursing Education.* Seattle: Washington University Press.

Bernzweig, E.P. (1996). *The Nurse's Liability for Malpractice: A Programmed Text,* 6th ed. St. Louis: C.V. Mosby.

Black, H.C. (2004). In Gardner, B.A. (ed.). *Black's Law Dictionary,* 8th ed. St. Paul: West Publishing.

Blais, K.K., Hayes, J.S., Kozier, B., & Erb, G. (2006). *Professional Nursing Practice: Concepts and Perspectives,* 5th ed. Upper Saddle River, NJ: Prentice-Hall.

Canadian Nurses Association. Canadian registered nurse examination. Retrieved on December 20, 2005, from cna-aiic.ca

Catalano, J.T. (2000). *Nursing Now! Today's Issue, Tomorrow's Trends,* 2nd ed. Philadelphia: FA Davis.

Charters, K.G. (2003). HIPAA's latest privacy rule. *Policy, Politics & Nursing Practice,* 4(1), 75–78.

Cushing, M. (1999). *Nursing Jurisprudence.* Upper Saddle River, NJ: Prentice-Hall.

Ellis, J.R., & Hartley, C.L. (2004). *Nursing in Today's World: Trends, Issues and Management,* 8th ed. Philadelphia: Lippincott, Williams & Wilkins.

Flarey, D. (1991). Advanced directives: In search of self-determination. *Journal of Nursing Administration,* 21 (11), 17.

Giese v. Stice. 567 NW 2d 156 (Nebraska, 1997).

Guido, G.W. (2001). *Legal and Ethical Issues in Nursing,* 3rd ed. Upper Saddle River, NJ: Prentice-Hall.

Hickey, J. (2002). *Clinical Practice of Neurological and Neurosurgical Nursing,* 5th ed. Philadelphia: Lippincott, Williams and Wilkins.

Iyer, P., & Camp, N. (2005). *Documentation: A Nursing Process Approach,* 4th ed. Flemington, NJ: MedLeague Support Services, Inc.

Kozier, B., Erb, G., Blais, K., & Wilkinson, J.M. (1995). *Fundamentals of Nursing: Concepts, Process and Practice,* 15th ed. Menlo Park, CA: Addison-Wesley.

National Council of State Boards of Nursing. (2005). Fast facts about alternative item formats and the NCLEX examination. Retrieved on December 27, 2005, from ncsbn.org

National Council of State Boards of Nursing. (2004). 2004 NCLEX-RN test plan. Retrieved on December 27, 2005, from ncsbn.org

National Council of State Boards of Nursing. (2004). Nursing regulation. Retrieved on December 16, 2005, from ncsbn.org

Northrop, C.E., & Kelly, M.E. (1987). *State of New Jersey v. Winter.* Legal Issues in Nursing. St. Louis: C.V Mosby.

Patient Self-Care Determination Act. (1989). S.R. 13566, Congressional Record.

Prosser, W.L., & Keeton, D. (1984). *The Law of Torts,* 5th ed. St. Paul: West Publishing.

Reigle, J. (1992). Preserving patient self-determination through advance directives. *Heart Lung,* 21(2), 196–198.

Tovar v. Methodist Healthcare. (2005). S.W. 3d WL 3079074 (Texas App., 2005).

Vernarec, E. (2000). Just say no to mandatory overtime. *RN* 63(12), 69–72.

Wendland v. Sparks. (1998). 574 N.W. 2d 327 (Iowa, 1998).

Young v. GastroIntestinal Center, Inc. (2005). S.W. 3d 2005 WL 675751 (Arkansas, 2005).

chapter 4

Questions of Values and Ethics

OBJECTIVES

After reading this chapter, the student should be able to:

- Discuss the way values are formed.

- Differentiate between personal ethics and professional ethics.

- Compare and contrast various ethical theories.

- Discuss virture ethics.

- Apply the seven basic ethical principles to an ethical issue.

- Analyze the impact sociocultural factors have on ethical decision making by nursing personnel.

- Discuss the influence organizational ethics have on nursing practice.

- Identify an ethical dilemma in the clinical setting.

- Discuss current ethical issues in health care and possible solutions.

OUTLINE

Values
Value Systems
How Values Are Developed
Values Clarification
Belief Systems
Morals and Ethics
Morals
Ethics
Ethical Theories
Ethical Principles
  Autonomy
  Nonmaleficence
  Beneficence
  Justice
  Fidelity
  Confidentiality
  Veracity
  Accountability

Ethical Codes
Virtue Ethics
Organizational Ethics
Ethical Dilemmas
**Resolving Ethical
Dilemmas Faced
by Nurses**
Assessment
Planning
Implementation
Evaluation
Current Ethical Issues
Practice Issues Related to
  Technology
  *Genetics and the
    Limitations of Technology*
  Professional Dilemmas
Conclusion

It is 1961. In a large metropolitan hospital, 10 health-care professionals are meeting to consider the cases of three individuals. Ironically, the cases have something in common. Larry Jones, age 66, Irma Kolnick, age 31, and Nancy Roberts, age 10, are all suffering from chronic renal failure and are in need of hemodialysis. Equipment is scarce, the cost of the treatment is prohibitive, and it is doubtful that treatment will be covered by health insurance. The hospital is able to provide this treatment to only one of these individuals. Who shall live, and who shall die? In a novel of the same name, Noah Gordon called this decision-making group *The Death Committee* (Gordon, 1963). Today, such groups are referred to as ethics committees.

In previous centuries, health care had neither the knowledge nor the technology to prolong life. The main role of nurses and physicians entailed supporting patients through times of illness, helping them toward recovery, or keeping them comfortable until death. There were few "who shall live, and who shall die?" decisions.

The polio epidemic that raged through Europe and the United States during 1947–1948 initiated the development of units for clients on manual ventilation (the "iron lung"). At this time, Danish physicians invented a method of manual ventilation by using a tube placed in the trachea of polio patients. This was the beginning of mechanical ventilation as we know it today.

During the 1950s, the development of mechanical ventilation required more intensive nursing care and client observation. The care and monitoring of clients proved to be more efficient when they were kept in a single care area; hence the term *intensive care*. The late 1960s brought greater technological advances, especially in the care of seriously ill clients with cardiovascular disease. These new therapies and monitoring methods made the intensive care unit possible (aacn.org, 2002).

Health care can now keep alive people who would die without intervention. The development of new drugs and advances in biomechanical technology permit physicians and nurses to challenge nature. This progress also brings new, perplexing questions. The ability to prolong life has created some heartbreaking situations for families and terrible ethical dilemmas for health-care professionals. How is the decision made when to turn off the life support machines that are keeping someone's beloved son or daughter alive after, for example, a motor vehicle accident? Families and professionals alike face some of the most difficult ethical decisions at times like this. How do we define death? How do we know when it has occurred? Perhaps we also need to ask, "What is life? Is there ever a time when life is no longer worth living?"

Health-care professionals have looked to philosophy, especially the branch that deals with human behavior, for resolution of these issues. The field of biomedical ethics (or, simply, bioethics), a subdiscipline of the area known as ethics—the philosophical study of morality—has evolved. In essence, bioethics is the study of medical morality, the moral and social implications of health care and science in human life (Mappes & DeGrazia, 2005).

To understand biomedical ethics, the basic concepts of values, belief systems, ethical theories, and morality are defined, followed by a discussion of the resolution of ethical dilemmas in health care.

VALUES

Webster's New World Dictionary (2000) defines *values* as the "estimated or appraised worth of something, or that quality of a thing that makes it more or less desirable, useful." Values, then, are judgments about the importance or unimportance of objects, ideas, attitudes, and attributes. Values become a part of a person's conscience and worldview. They provide a frame of reference and act as pilots to guide behaviors and assist people in making choices.

Value Systems

A value system is a set of related values. For example, one person may value (believe to be important) material aspects of life, such as money, objects, and social status. Another person may value more abstract concepts, such as kindness, charity, and caring. Values may vary significantly, based on an individual's culture and religious upbringing. An individual's system of values frequently affects how he or she makes decisions. For example, one person may base a decision on cost, and another person placed in the same situation may base the decision on a more abstract quality, such as kindness. There are different categories of values:

◆ *Intrinsic values* are those related to sustaining life, such as food and water (Steele & Harmon, 1983).

◆ *Extrinsic values* are not essential to life. Things, people, and ideas, such as kindness, understanding, and material items, are extrinsically valuable.

◆ *Personal values* are qualities that people consider valuable in their private lives. Such concepts as strong family ties and acceptance by others are personal values.

◆ *Professional values* are qualities considered important by a professional group. Autonomy, integrity, and commitment are examples of professional values.

People's behaviors are motivated by values. Individuals take risks, relinquish their own comfort and security, and generate extraordinary efforts because of their values (Edge & Groves, 2005). Traumatic brain injury clients may overcome tremendous barriers because they value independence. Racecar drivers may risk death or other serious injury because they value competition and winning.

Values also generate the standards by which people judge others. For example, someone who values work over leisure activities will look unfavorably on the coworker who refuses to work over the weekend. A person who believes that health is more important than wealth would approve of spending money on a relaxing vacation or perhaps joining a health club rather than putting the money in the bank.

Often people adopt the values of individuals they admire. For example, a nursing student may begin to value humor after observing it used effectively with clients. Values provide a guide for decision making and give additional meaning to life. Individuals develop a sense of satisfaction when they work toward achieving values they believe are important.

How Values Are Developed

Values are learned (Wright, 1987). Values can be taught directly, incorporated through societal norms, and modeled through behavior. Children learn by watching their parents, friends, teachers, and religious leaders. Through continuous reinforcement, children eventually learn about and then adopt values as their own. Because of the values they hold dear, people often make great demands on themselves, ignoring the personal cost. Here is an example:

David grew up in a family in which educational achievement was highly valued. Not surprisingly, he adopted this as one of his own values. At school, he worked very hard because some of the subjects did not come easily to him. When his grades did not reflect his great effort, he felt as though he had disappointed his family as well as himself. By the time David reached the age of 15, he had developed severe migraine headaches.

Values change with experience and maturity. For example, young children often value objects, such as a favorite blanket or stuffed animal. Older children are more likely to value a particular event, such as a scouting expedition. As they enter adolescence, they may value peer opinion over the opinions of their parents. Young adults often value certain ideals, such as beauty and heroism. The values of adults are formed from all of these experiences as well as from learning and thought.

The number of values that people hold is not as important as what values they consider important. Choices are influenced by values. The way people use their own time and money, choose friends, and pursue a career are all influenced by values.

Values Clarification

Values clarification is deciding what one believes is important. It is the process that helps people become aware of their own values. Values play an important role in everyday decision making. For this reason, nurses need to be aware of what they value and what they do not. This process helps them to behave in a manner that is consistent with their values.

Both personal and professional values influence nurses' decisions. Understanding one's own values simplifies solving problems, making decisions, and developing better relationships with others when one begins to realize how others develop their values. Raths, Harmin, and Simon (1979) suggested using a three-step model of choosing, prizing, and acting, with seven substeps, to identify one's own values (Table 4-1).

You may have used this method when making the decision to go to nursing school. Today, many career options are available. For some people, nursing is a first career; for others, it may be a second career. Using the model in Table 4-1, the valuing process is analyzed:

1. **Choosing.** After researching alternative career options, you freely chose nursing school. This choice was most likely influenced by factors such as educational achievement and abilities, finances, support and encouragement from others, time, and feelings about people.
2. **Prizing.** Once the choice was made, you were satisfied with it and told your friends about it.
3. **Acting.** *You* have entered school and begun the journey to your new career. Later in your career, you may decide to return to school for a bachelor's or master's degree in nursing.

As you progressed through school, you probably started to develop a new set of val-

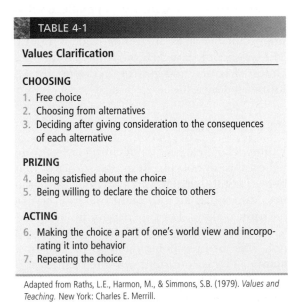

TABLE 4-1

Values Clarification

CHOOSING
1. Free choice
2. Choosing from alternatives
3. Deciding after giving consideration to the consequences of each alternative

PRIZING
4. Being satisfied about the choice
5. Being willing to declare the choice to others

ACTING
6. Making the choice a part of one's world view and incorporating it into behavior
7. Repeating the choice

Adapted from Raths, L.E., Harmon, M., & Simmons, S.B. (1979). *Values and Teaching.* New York: Charles E. Merrill.

ues—your professional values. Professional values are those established as being important in your practice. These values include caring, quality of care, and ethical behaviors.

BELIEF SYSTEMS

Belief systems are an organized way of thinking about why people exist in the universe. The purpose of belief systems is to explain such mysteries as life and death, good and evil, and health and illness. Usually these systems include an ethical code that specifies appropriate behavior. People may have a personal belief system, may participate in a religion that provides such a system, or both.

Members of primitive societies worshiped events in nature. Unable to understand the science of weather, for example, early civilizations believed these events to be under the control of someone or something that needed to be appeased, and they developed rituals and ceremonies to appease these unknown entities. They called these entities gods and believed that certain behaviors either pleased or angered the gods. Because these societies associated certain behaviors with specific outcomes, they created a belief system that enabled them to function as a group.

As higher civilizations evolved, belief systems became more complex. Archeology has provided evidence of the religious practices of ancient civilizations (Wack, 1992). The Aztec, Mayan, Incan, and Polynesian cultures each had a religious belief system comprising many gods and goddesses for the same functions. The Greek, Roman, Egyptian, and Scandinavian societies believed in a hierarchy of gods and goddesses. Although given different names by different cultures, it is very interesting that most of the deities had similar purposes. For example, Zeus was the Greek king of the gods, and Thor was the Norse god of thunder. Both used a thunderbolt as their symbol. Sociologists believe that these religions developed to explain what was then unexplainable. Human beings have a deep need to create order from chaos and to have logical explanations for events. Religion explains theologically what objective science cannot.

Along with the creation of rites and rituals, religions also developed codes of behaviors, or ethical codes. These codes contribute to the social order. There are rules regarding how to treat family members, neighbors, the young, and the old. Many religions also developed rules regarding marriage, sexual practices, business practices, property ownership, and inheritance.

The advancement of science certainly has not made belief systems any less important. In fact, the technology explosion has created an even greater need for these systems. Technological advances often place people in situations that justify religious convictions rather than oppose them. Many religions, particularly Christianity, focus on the will of a supreme being, and technology, for example, is considered a gift that allows health-care personnel to maintain the life of a loved one. Other religions, such as certain branches of Judaism, focus on free choice or free will, leaving such decisions in the hands of humankind. Many Jewish leaders believe that if genetic testing indicates, for instance, that an infant will be born with a disease such as Tay-Sachs, which causes severe suffering and ultimately death, an abortion may be an acceptable option.

Belief systems often help survivors in making decisions and living with them afterward. So far, more questions than answers have emerged from these technological advances. As science explains more and more previously unexplainable phenomena, people need beliefs and values to guide their use of this new knowledge.

MORALS AND ETHICS

Morals

Although the terms *morals* and *ethics* are often used interchangeably, *ethics* usually refers to a standardized code as a guide to behaviors, whereas *morals* usually refers to an individual's own code for acceptable behavior. Morals arise from an individual's conscience. They act as a guide for individual behavior and are learned through instruction and socialization. You may find, for example, that you and your clients dis-

agree on the acceptability of certain behaviors, such as premarital sex, drug use, or gambling. Even in your nursing class, you will probably encounter some disagreements because each of you has developed a personal code that defines acceptable behavior.

Ethics

Ethics is the part of philosophy that deals with the rightness or wrongness of human behavior. It is also concerned with the motives behind behaviors. *Bioethics,* specifically, is the application of ethics to issues that pertain to life and death. The implication is that judgments can be made about the rightness or goodness of health-care practices.

Ethical Theories

Several ethical theories have emerged to justify moral principles (Guido, 2001). *Deontological theories* take their norms and rules from the duties individuals owe each other by goodness of the commitments they make and the roles they take upon themselves. The term *deontological* comes from the Greek word *deon* (duty). This theory is attributed to the 18th-century philosopher Immanuel Kant (Kant, 1949). Deontological ethics considers the intention of the action, not the consequences of the action. In other words, it is the individual's good intentions or goodwill (Kant, 1949) that determines the worthiness or goodness of the action.

Teleological theories take their norms or rules for behaviors from the consequences of the action. This theory is also called *utilitarianism.* According to this concept, what makes an action right or wrong is its utility or usefulness. Usefulness is considered to be the amount of happiness the action carries. "Right" encompasses actions that have good outcomes, whereas "wrong" is composed of actions that result in bad outcomes. This theory had its origins with David Hume, a Scottish philosopher. According to Hume's approach, "Reason is and ought to be the slave of the passions" (Hume, 1978, p. 212). Based on this idea, ethics depends on what people want and desire. The passions determine what is right or wrong.

However, individuals who follow teleological theory disagree on how to decide on the "rightness" or "wrongness" of an action (Guido, 2001) because individual passions differ.

Principalism is an arising theory receiving a great deal of attention in the biomedical ethics community. This theory integrates existing ethical principles and tries to resolve conflicts by relating one or more of these principles to a given situation. Ethical principles actually influence professional decision making more than ethical theories.

Ethical Principles

Ethical codes are based on principles that can be used to judge behavior. Ethical principles assist decision making because they are a standard for measuring actions. They may be the basis for laws, but they themselves are not laws. *Laws* are rules created by a governing body. Laws can operate because the government has the power to enforce them. They are usually quite specific, as are the punishments for disobeying them. Ethical principles are not confined to specific behaviors. They act as guides for appropriate behaviors. They also take into account the situation in which a decision must be made. Ethical principles speak to the essence or fundamentals of the law rather than to the exactness of the law (Macklin, 1987). Here is an example:

Mrs. Van Gruen, 82 years old, was admitted to the hospital in acute respiratory distress. She was diagnosed with aspiration pneumonia and soon became septic, developing adult respiratory distress syndrome. She had a living will, and her attorney was her designated health-care surrogate. Her competence to make decisions was uncertain because of her illness. The physician presented the situation to the attorney, indicating that without a feeding tube and tracheostomy Mrs. Van Gruen would die. According to the laws governing living wills and health-care surrogates, the attorney could have made the decision to withhold all treatments. However, he believed he had an ethical obligation to discuss the situation with his client. The client requested that the tracheostomy and the feeding tube be inserted, which was done.

In some situations, two or more principles may conflict with each other. Making a decision under these circumstances is very difficult. Following are several of the ethical principles that are most important to nursing practice—autonomy, nonmaleficence, beneficence, justice, confidentiality, veracity, and accountability—and a discussion of some of the ethical dilemmas nurses encounter in clinical practice.

Autonomy

Autonomy is the freedom to make decisions for oneself. This ethical principle requires that nurses respect clients' rights to make their own choices about treatment. Informed consent before treatment, surgery, or participation in research is an example. To be able to make an autonomous choice, individuals need to be informed of the purpose, benefits, and risks of the procedures to which they are agreeing. Nurses accomplish this by providing information and supporting clients' choices.

Closely linked to the ethical principle of autonomy is the legal issue of competence. A client needs to be deemed competent in order to make a decision regarding treatment options. When clients refuse treatment, health-care personnel and family members who think differently often question the client's "competence" to make a decision. Of note is the fact that when clients agree with health-care treatment decisions, rarely is their competence questioned (AACN News, 2006).

Nurses are often in a position to protect a client's autonomy. They do this by ensuring that others do not interfere with the client's right to proceed with a decision. If a nurse observes that a client has insufficient information to make an appropriate choice, is being forced into a decision, or is unable to understand the consequences of the choice, then the nurse may act as a client advocate to ensure the principle of autonomy.

Sometimes nurses have difficulty with the principle of autonomy because it also requires respecting another's choice, even if the nurse disagrees with it. According to the principle of autonomy, a nurse cannot replace a client's decision with his or her own, even when the nurse honestly believes that the client has made the wrong choice. A nurse can, however, discuss concerns with clients and make sure clients have thought about the consequences of the decision they are about to make.

Nonmaleficence

The ethical principle of nonmaleficence requires that no harm be done, either deliberately or unintentionally. This rather complicated word comes from Latin roots: *non*, which means not; *male*, which means bad; and *facere*, which means to do.

The principle of nonmaleficence also requires that nurses protect from danger individuals who are unable to protect themselves because of their physical or mental condition. An infant, a person under anesthesia, and a person with Alzheimer's disease are examples of people with limited ability to protect themselves. Nurses are ethically obligated to protect their clients when they are unable to protect themselves.

Often, treatments meant to improve client health lead to harm. This is not intentional on the part of the nurse or other health-care personnel but is a direct result of treatment. Nosocomial infections as a result of hospitalization are harmful to a client. The nurses did not deliberately cause the infection. The side effects of chemotherapy or radiation therapy may result in harm. Chemotherapeutic agents cause a decrease in immunity that may result in a severe infection, whereas radiation may burn or damage the skin. For this reason, many clients opt not to pursue treatments.

The obligation to do no harm extends to the nurse who for some reason is not functioning at an optimal level. For example, a nurse who is impaired by alcohol or drugs is knowingly placing clients at risk. Other nurses who observe such behavior have an ethical obligation to protect the client according to the principle of nonmaleficence.

Beneficence

The word beneficence also comes from Latin: *bene*, which means well, and *facere*, which means to do.

The principle of beneficence demands that good be done for the benefit of others. For nurses, this means more than delivering competent physical or technical care. It requires helping clients meet all their needs, whether physical, social, or emotional. *Beneficence* is caring in the truest sense, and caring fuses thought, feeling, and action. It requires knowing and being truly understanding of the situation and the thoughts and ideas of the individual (Benner & Wrubel, 1989).

Sometimes physicians, nurses, and families withhold information from clients for the sake of beneficence. The problem with doing this is that it does not allow competent individuals to make their own decisions based on all available information. In an attempt to be beneficent, the principle of autonomy is violated. This is just one of many examples of the ethical dilemmas encountered in nursing practice. For instance:

Mrs. Chung has just been admitted to the oncology unit with ovarian cancer. She is scheduled to begin chemotherapy treatment. Her two children and her husband have requested that the physician ensure that Mrs. Chung not be told her diagnosis because they believe she would not be able to deal with it. The information is communicated to the nursing staff. After the first treatment, Mrs. Chung becomes very ill. She refuses the next treatment, stating that she did not feel sick until she came to the hospital. She asks the nurse what could possibly be wrong with her that she needs a medicine that makes her sick when she does not feel sick. Only people who get cancer medicine get this sick! Mrs. Chung then asks the nurse, "Do I have cancer?"

As the nurse, you understand the order that the client not be told her diagnosis. You also understand your role as a client advocate.

1. To whom do you owe your duty: the family or the client?
2. How do you think you may be able to be a client advocate in this situation?
3. What information would you communicate to the family, and how can you assist them in dealing with their mother's concerns?

Justice

The principle of justice obliges nurses and other health-care professionals to treat every person equally regardless of gender, sexual orientation, religion, ethnicity, disease, or social standing (Edge & Groves, 2005). This principle also applies in the work and educational setting. Everyone should be treated and judged by the same criteria according to this principle. Here is an example:

Found on the street by the police, Mr. Johnson was admitted through the emergency room to a medical unit. He was in deplorable condition: his clothes were dirty and ragged, he was unshaven, and he was covered with blood. His diagnosis was chronic alcoholism, complicated by esophageal varices and end-stage liver disease. Several nursing students overheard the staff discussing Mr. Johnson. The essence of the conversation was that no one wanted to care for him because he was dirty and smelly and brought this condition on himself. The students, upset by what they heard, went to their instructor about the situation. The instructor explained that every individual has a right to good care despite his or her economic or social position. This is the principle of justice.

The concept of *distributive justice* necessitates the fair allocation of responsibilities and advantages, especially in a society where resources may be limited (Davis, Arokar, Liaschenko, & Drought, 1997). Health-care costs have increased tremendously over the years, and access to care has become a social and political issue. In order to understand distributive justice, certain concepts need to be addressed: need, individual effort, ability to pay, contribution to society, and age (Davis, et al., p. 53).

Age has become an extremely controversial issue as it leads to quality of life questions, particularly technological care at the end of life. The other issue regarding age revolves around the technology in neonatal care. How do health-care providers place value on one person's quality of life over that of another? Should millions of dollars be spent preserving the life of an 80-year-old man who volunteers in his community, plays golf twice a week, and teaches reading to underprivileged children, or should that money be spent on a 26-week-old fetus that will most likely require intensive therapies and treatments for a lifetime, adding up to more millions of health-care dollars? In the social and business world, welfare payments are based on need, and jobs and promotions are usually distributed on an individual's contributions and achievements. Is it possible to apply these measures to health-care allocations?

Philosopher John Rawls addressed the issue of justice as fairness and justice as the foundation of social structures. According to Rawls, the idea of the original position should be used to negotiate the principles of justice. The original position based on Kant's social contract theory presents a hypothetical situation in which individuals act as a trustee for the interests of all individuals. The individuals, known as negotiators, are knowledgeable in the areas of sociology, political science, and economics.However, they are placed under certain limitations referred to as the *veil of ignorance.* These limitations represent the moral essentials of original position arguments.

The veil of ignorance eliminates information about age, gender, socioeconomic status, and religious convictions from the issues. Once this information is unavailable to the negotiators, the vested interests of involved parties disappears. According to Rawls, in a just society the rights protected by justice are not issues for political bargaining or subject to the calculations of social interests. Simply put, everyone has the same rights and liberties.

Fidelity

The principle of fidelity requires loyalty. It is a promise that the individual will fulfill all commitments made to himself or herself and to others. For nurses, fidelity includes the professional's loyalty to fulfill all responsibilities and agreements expected as part of professional practice. Fidelity is the basis for the concept of accountability—taking responsibility for one's own actions (Shirey, 2005).

Confidentiality

The principle of confidentiality states that anything said to nurses and other health-care providers by their clients must be held in the strictest confidence. Confidentiality presents both a legal and an ethical issue. Exceptions exist only when clients give permission for the release of information or when the law requires the release of specific information. Sometimes, just sharing information without revealing an individual's name can be a breach in confidentiality if the situation and the individual are identifiable. It is important to realize that what seems like a harmless statement can become harmful if other people can piece together bits of information and identify the client.

Nurses come into contact with people from different walks of life. Within communities, people know other people who know other people, and so on. Individuals have lost families, jobs, and insurance coverage because nurses shared confidential information and others acted on that knowledge (AIDS Update Conference, 1995).

In today's electronic environment, the principle of confidentiality has become a major concern. Many health-care institutions, insurance companies, and businesses use electronic media to transfer information. These institutions store sensitive and confidential information in computer databases. These databases need to have security safeguards to prevent unauthorized access. Health-care institutions have addressed the situation through the use of limited access, authorization passwords, and security tracking systems. However, even the most secure system developed is vulnerable and can be accessed by an individual who understands the complexities of computer systems.

Veracity

Veracity requires nurses to be truthful. Truth is fundamental to building a trusting relationship. Intentionally deceiving or misleading a client is a violation of this principle. Deliberately omitting a part of the truth is deception and violates the principle of veracity. This principle often creates ethical dilemmas. When is it permissible to lie? Some ethicists believe it is never appropriate to deceive another individual. Others think that if another ethical principle overrides veracity, then lying is permissible. Consider this situation:

Ms. Allen has just been told that her father has Alzheimer's disease. The nurse practitioner wants to come into the home to discuss treatment. Ms. Allen refuses, saying that the nurse practitioner should under no circumstances tell her father the diagnosis. She explains to the practitioner that she is sure he will kill himself if he learns that he has Alzheimer's disease. She bases this concern on statements he has made regarding this disease. The nurse practitioner replies that medication is available that might help her father. However, it is available only through a research study being conducted at a nearby university. To participate in the research, the client must be informed of the purpose of the study, the medication to be given and its side effects, and follow-up procedures. Ms. Allen continues to refuse to allow her father to be told his diagnosis because she is certain he will commit suicide.

The nurse practitioner faces a dilemma: does he abide by Ms. Allen's wishes based on the principle of beneficence, or does he abide by the principle of veracity and inform his client of the diagnosis. What would you do?

Accountability

Accountability is linked to fidelity and means accepting responsibility for one's actions. Nurses are accountable to their clients and to their colleagues. When providing care to clients, nurses are responsible for their actions, good and not so good. If something was not done, do not chart or tell a colleague that it was. An example of violating accountability is the story of Anna:

Anna was a registered nurse who worked nights on an acute care unit. She was an excellent nurse, but as the acuity of the clients' conditions increased, she was unable to keep up with both clients' needs and the technology, particularly intravenous lines (IVs). She began to chart that all the IVs were infusing as they should, even when they were not. Each morning, the day shift would find that the actual infused amount did not agree with what the paperwork showed. One night, Anna allowed an entire liter to be infused in 2 hours into a client with congestive heart failure. When the day staff came on duty, they found the client expired, the bag empty, and the tubing filled with blood. Anna's IV sheet showed 800 mL left in the bag. It was not until a lawsuit was filed that Anna took responsibility for her behavior.

The idea of a standard of care evolves from the principle of accountability. Standards of care provide a ruler for measuring nursing actions.

Ethical Codes

A *code of ethics* is a formal statement of the rules of ethical behavior for a particular group of individuals. A code of ethics is one of the hallmarks of a profession. This code makes clear the behavior expected of its members.

The Code of Ethics for Nurses with Interpretive Statements provides values, standards, and principles to help nursing function as a profession. The original code was developed in 1985. In 1995, the American Nurses Association Board of Directors and the Congress on Nursing Practice initiated the Code of Ethics Project (ANA, 2002). The code may be viewed online at nursingworld.org

The Canadian Nurses Association (CNA) also developed a code of ethics. The first code, adopted in 1954, was the International Council of Nursing Code for Nurses. In 1980, the CNA adopted a new code, named the Code of Ethics for Nursing. This code was revised in 1991. The Code of Ethics for Registered Nurses was adopted in 1997. This code replaced the 1991 revision. In 2002 the Code of Ethics for Registered Nurses was expanded and revised. The code may be obtained from the CNA Web site cna-nurses.ca/cna/documents/pdf/publications/CodeofEthics2002_e.pdf

Ethical codes are dynamic. They reflect the values of the profession and the society for which they were developed. Changes occur as society and technology evolve. For example, years ago no thought was ever given to do not resuscitate orders or withholding food and fluids. These things were not issues then, but the technological advances that have made it possible to keep people in a kind of twilight life, comatose and unable to participate in living in any way, have made these very important issues in health care.

It is not the purpose of ethical codes to change with every little breeze but to maintain a steady course, evolving as needed, but continuing to emphasize the basic ethical principles. Technology has increased our knowledge and skills, but our ability to make decisions regarding ourselves and those we care for is still guided by the principles of autonomy, nonmaleficence, beneficence, justice, confidentiality, fidelity, veracity, and accountability.

Virtue Ethics

Virtue ethics focuses on virtues, or moral character, rather than duties or rules that emphasize the consequences of actions. Take the following example:

Norman is driving along the road and finds a crying child sitting by a fallen bicycle. It is obvious that the child needs assistance. From one ethical standpoint (utilitarianism), helping the child will increase Norman's personal feelings of "doing good." The deontological stance states that by helping, Norman is behaving in accordance with a moral rule such as "Do unto others...." Virtue ethics looks at the fact that helping the person would be charitable or benevolent.

Plato and Aristotle are considered the founding fathers of virtue ethics. Its roots can be found in Chinese philosophy. During the 1800s it disappeared but in the late 1950s reemerged as an Anglo-American philosophy. Prior to this time, the focus had been more on the deontological and utilitarian philosophies. Neither of these philosophies considered the virtues of moral character and education and the question: "What type of person should I be, and how should I live" (Hooker, 2000; Driver, 2001).

Virtues include such qualities as honesty, generosity, altruism, and reliability. They are concerned with many other elements as well, such as emotions and emotional reactions, choices, values, needs, insights, attitudes, interests, and expectations. To embrace a virtue means that you are a person with a certain complex way of thinking. Nursing has practiced virtue ethics for many years.

Organizational Ethics

Organizational ethics focuses on the workplace and is aimed at the organizational level. Every organization, even one with hundreds of thousands of employees, consists of individuals. Each individual makes his and her own decisions about how to behave in the workplace. Each person has the opportunity to make the organization a more or less ethical place. These individual decisions can have a powerful effect on the lives of many others in the organization as well as in the surrounding community. Shirey (2005) explains that employees need to experience uniformity between what the organization states and what it practices.

Research conducted by the Ethics Research Center concluded the following:

◆ If positive outcomes are desired, ethical culture is what makes the difference;

◆ Leadership, especially senior leadership, is the most critical factor in promoting an ethical culture; and

◆ In organizations that are trying to strengthen their culture, formal program elements can help to do that (Harned, 2005, p. 1).

When looking for a professional position, it is important to consider the organizational culture. What are the values and beliefs of the organization? Do they blend with yours, or are they in conflict with your value system? To find out this information, look at the organization's mission, vision, and value statements. Speak with other nurses who work in the organization. Do they see consistency between what the organization states and what it actually expects from the employees? For example, if an organization states that it collaborates with the nurses in decision making, do nurses sit on committees that have input into the decision-making process?

Ethical Dilemmas

What is a dilemma? The word *dilemma* is of Greek derivation. A lemma was an animal resembling a ram and having two horns. Thus came the saying "stuck on the horns of a dilemma." The story of Hugo illustrates a hypothetical life-or-death dilemma with a touch of humor:

One day, Hugo, dressed in a bright red cape, walked through his village into the countryside. The wind caught the corners of the cape, and it was whipped in all directions. As he walked down the dusty road, Hugo happened to pass by a lemma. Hugo's bright red cape caught the lemma's attention. Lowering its head, with its two horns poised in attack position, the animal began to chase poor Hugo down the road. Panting and exhausted, Hugo reached the end of the road to find himself blocked by a huge stone wall. He turned to face the lemma, which was ready to charge. A decision needed to be made, and Hugo's life depended on this decision. If he moved to the left, the lemma would gore his heart. If he moved to the right, the lemma would gore his liver. Alas, no matter what his decision, our friend Hugo would be "stuck on the horns of da lemma."

Like Hugo, nurses are often faced with difficult dilemmas. Also, as Hugo found, an ethical dilemma can be a choice between two unpleasant alternatives.

An ethical dilemma occurs when a problem exists that forces a choice between two or more ethical principles. Deciding in favor of one principle will violate the other. Both sides have goodness and badness to them, but neither decision satisfies all the criteria that apply. Ethical dilemmas also have the added burden

of emotions. Feelings of anger, frustration, and fear often override rationality in the decision-making process. Consider the case of Mr. Sussman:

Mr. Sussman, 80 years old, was admitted to the neuroscience unit after suffering left hemispheric bleeding. He had a total right hemiplegia and was completely nonresponsive, with a Glasgow Coma Scale score of 8. He had been on IV fluids for 4 days, and the question was raised of placing a percutaneous endoscopic gastrostomy (PEG) tube for enteral feedings. The elder of the two children asked what the chances of recovery were. The physician explained that Mr. Sussman's current state was probably the best he could attain but that "miracles happen every day" and stated that tests could help in determining the prognosis. The family asked that these tests be performed. After the results were in, the physician explained that the prognosis was grave and that IV fluids were insufficient to sustain life. The PEG tube would be a necessity if the family wished to continue with food and fluids. As the physician went down the hall, the family pulled in the nurse, Gail, who had been with Mr. Sussman during the previous 3 days and asked, "If this was your father, what would you do?" This situation became an ethical dilemma for Gail as well.

If you were Gail, what would you say to the family? Depending on your answer, what would be the possible principles that you might violate?

RESOLVING ETHICAL DILEMMAS FACED BY NURSES

Ethical dilemmas can occur in any aspect of life, personal or professional. This section focuses on the resolution of professional dilemmas. The various models for resolving ethical dilemmas consist of 5 to 14 sequential steps. Each step begins with the complete understanding of the dilemma and concludes with the evaluation of the implemented decision.

The nursing process provides a helpful mechanism for finding solutions to ethical dilemmas. The first step is assessment, including identification of the problem. The simplest way to do this is to create a statement that summarizes the issue. The remainder of the process evolves from this statement (Box 4-1).

Assessment

Ask yourself, "Am I directly involved in this dilemma?" An issue is not an ethical dilemma

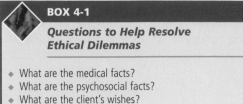

BOX 4-1

Questions to Help Resolve Ethical Dilemmas

◆ What are the medical facts?
◆ What are the psychosocial facts?
◆ What are the client's wishes?
◆ What values are in conflict?

for nurses unless they are directly involved or have been asked for their opinion about a situation. Some nurses involve themselves in situations even when their opinion has not been solicited. This is generally unwarranted, unless the issue is a violation of the professional code of ethics.

Nurses are frequently in the position of hearing both sides of an ethical dilemma. Often, all that is wanted is an empathetic listener. At other times, when guidance is requested, nurses can help people work through the decision-making process (remember the principle of autonomy).

Collecting data from all the decision makers helps identify the reasoning process being used by these individuals as they struggle with the issue. The following questions assist in the information-gathering process:

◆ *What are the medical facts?* Find out how the physicians, physical and occupational therapists, dietitians, and fellow nurses view the client's condition and treatment options. Speak with the client if possible, and determine his or her understanding of the situation.

◆ *What are the psychosocial facts?* In what emotional state is the client right now? The client's family? What kind of relationship exists between the client and his or her family? What are the client's living conditions? Who are the individuals who form the client's support system? How are they involved in the client's care? What is the client's ability to make medical decisions about his or her care? Do financial considerations need to be taken into account? What concepts or things does the client value? What does the client's family value?

The answers to these questions will provide a better understanding of the situation. Ask more questions, if necessary, to complete the picture. The social facts of a situation also include institutional policies, legal aspects, and economic factors. The personal belief systems of physicians and other health-care professionals also influence this aspect.

◆ *What are the cultural beliefs?* Cultural beliefs play a major role in ethical decisions. Some cultures will not allow surgical interventions as they fear that the "life force" may escape. Many cultures forbid organ donation. Other cultures focus on the sanctity of life, thereby requesting all methods for sustaining life be used regardless of the futility.

◆ *What are the client's wishes?* Remember the ethical principle of autonomy. With very few exceptions, if the client is competent, his or her decisions take precedence. Too often, the family's or physician's worldview and belief system overshadow that of the client. Nurses can assist by maintaining the focus on the client. If the client is unable to communicate, try to discover whether the individual has discussed the issue in the past. If the client has completed a living will or designated a health-care surrogate, this will help determine the client's wishes. By interviewing family members, the nurse can often learn about conversations in which the client has voiced his or her feelings about treatment decisions. Through guided interviewing, the nurse can encourage the family to tell anecdotes that provide relevant insights into the client's values and beliefs.

◆ *What values are in conflict?* To assess values, begin by listing each person involved in the situation. Then identify the values represented by each person. Ask such questions as, "What do you feel is the most pressing issue here?" and "Tell me more about your feelings regarding this situation." In some cases, there may be little disagreement among the people involved, just a different way of expressing beliefs. In others, however, a serious value conflict may exist.

Planning

For planning to be successful, everyone involved in the decision must be included in the process. Thompson and Thompson (1985) listed three specific and integrated phases of this planning:

1. *Determine the goals of treatment.* Is cure a goal, or is the goal to keep the client comfortable? Is life at any cost the goal, or is `the goal a peaceful death at home? These goals need to be client-focused, reality-centered, and attainable. They should be consistent with current medical treatment and, if possible, be measurable according to an established time frame.

2. *Identify the decision makers.* As mentioned earlier, nurses may or may not be decision makers in these health-related ethical dilemmas. It is important to know who the decision makers are and what their belief systems are. When the client is a capable participant, this task is much easier. However, people who are ill are often too exhausted to speak up for themselves or to ensure that their voices are heard. When this happens, the client needs an advocate. Family, friends, spiritual advisers, and nurses often act as advocates for clients. If the client is unable to speak for himself or herself, then someone else must speak. A family member may need to be designated as the primary decision maker, a role often called the *health-care surrogate.*

The creation of living wills, establishment of advance directives, and appointment of a health-care surrogate while a person is still healthy often ease the burden for the decision makers during a later crisis. Clients can exercise autonomy through these mechanisms, even though they may no longer be able to communicate their wishes directly. When these documents are not available, the information gathered during the assessment of social factors helps identify those individuals who may be able to act in the client's best interest.

3. *List and rank all the options.* Performing this task involves all the decision makers. It is sometimes helpful to begin with the least desired choice and methodically work toward the preferred treatment choice that is most likely to lead to the desired outcome. Asking all participating parties to discuss what they believe are reasonable outcomes to be attained with the use of available medical treatment often helps in the decision process. By listening to others in a controlled situation, family members and health-care professionals discover that they actually want the same result as the client and just had different ideas about how to achieve their goal.

Implementation

During the implementation phase, the client or the surrogate (substitute) decision makers and members of the health-care team reach a mutually acceptable decision. This occurs through open discussion and sometimes negotiation. An example of negotiation follows:

Elena's mother has metastatic ovarian cancer. She and Elena have discussed treatment options. Her physician suggested the use of a new chemotherapeutic agent that has demonstrated success in many cases. But Elena's mother emphatically states that she has "had enough" and would just like to spend her remaining time doing whatever she chooses. Elena would like her mother to try the drug. To resolve the dilemma, the oncology nurse practitioner and the physician sit down to talk with Elena and her mother. Everyone reviews the facts and expresses their feelings about the situation. Seeing Elena's distress over her decision, Elena's mother says, "OK, I will try the Taxol for a month. If there is no improvement after this time, I want to stop all treatment and live out the time I have with my daughter and her family." All agreed that this was a reasonable decision.

The role of the nurse during the implementation phase is to ensure that communication does not break down. Ethical dilemmas are often emotional issues, filled with guilt, sorrow, anger, and other strong emotions. These strong feelings can cause communication failures among decision makers. Remind yourself, "I am here to do what is best for this client."

Keep in mind that an ethical dilemma is not always a choice between two attractive alternatives. Many are between two unattractive, even unpleasant, choices. Elena's mother's options did not include the choice she really wanted: good health and a long life.

Once an agreement is reached, the decision makers must live with it. Sometimes, an agreement is not reached because the parties cannot reconcile their conflicting belief systems or values. At other times, caregivers are unable to recognize the worth of the client's point of view. Occasionally, the client or the surrogate may make a request that is not institutionally or legally possible. In some cases, a different institution or physician may be able to honor the request. In other cases, the client or surrogate may request information from the nurse regarding illegal acts. When this happens, the nurse should sit down with the client and family and ask them to consider the consequences of their proposed actions. It may be necessary to bring other counselors into the discussion (with the client's permission) to negotiate an agreement.

Evaluation

As in the nursing process, the purpose of evaluation in resolving ethical dilemmas is to determine whether the desired outcomes have occurred. In the case of Mr. Sussman, some of the questions that could be posed by Gail to the family are as follows:

◆ "I have noticed the amount of time you have been spending with your father. Have you observed any changes in his condition?"

◆ "I see Dr. Washburn spoke to you about the test results and your father's prognosis. How do you feel about the situation?"

◆ "Now that Dr. Washburn has spoken to you about your father's condition, have you considered future alternatives?"

Changes in client status, availability of medical treatment, and social facts may call for reevaluation of a situation. The course of treatment may need to be altered. Continued communication and cooperation among the decision makers are essential.

Another model, the MORAL model created by Thiroux (1977) and refined for nursing by Halloran (1982), is gaining popularity. The

---

BOX 4-2

The Moral Model

◆ M   Massage the dilemma
◆ O   Outline the options
◆ R   Resolve the dilemma
◆ A   Act by applying the chosen option
◆ L   Look back and evaluate the complete process, including the actions taken

---

MORAL acronym reminds nurses of the sequential steps needed for resolving an ethical dilemma. This ethical decision-making model is easily implemented in all client care settings (Box 4-2).

Current Ethical Issues

During fall 1998, the well known Dr. Jack Kevorkian (sometimes called Dr. Death in the press) openly admitted that at the patient's request, he gave the patient a lethal dose of medication causing the individual's death. His statement raised the consciousness of the American people and the health-care system about the issues of euthanasia and assisted suicide. Do individuals have the right to consciously end their own lives when they are suffering from terminal conditions? If they are unable to perform the act themselves, should others assist them in ending their lives? Should assisted suicide be legal? We do not have answers to these difficult questions, yet clients and their families across the country face these same questions every day.

More recently, the Terri Schiavo case gained tremendous media attention, probably becoming the most important case of clinical ethics in more than a decade. Her illness and death created a major medical, legal, theological, ethical, political, and social controversy. The case brought to the forefront the deep divisions and fears that reside in our society regarding life and death, the role of the government and courts in life decisions, and the treatment of disabled persons. Many aspects of this case will never be clarified, however many questions raised by this case need to be addressed for future ethical decsion making. Some of these are:

1. What is the true definition of a persistent vegetative state?
2. How is cognitive recovery determined?
3. What role do the courts play when there is a familial dispute? Who has the right to make decisions when an individual is married?
4. What are the duties of surrogate decision makers? (Hook & Mueller, 2005)

The primary goal of nursing and other health-care professions is to keep people alive and well or, if this cannot be done, to help them live with their problems and die peacefully. To accomplish this, health-care professionals struggle to improve their knowledge and skills so that they can care for their clients, provide them with some quality of life, and bring them back to the state known as wellness. The costs involved in achieving this goal can be astronomical.

Questions are being raised more and more often about who should receive the benefits of this technology. Managed care and the competition for resources are also creating ethical dilemmas. Other difficult questions, such as who should pay for care when the illness may have been due to poor health-care practices such as smoking or substance abuse, are also being debated.

Practice Issues Related to Technology

Genetics and the Limitations of Technology

When facing issues of technology, the principles of beneficence and nonmaleficence may be in conflict. A specific technology administered with the intention of "doing good" may result in enormous suffering. Causing this type of torment is in direct conflict with the idea of "do no harm" (Burkhardt & Nathaniel, 2001). At times, this is an accepted consequence, such as the use of chemotherapy. However, the ultimate outcome in this case is that recovery is expected. In situations in which little or no improvement is expected, the issue of whether the good outweighs the bad prevails. Suffering induced by technology may include physical, spiritual, and emotional components for both the client and the families.

Today, many low birth weight infants and infants with birth defects who not so long ago would have been considered incompatible with life are maintained on machines in highly sophisticated neonatal units. This process may keep babies alive only to die several months later or may leave them with severe chronic disabilities. Children with chronic disabilities require additional medical, educational, and social services. These services are expensive and often require families to travel long distances to obtain them (Urbano, 1992).

Genetic diagnosis and gene therapy present new ethical issues for nursing. *Genetic diagnosis* is a process that involves analyzing parents or an embryo for a genetic disorder. This is usually done before in vitro fertilization with couples who have a high risk of conceiving a child with a genetic disorder. The embryos are tested and only those that are free of genetic flaws are implanted.

Genetic screening is used only as a tool to determine whether couples hold the possibility of giving birth to a genetically impaired infant. For example, in older couples it is commonplace to test for Down syndrome. In other cases, say, if a couple has one child with a genetic disorder, genetic specialists test the parents or the fetus for the presence of the gene. This leads to issues pertaining to reproductive rights. It also opens new issues: What is a disability versus a disorder, and who decides this? Is a disability a disease, and does it need to be cured or prevented? The technology is also used to determine whether individuals are predisposed to certain diseases, such as breast cancer or Huntington's chorea. This has created additional ethical issues regarding genetic screening. Take the following example:

Bianca, age 33, is diagnosed with breast cancer. She has two daughters, ages 6 and 4. Both her mother and grandmother had breast cancer. Neither survived more than 5 years post treatment. She undergoes a lumpectomy followed by radiation and chemotherapy. Her cancer is found to be nonhormonally-dependent. Due to her age and family history, Bianca's oncologist recommends that she see a geneticist and have genetic testing for the *BRCA-1* and *BRCA-2* genes. Bianca makes an appointment to discuss the testing. She meets with the nurse who has additional education in genetics and discusses the following questions:

1. "If I am positive for the genes, what are my options? Do I have a bilateral mastectomy with reconstruction?"
2. "Will I be able to get health insurance coverage, or will the companies consider this to be a preexisting condition?"
3. "What are the future implications for my daughters?"

If you were the nurse, how would you address these concerns?

Genetic engineering is the ability to change the genetic structure of an organism. Through this process, researchers have created more disease-resistant fruits and vegetables and certain medications, such as insulin. This process theoretically allows for the genetic alteration of embryos, eliminating genetic flaws and creating healthier babies. This technology enables researchers to make a brown-haired individual blonde, to change brown eyes to blue, and make a short person taller. Imagine being able to "engineer" your child. Imagine, as Aldous Huxley did in *Brave New World* (1932), being able to create a society of perfect individuals: "We also predestine and condition. We decant our babies as socialized human beings, as Alphas or Epsilons, as future sewage workers or future . . . he was going to say future World controllers but correcting himself said future directors of Hatcheries, instead" (p. 12).

The ethical implications pertaining to genetic technology are profound. For example, some questions recently raised by the Human Genome Project relate to:

◆ Fairness in the use of the genetic information.

◆ Privacy and confidentiality of obtained genetic information.

◆ Genetic testing of an individual for a specific condition due to family history:

◆ Should testing be performed if no treatment is available?
◆ Should parents have the right to have minors tested for adult-onset diseases?
◆ Should parents have the right to use gene therapy for genetic enhancement?

The Human Genome Project is dedicated to mapping and identifying the genetic composi-

tion of humans. Scientists hope to identify and eradicate many of the genetic disorders affecting individuals. Initiated in 1990, the Human Genome Project was projected to be a 13-year effort coordinated by the U.S. Department of Energy and the National Institutes of Health. However, the swift technological advances accelerated the time frame, and in February 2001 the scientists announced they had cracked the human genetic code and accomplished the following goals (Human Genome Project Information, 2002):

◆ Identified all of the genes in human DNA.

◆ Determined the sequences of the three billion chemical bases that make up human DNA.

◆ Stored this information in databases.

◆ Developed tools for data analysis.

◆ Addressed the ethical, legal, and social issues that may arise from the project.

Rapid advances in the science of genetics and its applications present new and complex ethical and policy issues for individuals, healthcare personnel, and society. Economics come into play because, currently, only those who can afford the technology have access to it. Efforts need to be directed toward creating standards that identify the uses for genetic data and the protection of human rights and confidentiality. This is truly the new frontier.

A primary responsibility of nursing is to help clients and families cope with the purposes, benefits, and limitations of the new technologies. Hospice nurses and critical care nurses help clients and their families with end-of-life decisions. Nurses will need to have knowledge about the new genetic technologies because they will fill the roles of counselors and advisers in these areas. Many nurses now work in the areas of in vitro fertilization and genetic counseling.

Professional Dilemmas

Most of this chapter has dealt with client issues, but ethical problems may involve leadership and management issues as well. What do you do about an impaired coworker? Personal loyalties often cause conflict with professional ethics, creating an ethical dilemma. For this reason, most nurse practice acts now address this problem and require the reporting of impaired professionals and providing rehabilitation for them.

Other professional dilemmas may involve working with incompetent personnel. This may be frustrating for both staff and management. Regulations created to protect individuals from unjustified loss of position and the enormous amounts of paperwork, remediation, and time that must be exercised to terminate an incompetent health-care worker often make management look the other way.

Employing institutions that provide nursing services have an obligation to establish a process for the reporting and handling of practices that jeopardize client safety (ANA, 1994). The behaviors of incompetent staff place both clients and other staff members in jeopardy,

and, eventually, the incompetency may lead to legal action that may have been avoidable if a different approach had been taken.

CONCLUSION

Ethical dilemmas are becoming more common in the changing health-care environment. More questions are being raised, and fewer answers are available. New guidelines need to be developed to assist in finding more answers. Technology has provided enormous power to alter the human organism and to keep the human organism alive, but economics may force an answers to the questions of what living is and when people should be allowed to die. Will society become the brave new world of Aldous Huxley? Again and again the question is raised, "Who shall live, and who shall die?" What is *your* answer?

STUDY QUESTIONS

1 What is the difference between intrinsic and extrinsic values? Make a list of your intrinsic values.

2 Consider a decision you made recently that was based on your values. How did you make your choice?

3 Describe how you could use the valuing process of choosing, prizing, and acting in making the decision considered in Question 2.

4 Which of your personal values would be primary if you were assigned to care for a microcephalic infant whose parents have decided to withhold all food and fluids?

5 The parents of the microcephalic infant in Question 4 confront you and ask, "What would you do if this were your baby?" What do you think would be most important for you to consider in responding to them?

6 Your friend is single and feels that her "biological clock" is ticking. She decides to undergo in vitro fertilization using donor sperm. She tells you that she has researched the donor's background extensively and wants to show you the "template" for her child. She asks for your professional opinion about this situation. How would you respond? Identify the ethical principles involved.

7 Over the past several weeks, you have noticed that your closest friend, Jimmy, has not been himself at work. He is erratic and has been making poor client-care decisions. On two separate occasions, you quietly intervened and "fixed"

(Continued on following page)

his errors. You have also noticed that he volunteers to give the pain medications to other nurses' clients, and you see him standing very close to other nurses when they remove controlled substances from the Medication Distribution Center. Today you watched him go to the Medication Distribution Center immediately after another colleague and then saw him go into the men's room. Within about 20 minutes his behavior has completely changed. You suspect that he may be taking controlled substances. You and Jimmy have been friends for more than 20 years. You grew up together and went to nursing school together. You realize that if you approach him, you may jeopardize this close friendship that means a great deal to you. Using the MORAL ethical decision-making model, devise a plan to resolve this dilemma.

CRITICAL THINKING EXERCISE

Andy is assigned to care for a 14-year-old girl, Amanda, admitted with a large tumor located in the left groin area. During an assessment, Amanda shares her personal feelings with Andy. She tells him that she feels "different" from her friends. She is ashamed of her physical development because all her girlfriends have "breasts" and boyfriends. She is very flat-chested and embarrassed. Andy listens attentively to Amanda and helps her focus on some of her positive attributes and talents.

A CT scan is ordered and reveals that the tumor extends to what appears to be the ovary. A gynecological surgeon is called in to evaluate the situation. An ultrasonic-guided biopsy is performed. It is discovered that the tumor is an enlarged lymph node and that the "ovary" is actually a testes. Amanda has both male and female gonads.

When this information is given to Amanda's parents, they do not want her to know. They feel that she has been raised as "our daughter." They ask the surgeon to remove the male gonads and leave only the female gonads. That way, "Amanda will never need to know." The surgeon refuses to do this. Andy shares his discussion with Amanda with her parents. He believes that they should discuss the situation with Amanda as they are denying her choices. The parents are adamant about Amanda not knowing anything. Andy returns to Amanda's room, and Amanda begins asking all types of questions regarding the tests and the treatments. In answering, Andy hesitates, and Amanda picks up on this, demanding that he tell her the truth.

1. How should Andy respond?

2. What are the ethical principles in conflict?

3. What are the long-term effects of Andy's decision?

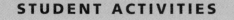

STUDENT ACTIVITIES

1. In your clinical setting, identify a possible ethical dilemma:

   a. Describe the situation.

   b. Identify the individuals involved.

   c. Identify the ethical principles involved. Which ones are in conflict?

   d. Choose an ethical decision-making model, and map the process for implementing a resolution to the dilemma.

2. Make arrangements to attend a meeting of the hospital ethics committee.

   a. Who is on the committee?

   b. Are family members or clients allowed to attend the meeting?

   c. Was an ethical decision-making model applied to the resolution of the issues?

   d. Was the outcome what you expected? Explain your answer.

REFERENCES

AIDS Update Conference. (1995). Hollywood Memorial Hospital, Hollywood, FL.

American Association of Critical Care Nurses (AACN). At loggerheads: Questioning patient autonomy. Retrieved on January 11, 2006, from aacn.org/AACN/aacn-news.nsf/GetArticle/ArticleThree184?

American Nurses Association (ANA). (2002). Code of Ethics Project. Washington, DC: ANA.

American Nurses Association (ANA). (1994). Guidelines on reporting incompetent, unethical, or illegal practices. Washington, DC: ANA.

Benner, P., & Wrubel, J. (1989). *The Primacy of Caring: Stress and Coping in Health and Illness.* Menlo Park, CA: Addison Wesley.

Burkhardt, M.A., & Nathaniel, A.K. (2001). *Ethics and Issues in Contemporary Nursing.* Albany, NY: Delmar.

Canadian Nurses Association (CNA). (2002). Code of ethics for registered nurses. Retrieved on January 11, 2006, from cna-nurses.ca/cna/documents/pdf/publications/CodeofEthics2002_e.pdf

Davis, A.J., Arokar, M.A., Liaschenko, J., & Drought, T.S. (1997). *Ethical Dilemmas and Nursing Practice,* 4th ed. Stamford, CT: Appleton & Lange.

Driver, J. (2001). *Uneasy Virtue.* New York: Cambridge University Press.

Edge, R.S., & Groves, J.R. (2005). *The Ethics of Healthcare: A Guide for Clinical Practice.* 3rd ed. Albany, NY: Thomson–Delmar Learning.

Gordon, N. (1963). *The Death Committee.* New York: Fawcett Crest.

Guido, G.W. (2001). *Legal and Ethical Issues in Nursing,* 3rd ed. Saddle River, NJ: Prentice-Hall.

Halloran, M.C. (1982). Rational ethical judgments utilizing a decision-making tool. *Heart Lung,* 11(6), 566–570.

Harned, P. (2005). National business ethics survey, 2005. Ethics Today Online, 4(2). Retrieved on January 13, 2005, from ethics.org/today/et_current.html pres

Hook, C.C. & Mueller, P.S. (2005). The Terri Schiavo Saga: The making of a tragedy and lessons learned. Retrieved on April 20, 2006 from mayoclinicproceedings.com/inside.asp?AID=1054&UID=8934

Hooker, B. (2000). *Ideal Code, Real World.* Oxford, UK: Oxford University Press.

Human Genome Project. Retrieved on July 19, 2002, from ornl.gov/hgmis/about

Hume, D. (1978). A treatise of human nature. In Johnson, O.A. *Ethics,* 4th ed. New York: Holt, Rinehart, and Winston, p. 212.

Huxley, A. (1932). *Brave New World.* New York: Harper Row Publishers.

Kant, I. (1949). *Fundamental Principles of the Metaphysics of Morals.* New York: Liberal Arts.

Macklin, R. (1987). *Mortal Choices: Ethical Dilemmas in Modern Medicine.* Boston: Houghton Mifflin.

Mappes, T.A., & DeGrazia, D. (2005). *Biomedical Ethics,* 6th ed. St. Louis: McGraw-Hill.

Raths, L.E., Harmin, M., & Simon, S.B. (1979). *Values and Teaching.* New York: Charles E. Merrill.

Shirey, M.R. (2005). Ethical climate in nursing practice: The leader's role. *Journal of Nursing Administration,* 7(2), 59–67.

Steele, S.M., & Harmon, V. (1983). *Values Clarification in Nursing.* New York: Appleton-Century-Crofts.

Thiroux, J. (1977). *Ethics: Theory and Practice.* Philadelphia: MacMillan.

Thompson, J., & Thompson, H. (1985). *Bioethical Decision Making for Nurses.* New York: Appleton-Century-Crofts.

Urbano, M.T. (1992). *Preschool Children with Special Health-Care Needs.* San Diego: Singular Publishing.

Wack, J. (1992). *Sociology of Religion.* Chicago: University of Chicago Press.

Webster's New World Dictionary. (2000). New York: Simon & Schuster.

Wright, R.A. (1987). *Human Values in Health Care.* St. Louis: McGraw-Hill.

Organizations, Power, and Empowerment

OBJECTIVES

After reading this chapter, the student should be able to:

◆ Recognize the various ways in which health-care organizations differ.

◆ Define power and empowerment.

◆ Identify sources of power in a health-care organization.

◆ Describe several ways in which nurses can be empowered.

OUTLINE

CHAPTER 5 SELF-ASSESSMENT
How Empowered Do You Feel?

Choose an organization in which you actively participate—school, job, religious organization, or large social club—and rate your sense of empowerment in that organization:

1. Do you feel that you are an important member of this organization?
   Yes _____ No _____

2. If you made a suggestion for change, would this suggestion be given serious consideration?
   Yes _____ No _____

3. Do you feel that you have a voice in deciding the direction of the organization?
   Yes _____ No _____

4. Do you have a say in the way in which you function/participate/work in this organization?
   Yes _____ No _____

5. Can you decide or at least influence your future direction/roles in the organization?
   Yes _____ No _____

The subjects of this chapter—organizations, power, and empowerment—are not as remote from a nurse's everyday experience as you may first think. It is difficult to focus on these "big picture" factors when caught up in the busy day-to-day work of a staff nurse, but they have an impact on your practice as you will see in this chapter. Consider two scenarios, which are analyzed later in the chapter.

SCENARIO ◆ 1

In school, Hazel Rivera had always received high praise for the quality of her nursing care plans. "Thorough, comprehensive, systematic, holistic—beautiful!" was the comment she received on the last one she wrote before graduation.

Now Hazel is a staff nurse on a busy orthopedic surgery unit. Although her time to write comprehensive care plans during the day is limited, Hazel often stays after work to complete them. Her friend Carla refuses to stay late with her. "If I can't com-plete my work during the shift, then they have given me too much to do," she said.

At the end of their 3-month probationary period, Hazel and Carla received written evaluations of their progress and comments about their value to the organization. To Hazel's surprise, her friend Carla received a higher rating than she did. What happened?

SCENARIO ◆ 2

The nursing staff of the critical care department of a large urban hospital formed an evidence-based practice group about a year ago. They had made many changes in their practice, based on reviews of the research on several different procedures, and they were quite pleased with the results.

"Let's look at the bigger picture next month," their nurse manager suggested at one of their meetings. "This time, let's look at the research on different models of client care. We might get some good ideas for our unit." The staff nurses agreed. It would be a nice change to look at the way they organized client care in their department.

The nurse manager found a wealth of information on different models for organizing nursing care. One research study about a model for caring for the chronically critically ill (Rudy, et al., 1995) particularly interested them because they had had many clients in that category.

Several nurses volunteered to form an ad hoc committee to design a similar unit for the chronically critically ill within their critical care department. When the plan was presented, both the nurse manager and the staff thought it was excellent. The nurse manager offered to present the plan to the vice president for nursing. The staff eagerly awaited the vice president's response.

The nurse manager returned with discouraging news. The vice president did not support their concept and said that, although they were free to continue developing the idea, they should not assume that it would ever be implemented. What happened?

Were the disappointments experienced by Hazel Rivera and the critical care department staff predictable? Could they have been avoided? Without a basic understanding of organizations and of the part that power plays in health-care institutions, people are doomed to be continually surprised by the responses to their well-intentioned efforts. As you read this chapter, you will learn why Hazel Rivera and the critical care department staff were disappointed.

This chapter begins by looking at some of the characteristics of the organizations in which nurses work and how these organizations operate. Then it focuses on the subject of power within organizations: what it is, how it is obtained, and how nurses can become empowered.

UNDERSTANDING ORGANIZATIONS

One of the attractive features of nursing as a career is the wide variety of settings in which

nurses can work. From rural migrant health clinics to organ transplant units, nurses' skills are needed wherever there are concerns about people's health. Relationships with clients may extend for months or years, as they do in school health or in nursing homes, or they may be brief and never repeated, as often happens in doctors' offices, clinics, and emergency departments.

Types of Health-Care Organizations

Although some nurses work as independent practitioners, as consultants, or in the corporate world, the majority are employed by health-care organizations. These organizations can be classified into three types on the basis of their sponsorship and financing:

1. **Private not-for-profit.** Many health-care organizations were founded by civic, charitable, or religious groups. Some have been in existence for generations. Many hospitals, long-term care facilities, home-care services, and community agencies began this way. Although they need money to pay their staff and expenses, they do not have to generate a profit.
2. **Publicly supported.** Government-operated service organizations range from county public health departments to complex medical centers, such as those operated by the Veterans Administration, a federal agency.
3. **Private for-profit.** Increasing numbers of health-care organizations are operated for profit like any other business. These include large hospital and nursing home chains, health maintenance organizations, and many freestanding centers that provide special services, such as surgical and diagnostic centers.

The differences between these categories have become blurred for many reasons:

◆ All compete for clients, especially for clients with health-care insurance or the ability to pay their own health-care bills.

◆ All experience the effect of cost constraints.

◆ All may provide services that are eligible

for government reimbursement, particularly Medicaid and Medicare funding, if they meet government standards.

Organizational Cultures

The size and complexity of many health-care organizations make them difficult to understand. One way to begin is to find a colorful image or metaphor that sums up their characteristics in a few well-chosen words. Morgan (1997) suggested using animals or other familiar images to describe an organization. For example, an aggressive organization that crushes its competitors could be likened to a bull elephant, whereas a timid organization in danger of being crushed by that bull elephant could be described as a mouse. Using another metaphor, an organization adrift without a clear idea of its future could be described as a "rudderless boat on a stormy sea," whereas an organization with its sights set clearly on exterminating its competition could be described as a "guided missile."

People seek some stability, consistency, and meaning in their work. To achieve this, some type of culture will develop within an organization (Schein, 2004). This culture is a pattern of shared values and assumptions that is taught (often indirectly or unconsciously) to new employees as the right way to assess client needs, provide care, and relate to one's fellow caregivers. As with the cultures of societies and communities, it is easy to observe the superficial aspects of an organization's culture, but much of it remains hidden. Edgar Schein, a well-known scholar of organizational culture, divided these aspects of organiztional culture into three levels:

1. **Artifact level:** visible characteristics such as client room layout, patient record forms, etc.
2. **Espoused beliefs:** stated, often written, goals; philosophy of the organization.
3. **Underlying assumptions:** unconscious but powerful beliefs and feelings such as a commitment to effect a cure, no matter what it may cost (Schein, 2004).

Organizational cultures differ a great deal. Some are very traditional, preserving their customary ways of doing things even when these processes no longer work well. Others are very progressive, eternally chasing the newest management fad or buying the latest high-tech equipment. Some seem to be warm, friendly, and open to new people and new ideas. Others are cold, defensive, and indifferent or even hostile to the outside world (Tappen, 2001). These very different organizational cultures have a powerful effect on the employees and the people served by the organization. The culture shapes people's behavior, especially their responses to each other, a particularly important factor in health care.

The culture of an organization is intangible; you cannot see it or touch it but you will recognize it when you bump up against it. To find out what the culture of an organization is when you are applying for a new position or trying to familiarize yourself with your new workplace, you can ask several people who work there or are familiar with the organization to describe it in just a few words.

Does it matter in what type of organization you work? The answer is emphatically *"yes."* For example, the extreme value placed on "busy-ness" in hospitals, i.e., being seen doing something at all times, leads to manager actions such as floating a staff member to a "busier" unit if she or he is found reading new research or looking up information on the Web (Scott-Findley & Golden-Biddle, 2005). Even more important, a hospital with a positive work environment is not only a better place for nurses to work but safer for clients. Hospitals with a richer skill mix (i.e., a higher proportion of registered nurses), better prepared nurses, and fewer temporary or agency staff actually have lower client death rates (Estabrooks, et al., 2005). Why is this? Here is one reason:

A shift from a culture of blame to a blameless culture is critical to reducing medication errors because the first step in preventing them is to determine why they occur. Nurses need to feel safe to report errors and near misses before they will do so freely (Hofler, 2005; Simpson, 2005).

Once you have grasped the totality of an organization in terms of its overall culture, you are ready to analyze it in a little more detail.

Goals

It is also helpful to identify the organization's goals, structure, and processes.

Try answering this true-or-false question:

Question: The primary goal of any health-care organization is to keep people healthy, restore them to health, or assist them in dying as comfortably as possible. True or false?

Answer: False. The previous statement is only partially correct. Most health-care organizations have several goals.

What other goals might a health-care organization have? Following are some examples:

◆ **Survival.** Organizations have to maintain their own existence. Many health-care organizations are "cash-strapped," causing them to limit hiring, streamline work, and reduce costs, putting enormous pressure on remaining staff (Roark, 2005). This goal is threatened when, for example, reimbursements are reduced, competition increases, the organization fails to meet standards, or clients are unable to pay their bills (Trinh & O'Connor, 2002).

◆ **Growth.** The chief executive officers (CEOs) also want their organizations to grow by expanding into new territories, adding new services, and bringing in new clients.

◆ **Profit.** For-profit organizations are expected to return some profit to their owners. Not-for-profit organizations have to be able to pay their bills and to avoid slipping into too much debt. This is sometimes difficult for an organization.

◆ **Status.** The leaders or owners of many health-care organizations also want to be known as the best in their field; for example, by having the best open-heart surgeon, providing "the best nursing care in the world" (Frusti, Niesen, & Campion, 2003, p. 34), or providing the most attractive client rooms in town.

◆ **Dominance.** Some organizations also want to drive others out of the health-care business or to acquire them, surpassing the goal of survival and moving toward dominance of a particular market by driving out the competition.

These additional goals are not discussed in public as often as the first, more lofty, statement of goals in the true-or-false question. However, they drive an organization, especially the way an organization handles its finances and treats its employees.

These goals may have profound effects on every one of the organization's employees, nurses included. For an example, return to the story of Hazel Rivera. Why did she receive a less favorable rating than her friend Carla?

After comparing ratings with her friend Carla, Hazel scheduled a meeting with her nurse manager to discuss her evaluation. The nurse manager explained the rating: Hazel's care plans were very well done, and she genuinely appreciated Hazel's efforts to make them so. The problem was that Hazel had to be paid overtime for this work according to the union contract, and this reduced the amount of overtime pay the nurse manager had available when the client care load was especially high. "The corporation is very strict about staying within the budget," she said. "In fact, my rating is higher when I don't use up all of my budgeted overtime hours." When Hazel asked what she could do to improve her rating, the nurse manager offered to help her streamline the care plans and manage her time better so that the care plans could be done during her shift.

Structure

The Traditional Approach

Virtually all health-care organizations have a hierarchical structure of some kind (Box 5-1). In a *traditional hierarchical structure,* employees are ranked from the top to the bottom, as if they were on the various steps of a ladder (Fig. 5-1). The number of people on the bottom rungs of the ladder is almost always much greater than the number at the top. The president or CEO is usually at the top of this ladder; the maintenance crew is usually at the bottom. Nurses fall somewhere in the middle of most health-care organizations, higher than the cleaning people, aides, and technicians but lower than physicians and administrators.

The people at the top of the ladder have authority to issue orders, spend the organization's money, and hire and fire people. Much of this authority is delegated to people below them, but they retain the right to reverse a decision or regain control of these activities whenever they deem it necessary.

The people at the bottom have little authority and usually play no part in deciding how

---

BOX 5-1

What Is a Bureaucracy?

Although it seems as if everyone complains about "the bureaucracy," not everyone is clear about what a bureaucracy really is. Max Weber defined a *bureaucratic organization* as having the following characteristics:

◆ **Division of labor.** Specific parts of the job to be done are assigned to different individuals or groups. For example, nurses, physicians, therapists, dietitians, and social workers all provide portions of the health care needed by an individual client.

◆ **Hierarchy.** All employees are organized and ranked according to their level of authority within the organization. For example, administrators and directors are at the top of most hospital hierarchies, whereas aides and maintenance workers are at the bottom.

◆ **Rules and regulations.** Acceptable and unacceptable

behavior and the proper way to carry out various tasks are defined, often in writing. For example, procedure books, policy manuals, bylaws, statements, and memos prescribe many types of behavior, from acceptable isolation techniques to vacation policies.

◆ **Emphasis on technical competence.** People with certain skills and knowledge are hired to carry out specific parts of the total work of the organization. For example, a community mental health center has psychiatrists, social workers, and nurses to provide different kinds of therapies and clerical staff to do the typing and filing. Some bureaucracy is characteristic of the formal operation of every organization, even the most deliberately informal, because it promotes smooth operations within a large and complex group of people.

Weber, M. (1969). Bureaucratic organization. In Etzioni, A. (ed.). *Readings on Modern Organizations.* Englewood Cliffs, NJ: Prentice-Hall. Adapted by permission of Pearson Education, Inc., Upper Saddle River, NJ.

---

money is spent or who will be hired or fired but are responsible for carrying out the directions from people above them on the ladder. The people at the bottom are not entirely without power or the ability to influence people higher up on the ladder, however. If there was no one at the bottom, the work would not get done. In reality, the people at the top depend on the people lower on the ladder to do most of the work.

Some amount of bureaucracy is characteristic of the formal operation of every organization, even the most deliberately informal, because it promotes smooth operations within a large and complex group of people.

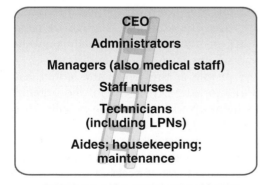

FIGURE 5-1 ◆ The organizational ladder.

More Innovative Structures

There is much interest in restructuring organizations, not only to save money but also to make the best use of a health-care organization's most valuable resource, its people. This begins with hiring the right people. It also involves providing them with the resources they need to function and the kind of leadership that can inspire the staff and unleash their creativity (Rosen, 1996).

Increasingly, people recognize that organizations need to be both efficient and adaptable and innovative. Organizations need to be prepared for uncertainty, for rapid changes in their environment, and for quick, creative responses to these challenges. In addition, they need to provide an internal climate that not only allows but also motivates employees to work to the best of their ability. They need to stop thinking of the managers as the brains of the organization and employees as the muscle (Parker & Gadbois, 2000, p. 428).

Innovative organizations have adapted an increasingly *organic* structure that is more dynamic, more flexible, and less centralized than the static traditional hierarchical structure (Yourstone & Smith, 2002). In these organically structured organizations, decisions are made by the people who will implement them, not by their bosses and not by their bosses' boss.

The organic network emphasizes increased flexibility of the organizational structure, decentralized decision making, and autonomy for working groups or teams. Rigid unit structures are reorganized into autonomous teams made up of professionals from different departments and disciplines. Each team is given a specific task or function to perform (e.g., intravenous team, a hospital infection control team, a child protection team in a community agency). The teams are responsible for their own self-correction and self-control, although they may also have a designated leader. Together, team members make decisions about work assignments and how to deal with problems that arise. In other words, the teams supervise and manage themselves.

Supervisors, administrators, and support staff have different functions in an organic network. Instead of spending their time observing and controlling other people's work, they become planners and resource people. They are responsible for providing the conditions required for the optimal functioning of the teams, and they are expected to ensure that the support, information, materials, and funds needed to do the job well are available to the teams. They also act as coordinators between the teams so that the teams are cooperating rather than blocking each other, working toward congruent goals, and not duplicating effort.

Very large organizations can also be separated into functional *divisions* that can be integrated internally when integration of the organization as a whole becomes almost impossible because of its great size, complexity, and diversity. However, communication among these divisions can become more difficult. This is the downside of organic structure. If it is not done well, there is a potential for creating chaos and confusion instead of creativity (Senge et al., 1999).

Organic networks have been compared with spider plants, with their central cluster and offshoots (Morgan, 1997). Each cluster represents a discipline (e.g., nursing, social work, occupa-

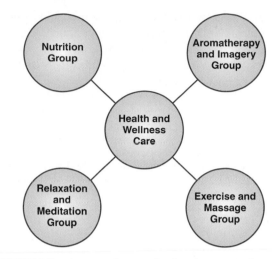

FIGURE 5-2 ◆ An organic organizational structure for a nontraditional wellness center. (Based on Morgan, A. [1993]. *Imaginization: The Art of Creative Management.* Newbury Park, CA: Sage.)

tional therapy) or a service (e.g., psychiatry, orthopedics). For example, Figure 5-2 shows an organic network for a wellness center. Each cluster represents a separate set of services. A client might use just one or all of them to develop a personal plan for wellness. Staff members may move from one cluster to another, or the entire configuration of interconnected clusters may be reorganized as the organization shapes and is shaped by the environment.

Processes

Organizations have formal processes for getting things done and informal ways to get around the formal processes (Perrow, 1969). The *formal* processes are the written policies and procedures that all health-care organizations have. The *informal* processes are neither written nor discussed most of the time. They exist in organizations as a kind of "shadow" organization that is harder to see but equally important to recognize and understand (Purser & Cabana, 1999).

The informal process is often much simpler and faster than the formal one. Because the informal ways of getting things done are seldom discussed (and certainly not as a part of a new employee's orientation), it may take some time for you to figure out what they are and how to use them. Once you know they exist, they may be easier for you to identify. The following is an example:

Jocylene noticed that Harold seemed to get STAT laboratory results back on his clients faster than she did. Although the results she requested came back quickly, the turnaround time for Harold's clients seemed almost instantaneous. At lunch one day, Jocylene asked Harold why that happened. "That's easy," he said. "The people in our lab feel unappreciated. I always tell them how helpful they are. Also, if you call and let them know that the specimens are coming, they will get to them faster. They can't monitor their e-mail constantly." Harold has just explained an informal process to Jocylene.

Sometimes, people are unwilling to discuss the informal processes. However, careful observation of the most experienced, "system-wise" individuals in an organization will eventually reveal these processes. This will help you do things as efficiently as they do.

POWER

There are times when one's attempts to influence others are overwhelmed by other forces or individuals. Where does this power come from? Who has it? Who does not?

In an earlier section on hierarchy, it was noted that, although people at the top of the hierarchy have most of the *authority* in the organization, they do not have all of the power. In fact, the people at the bottom of the hierarchy also have some sources of *power*. This section explains how this can be true. First, power is defined, and then the sources of power available to people on the lower rungs of the ladder are considered.

Definition

Power is the ability to influence other people despite their resistance. In other words, one person or group can impose its will on another person or group (Haslam, 2001). The use of power can be positive, as when the nurse manager gives a staff member an extra day off in exchange for working during the weekend, or negative, as when a nurse administrator transfers a "bothersome" staff nurse to another unit after the staff nurse pointed out a physician error (Talarico, 2004).

Sources

There are numerous sources of power. Many of them are readily available to nurses, but some of them are not. The following is a list derived primarily from the work of French, Raven, and Etzioni (Barraclough & Stewart, 1992):

◆ **Authority.** The power granted to an individual or a group by virtue of position (within the organizational hierarchy, for example).

◆ **Reward.** The promise of money, goods, services, recognition, or other benefits.

◆ **Expertise.** The special knowledge an individual is believed to possess. As Sir Francis Bacon said, "Knowledge is power" (Bacon, 1597, quoted in Fitton, 1997, p. 150).

◆ **Coercion.** The threat of pain or of harm, which may be physical, economic, or psychological.

Following is a survey of various groups of people in a health-care organization in terms of the types of power that may be available to them:

◆ *Managers* are able to reward people with salary increases, promotions, and recognition. They can also cause economic or psychological pain for the people who work for them, particularly through their authority to evaluate and fire people.

◆ *Clients* at first appear to be relatively powerless in a health-care organization. However, if clients refused to use the services of a particular organization, that organization would eventually cease to exist. Clients reward health-care workers by praising them to their supervisors. They can also cause discomfort by complaining about them.

◆ *Assistants and technicians* may appear to be relatively powerless because of their low position in the hierarchy. Imagine, however, how the work of the organization (e.g., hospital, nursing home) would be impeded if all the nursing aides failed to appear one morning.

◆ *Nurses* have expertise, power, and authority over licensed practical nurses, aides, and other personnel by virtue of their position in the hierarchy. They are critical to the operation of most health-care organizations and could cause considerable trouble if they refused to work, another source of nurse power.

Fralic (2000) offered a good example of the power of information that nurses have always had: Florence Nightingale showed very graphically in the 1800s that wherever her nurses were, far fewer died, and wherever they were not, many more died.

Think of the power of that information. Immediately, people were saying, "What would you like, Miss Nightingale? Would you like more money? Would you like a school of nursing? What else can we do for you?" She had solid data, she knew how to collect it, and she knew how to interpret and distribute it in terms of things that people valued. (p. 340)

EMPOWERING NURSES

This final section looks at several ways in which nurses, either individually or collectively, can maximize their power and increase their feelings of empowerment.

First, the concepts of power and empowerment need to be defined. *Power* is the actual or potential ability to "recognize one's will even against the resistance of others," according to Max Weber (quoted in Mondros & Wilson, 1994, p. 5). *Empowerment* is a psychological state, a feeling of competence, control, and entitlement. Given these definitions, it is possible to be powerful and yet not feel empowered. *Power* refers to ability, and *empowerment* refers to feelings. Both are of interest to nursing leaders and managers.

Feeling empowered includes the following:

◆ **Self-determination.** Feeling free to decide how to do your work.

◆ **Meaning.** Caring about your work, enjoying it, and taking it seriously.

◆ **Competence.** Confidence in your ability to do your work well.

◆ **Impact.** Feeling that people listen to your ideas, that you can make a difference (Spreitzer & Quinn, 2001).

The following contribute to nurse empowerment:

◆ **Manageable workoad.** Reasonable work assignments.

◆ **Reward and recognition.** Appreciation received for a job well done.

◆ **Fairness.** Consistent, equitable treatment of all staff (Spence, Laschinger, & Finegan, 2005).

Alternately, work overload and lack of meaning, recognition, or reward produce emotional exhaustion and burnout (Spence, Laschinger, & Finegan, 2005). Nurses, like most people, want to have some power and to feel empowered. They want to be heard, to be recognized, to be valued, and to be respected. They do not want to feel unimportant or insignificant to society or to the organization in which they work.

Professional Organizations

Although the purpose of the American Nurses Association and that of other professional organizations are discussed in Chapter 16, these organizations are considered here specifically in terms of how they can empower nurses.

A collective voice, expressed through these organizations, can be stronger and more easily heard than one individual voice. By joining together in professional organizations, nurses make their viewpoint known and their value recognized. The power base of nursing professional organizations is derived from the number of members and from their expertise in health matters.

Why there is power in numbers may need some further explanation. Large numbers of active, informed members of an organization represent large numbers of potential voters to state and national legislators, most of whom wish to be remembered favorably in forthcoming elections. Large groups of people also have a louder voice: they can write more letters, speak to more friends and family members, make more telephone calls, and generally attract more attention than small groups can.

Professional organizations can empower nurses in a number of ways:

◆ Collegiality, the opportunity to work with peers on issues of importance to the profession.

◆ Commitment to improving the health and well-being of the people served by the profession.

◆ Representation in state legislatures and in Congress when issues of importance to nursing arise.

◆ Representation during collective bargaining, the protection of nurses' rights and privileges as employed professionals.

◆ Enhancement of nurses' competence through publications and continuing education.

◆ Recognition of achievement through certification programs, awards, and the media.

Collective Bargaining

Like professional organizations, collective bargaining uses the power of numbers, in this case for the purpose of equalizing the power of employees and employer to improve working conditions, gain respect, increase job security, and have greater input into collective decisions (empowerment) and pay increases (Tappen, 2001). When people join for a common cause, they are often more powerful than when they attempt to bring about change individually. Large numbers of people have the potential to cause more psychological or economic pain than an individual can. For example, the resignation of one nursing assistant or one nurse may cause a temporary problem, but it is usually resolved rather quickly by hiring another individual. If 50 or 100 aides or nurses resign, however, the organization can be virtually paralyzed and will have much more difficulty replacing these essential workers. Collective bargaining takes advantage of this power in numbers.

An effective collective bargaining contract can provide considerable protection to employees. However, the downside of collective bargaining (as with most uses of coercive power) is that it may encourage conflict rather than cooperation between employees and managers, an "us" against "them" environment (Haslam, 2001). Many nurses are also concerned about the effect that going out on strike might have on their clients' welfare and on their own economic security. Most administrators and managers prefer to operate within a union-free environment (Hannigan, 1998).

Participation in Decision Making

Actions can also be taken by managers and higher-level administrators to empower nursing staff. The amount of power available to or exercised by a given group (e.g., nurses) *within* an organization can vary considerably from one organization to the next. Three sources of power are particularly important in health-care organizations:

◆ **Resources.** The money, materials, and human help needed to accomplish the work.

◆ **Support.** Authority to take action without having to obtain permission.

◆ **Information.** Client care expertise and information about the organization's goals and activities of other departments.

In addition, nurses also need access to *opportunities*: opportunities to be involved in decision making, to be involved in vital functions of the organization, to grow professionally, and to move up the organizational ladder (Sabiston & Laschinger, 1995). Without these, employees cannot be empowered (Bradford & Cohen, 1998). Nurses who are part-time, temporary, or contract employees are less likely to feel empowered than full-time permanent employees, who feel more secure in their positions and connected to the organization (Kuokkanen & Katajisto, 2003).

Shared Governance

Genuine sharing of decision making is difficult to accomplish, partly because managers are reluctant to relinquish control or to trust their staff members to make wise decisions. Yet genuine empowerment of the nursing staff cannot occur without this sharing. Having some control over one's work and the ability to influence decisions are essential to empowerment (Monojlovich & Laschinger, 2002). For example, if staff members do not control the budget for their unit, they cannot implement a decision to replace aides with registered nurses without approval from higher-level management. If they want increased autonomy in decision making about the care of individual clients, they cannot do so if opposition by another group, such as the physicians, is given greater credence by the organization's administration.

Return to the example of the staff of the critical care department (Scenario 2). Why did the vice president for nursing tell the nurse manager that the plan would not be implemented?

Actually, the vice president for nursing thought the plan had some merit. He believed that the proposal to implement a nurse-managed model of care for the chronically critically ill could save a little money, provide a higher quality of client care, and result in increased nursing staff satisfaction. However, the critical care department was the centerpiece of the hospital's agreement with a nearby medical school. In this agreement, the medical school provided the services of highly skilled intensivists in return for the learning opportunities afforded their students. In its present form, the nurses' plan would not allow sufficient autonomy for the medical students, a situation that would not be acceptable to the medical school. The vice president knew that the board of trustees of the hospital believed their affiliation with the medical school brought a great deal of prestige to the organization and that they would not allow anything to interfere with this relationship.

"If shared governance were in place here, I think we could implement this or a similar model of care," he told the nurse manager.

"How would that work?" she asked.

"If we had shared governance, the nursing practice council would review the plan and, if they approved it, forward it to a similar medical practice council. Then committees from both councils would work together to figure out a way for this to benefit everyone. It wouldn't necessarily be easy to do, but it could be done if we had real collegiality between the professions. I have been working toward this model but haven't convinced the rest of the administration to put it into practice yet. Perhaps we could bring this up at the next nursing executive meeting. I think it is time I shared my ideas on this subject with the rest of the nursing staff."

In this case, the goals and processes existing at the time the nurses developed their proposal did not support their idea. However, they could see a way for it to be accomplished in the future. Implementation of real shared governance would make it possible for the critical care nurses to accomplish their goal.

Shared governance is a term used to describe formal ways in which access to these sources of power and opportunity is made available to staff nurses. In shared governance, staff nurses are included in the highest levels of decision making within the nursing department through representation on various councils that govern practice and management issues. These councils set the standard for staffing, promotion, and so forth. Staff nurses are also involved in decisions that affect their particular unit (Westrope, Vaughn, Bott, & Taunton, 1995). In many cases, a change in the organizational culture is necessary before shared governance can work (Currie & Loftus-Hills, 2002).

RESEARCH EXAMPLE

Can nurse managers empower their staff? The answer is yes, according to nurse researchers who surveyed 537 staff nurses in two large hospitals. Fostering autonomy and showing confidence in the staff were especially empowering. Empowered staff worked more effectively and had lower levels of job-related tension.

Laschinger, H.K.S., Wong, C., McMahon, L., & Kaufman, C. (1999). Leader behavior impact on staff nurse empowerment, job tension, and work effectiveness. *Journal of Nursing Administration,* 29(5), 28–39.

Enhancing Expertise

Most health-care professionals, including nurses, are empowered to some extent by their own professional knowledge and competence. You can take steps to enhance your own competence, thereby increasing your own sense of empowerment (Fig. 5-3)

◆ Participate in interdisciplinary team conferences and client-centered conferences on your unit.

Participate in interdisciplinary conferences

Attend continuing education offerings

Attend professional organization meetings

Read books and journals related to
your nursing practice

Problem-solve and brainstorm
with colleagues

Return to school to earn a higher degree

FIGURE 5-3 ◆ How to increase your expert power.

◆ Attend continuing education offerings to enhance your expertise.

◆ Attend local, regional, and national conferences sponsored by relevant nursing and specialty organizations.

◆ Read journals and books in your specialty area.

◆ Participate in nursing research projects related to your clinical specialty area.

◆ Discuss with colleagues in nursing and other disciplines how to handle a difficult clinical situation.

◆ Observe the practice of experienced nurses.

◆ Return to school to earn a bachelor's degree and higher degrees in nursing.

You can probably think of more, but this list at least gives you some ideas. You can also share the knowledge and experience you have gained with other people. This means not only using your knowledge to improve your own practice but also communicating what you have learned to your colleagues in nursing and in other health-care professions. It also means letting your supervisors know that you have enhanced your professional competence. You can share your knowledge with your clients, empowering them as well. You may even reach the point at which you have learned more about a particular subject than most nurses have and want to write about it for publication.

CONCLUSION

Although most nurses are employed by health-care organizations, too few have taken the time to analyze the operation of their employing organizations and the effect it has on their practice. Understanding organizations and the power relationships within them will increase the effectiveness of your leadership.

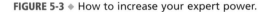

STUDY QUESTIONS

1 Describe the organizational characteristics of a facility in which you currently have a clinical assignment. Include the following:
a. The type of organization it is.
b. The organizational culture.
c. How the organization is structured.
d. The formal and informal goals and processes of the organization.

2 Define power, and describe how power affects the relationships between people of different disciplines (e.g., nursing, medicine, microbiology, administration, finance, social work) in a health-care organization.

3 Discuss ways in which nurses can become more empowered. How can you use your leadership skills to do this?

CRITICAL THINKING EXERCISE

Tanya Washington will finish her associate's degree nursing program in 6 weeks. Her preferred clinical area is parent-child nursing, and she hopes to become a pediatric nurse practitioner one day. Tanya has received two job offers, both from urban hospitals with large pediatric populations. Because several of her friends are already employed by these facilities, she asked them for their impressions.

"Central Hospital is a good place to work," said one friend. "It is a dynamic, growing institution, always on the cutting edge of change. Any new idea that seems promising, Central is the first to try it. It's an exciting place to work."

"City Hospital is also a good place to work," said her other friend. "It is a strong, stable institution where traditions are valued. Any new idea must be carefully evaluated before it is adapted. It's been a pleasure to work there."

1. How would the organizational climate of each hospital affect a new graduate?

2. Which organizational climate do you think would be best for a new graduate, Central's or City's?

3. Would your answer differ if Tanya were an experienced nurse?

4. What do you need to know about Tanya before deciding which hospital would be best for her?

5. What else would you like to know about the hospitals?

REFERENCES

Barraclough, R.A., & Stewart, R.A. (1992). Power and control: Social science perspectives. In Richmond, V.P., & McCroskey, J.C. (eds.). *Power in the Classroom: Communication, Control and Concern.* Hillsdale, NJ: Lawrence Erlbaum.

Bradford, D.L., & Cohen, A.R. (1998). *Power Up: Transforming Organizations Through Shared Leadership.* New York: John Wiley & Sons.

Currie, L., & Loftus-Hills, A. (2002). The nursing view of clinical governance. *Nursing Standard,* 16(27), 40–44.

Estabrooks, C.A., Midodzi, W.K., Cummings, G.G., Ricker, K.L., & Giovanetti, P. (2005). The impact of hospital nursing characteristics on 30-day mortality. *Nursing Research,* 54(2), 74–84.

Fitton, R.A. (1997). *Leadership: Quotations From the World's Greatest Motivators.* Boulder, CO: Westview Press.

Fralic, M.F. (2000). What is leadership? *Journal of Nursing Administration,* 30(7/8), 340–341.

Frusti, D.K., Niesen, K.M., & Campion, J.K. (2003). Creating a culturally competent organization. *Journal of Nursing Administration,* 33(1), 33–38.

Hannigan, T.A. (1998). *Managing Tomorrow's High-Performance Unions.* Westport, CN: Greenwood Publishing.

Haslam, S.A. (2001). *Psychology in Organizations.* Thousand Oaks, CA: Sage.

Hofler, L.D. (2005). Public reporting, patient safety and quality improvement. *Journal of Nursing Administration,* 35(4), 161–162.

Kuokkanen, L., & Katajisto, J. (2003). Promoting or impeding empowerment? *Journal of Nursing Administration,* 33(4), 209–215.

Manojlovich, M., & Laschinger, H.K. (2002). The relationship of empowerment and selected personality characteristics to nursing job satisfaction. *Journal of Nursing Administration,* 32(11), 586–595.

Mondros, J.B., & Wilson, S.M. (1994). *Organizing for Power and Empowerment.* New York: Columbia University Press.

Morgan, A. (1997). *Images of Organization.* Thousand Oaks, CA: Sage.

Morgan, A. (1993). *Imaginization: The Art of Creative Management.* Newbury Park, CA: Sage.

Parker, M., & Gadbois, S. (2000). Building community in the healthcare workplace. *Journal of Nursing Administration,* 30(9), 426–431.

Perrow, C. (1969). The analysis of goals in complex organizations. In Etzioni, A. (ed.). *Readings on Modern Organizations*. Englewood Cliffs, NJ: Prentice-Hall.

Purser, R.E., & Cabana, S. (1999). *The Self-Managing Organization*. New York: Free Press (Simon & Schuster).

Roark, D.C. (2005). Managing the healthcare supply chain. *Nursing Management*, 36(2), 36–40.

Rosen, R.H. (1996). *Leading People: Transforming Business From the Inside Out*. New York: Viking Penguin.

Rudy, E.B., Daly, B.J., Douglas, S., Montenegro, H.D., Song, R., & Dyer, M.A. (1995). Patient outcomes for the chronically critically ill: Special care unit versus intensive care unit. *Nursing Research*, 44, 324–331.

Sabiston, J.A., & Laschinger, H.K.S. (1995). Staff nurse work empowerment and perceived autonomy. *Journal of Nursing Administration*, 28(9), 42–49.

Schein, E.H. (2004). *Organizational Culture and Leadership*. New York: Jossey-Bass.

Scott-Findley, S., & Golden-Biddle, K. (2005). Understanding how organizational culture shapes research use. *Journal of Nursing Administration*, 35(7/8), 359–365.

Senge, P, Kleiner, A., Roberts, C., Ross, R., Roth, G., & Smith, B. (1999). *The Dance of Change*. New York: Currency/Doubleday.

Simpson, R.L. (2005). Error reporting as a preventive force. *Nursing Management*, 36(6), 21–24.

Spence, Laschinger, H.K. & Finegan, J. (2005). Empowering nurses for work engagement and health in hospital settings. *Journal of Nursing Administration*, 35910, 439–441.

Spreitzer, G.M., & Quinn, R.E. (2001). *A Company of Leaders*. San Francisco: Jossey-Bass.

Talarico, K.M. (2004/April 27) A look at power in nursing. *Vital Signs*, 6–7, 21.

Tappen, R.M. (2001). *Nursing Leadership and Management: Concepts and Practice*, 4th ed. Philadelphia: FA Davis.

Trinh, H.Q., & O'Connor, S.J. (2002). Helpful or harmful? The impact of strategic change on the performance of U.S. urban hospitals. *Health Services Research*, 37(1), 145–171.

Weber, M. (1969). Bureaucratic organization. In Etzioni, A. (ed.). *Readings on Modern Organizations*. Englewood Cliffs, NJ: Prentice-Hall.

Westrope, R.A., Vaughn, L., Bott, M., & Taunton, R.L. (1995). Shared governance: From vision to reality. *Journal of Nursing Administration*, 25(2), 45–54.

Yourstone, S.A., & Smith, H.L. (2002). Managing system errors and failures in health care organizations: Suggestions for practice and research. *Health Care Management Review*, 27(1), 50–61.

Working Within
the Organization

chapter **6**

Getting People to
Work Together

OBJECTIVES

*After reading this chapter, the student should
be able to:*

◆ Describe the basic listening sequence
and principles for effective
communication.

◆ Identify barriers to effective
communication.

◆ Discuss strategies for communication
with colleagues and clients in health-
care settings.

◆ Provide positive and negative
feedback in a constructive manner.

◆ Respond to feedback in a constructive
manner.

◆ Evaluate the conduct of performance
appraisals.

◆ Participate in formal peer review.

OUTLINE

Claude has been working on a busy oncology floor for several years. He usually has a caseload of six to eight clients on his shift, and he believes that he provides safe, competent care. While Claude was on his way to medicate a client suffering from osteosarcoma, a colleague called to him, "Claude, come with me, please." Claude responded, "I need to medicate Mr. J. in Room 203. I will come right after that. Where will you be?" "Never mind!" his colleague answered. "I'll find someone who's more helpful. Don't ask me for help in the future." This was not the response Claude had expected. He thought he had expressed both an interest in his client and a willingness to help his colleague. What was the problem?

After Claude gave Mr. J. his pain medication, he went back to his colleague. "Sonja, what's the matter?" he asked. Sonja replied, "Mrs. V. fell in the bathroom. I needed someone to stay with her while I got her walker." "Why didn't you tell me it was urgent?" asked Claude. "I was so upset that I wasn't thinking about what else you were doing," answered Sonja. Claude added, "And I didn't ask you why you needed me. I guess we need to work on our communication, don't we?"

In the busy and sometimes chaotic world of nursing practice, nurses work continuously with all sorts of people. This variety makes the job dynamic and challenging. Just when it appears that things have settled down, something else happens that requires immediate attention. All of these busy people need to communicate effectively with each other. This chapter helps new nurses communicate more effectively with their colleagues and work with people of all kinds, even in situations that are filled with multiple demands and constant change.

COMMUNICATION

People often assume that communication is simply giving information to another person. Communication involves the spoken word as well as the nonverbal message, the emotional state of people involved, and the cultural background that affects their interpretation of the message (Fontaine & Fletcher, 2002). Superficial listening often results in misinterpretation of the message. An individual's attitude also influences what is heard and how the message is interpreted. Active listening is necessary to pick up all these levels of meaning in a communication.

It is important for nurses to observe nonverbal behavior when communicating with colleagues and clients and to try to make their own nononverbal behavior congruent with their verbal communications. Telling people you understand their problem when you appear thoroughly confused or inattentive is an example of incongruence between verbal and nonverbal communication.

THE BASIC LISTENING SEQUENCE

Listening is the most critical of all communication skills. To be a good listener, one needs to listen for both the information (content) and emotion (feelings) conveyed. A good listener also shows attentiveness through eye contact and body language and gives the speaker some feedback to indicate that what is being said is understood (Rees, 2005) (Box 6-1). Contrast this to the poor listener who interrupts, misinterprets what is said, or misses it entirely due to inattention (Rees, 2005).

PRINCIPLES FOR EFFECTIVE COMMUNICATION

To communicate effectively with others, consider the following principles (Table 6-1).

1. Be sure that the message is understood. Ask for feedback from the receiver to clarify any confusion. Bring focus to the

---

BOX 6-1

Basic Listening Sequence

Listen to the:
  Information
  Emotion
Demonstrate attentiveness through:
  Eye contact
  Body language
Verify understanding by:
  Asking occasional questions
  Repeating important points
  Summarizing

Adapted from Rees, F. (2005). *25 Activities for Developing Team Leaders.* San Francisco: Pfeiffer.

TABLE 6-1	
Principles for Effective Communication	
PRINCIPLE ONE:	Aim for clarity and focus.
PRINCIPLE TWO:	Use direct and exact language.
PRINCIPLE THREE:	Encourage feedback.
PRINCIPLE FOUR:	Acknowledge the contributions of others.
PRINCIPLE FIVE:	Use the most direct channels of communication available.

Tappen, R.M. (2001). *Nursing Leadership and Management Concept and Practice* (3rd ed.). Philadelphia: FA Davis, with permission.

interaction. Repeating key words or phrases as questions or using open-ended questions can accomplish this. For example: "You have been telling me that Susan is not providing safe care to her patients. Can you tell me specifically what you have identified as unsafe care?"

2. Use direct and exact language. In both written and spoken messages, use language that is easily understood by all involved.

3. Encourage feedback. This is the best way to help people understand each other and work together better. Remember, though, that feedback may not be complimentary. This is discussed later in the chapter.

4. Acknowledge the contributions of others. Everyone wants to feel that he or she has worth.

5. Use the most direct channel of communication available. The greater the number of individuals involved in filtering a message, the less likely the message will be received correctly. Remember the children's game Whisper Down the Lane? Messages sent through a number of senders become more and more distorted. Information that is controversial or distressing should definitely be delivered in person so that the receiver can ask questions or receive further clarification. A memo delivered "To all nursing staff" in which cutbacks in staffing are announced would deliver a message very different from that in a meeting in which staff are allowed to talk and ask questions.

ASSERTIVENESS IN COMMUNICATION

Assertive behaviors allow people to stand up for themselves and their rights without violating the rights of others. Several authors have stated that nurses lack assertiveness, claiming that nurses would rather be silent than voice opinions that may result in confrontation (Tappen, 2001). Assertiveness is different from aggressiveness. People use aggressive behaviors to force their wishes or ideas on others. In assertive communication, an individual's position is stated clearly and firmly, using "I" statements. For example:

The nurse manager noticed that Steve's charting has been of lower quality than expected during the past few weeks. She approached Steve and said, "JCAHO surveyors are coming in several months. I have been reviewing records and noticed that on several of your charts some pertinent information is missing. I have scheduled time today and tomorrow from 1:00 to 2:00 in the afternoon for us to review the charts. This allows you time to make the necessary corrections and return the charts to me."

By using "I" statements, the nurse manager is confronting the issue without being accusatory. Assertive communication always requires congruence between verbal and nonverbal messages. Had she shook her finger close to Steve's face or used a loud voice, the nurse manager might think she was being assertive when in fact her manner would have been aggressive.

There is a misconception that people who communicate assertively always get what they want. Being assertive involves both rights and responsibilities. Assertive communicators have the right to speak up, but they also must be prepared to listen to the response.

BARRIERS TO EFFECTIVE COMMUNICATION IN THE WORKPLACE

People often are unwilling or unable to accept responsibility or to perform a specific task because they do not fully understand what is expected of them. Professional nurses are required to communicate client information to other members of the nursing team. Although this may sound easy, there are many potential barriers to communication. These barriers may be physical, psychological, semantic, or even gender-related.

Physical Barriers

Physical barriers to communication include extraneous noise, too much activity in the area where the communication is taking place, and physical separation of the people trying to engage in verbal interaction.

Psychological Barriers

Psychological "noise," such as increased anxiety, may interfere with the ability to pay attention to the other speaker. Social values, emotions, judgments, and cultural influences also impede communication. Previous life experiences and preconceived ideas about other cultures also influence how people communicate.

Semantic Barriers

Semantic refers to the meaning of words. Sometimes, no matter how great the effort, the message just does not get across. For example, words such as *neat, cool,* and *bad* may convey meanings other than those intended. Many individuals have learned English as a second language and therefore understand only the literal meaning of certain words. For example, to many people, *cool* means interesting, unique, clever, or even sharp (e.g., "This is a cool way to find the vein."). To someone for whom the word *cool* refers only to temperature (e.g., "It is cool outside"), the preceding statement would make very little sense.

Gender Barriers

Men and women develop dissimilar communication skills and are inclined to communicate differently. Often, they give different meanings to conveyed information or feelings. This may be related to psychosocial development. Boys learn to use communication as a way to negotiate and to develop independence, whereas

girls use communication to confirm, minimize disparities, and create or strengthen closeness (Blais, Hayes, Kozier, Erb, 2002).

COMMUNICATION WITH COLLEAGUES

Information Systems and E-Mail

Computerized Systems

Communication through the use of computer technology is rapidly growing in nursing practice. A study conducted by KPMG–Peat Marwick of health-care systems that used bedside terminals found that medication errors and use of client call bells decreased and nurse productivity increased. The use of electronic patient records allows health-care providers to retrieve and distribute patient information precisely and quickly. Decisions regarding client care can be made more efficiently with less waiting time. Information systems in many organizations also provide opportunities to access current, high-quality clinical and research data to support evidence-based practice. Unfortunately, these rich resources are still underutilized by most nurses (Dee, 2005). Additional benefits of computerized systems for health-care applications are listed in Box 6-2 (Arnold & Pearson, 1992; Hebda, Czar, & Mascara, 1998).

BOX 6-2

Potential Benefits of Computer-Based Client Information Systems

- Increased hours for direct patient care.
- Patient data accessible at bedside.
- Improved accuracy and legibility of data.
- Immediate availability of all data to all members of the team.
- Increased safety related to positive patient identification, improved standardization, and improved quality.
- Decreased medication errors.
- Increased staff satisfaction.

Adapted from Arnold, J., & Pearson, G. (eds.). (1992). *Computer Applications in Nursing Education and Practice.* New York: National League for Nursing.

E-Mail

Today, most institutions use e-mail. Using e-mail competently and effectively requires writing skills; the same communication principles apply to both e-mail and letter writing. Remember, when communicating by e-mail, you are not only making an impression but also leaving a written record (Shea, 2000).

The rules for using e-mail in the workplace are somewhat different than for using e-mail among friends. Much of the humor and wit found in personal e-mail is not appropriate for the work setting. Professional e-mail may remain informal. However, the message must be clear, concise, and courteous. Think about what you need to say before you write it. Then write it, read it, and reread it. Once you are satisfied that the message is clear and concise, then send it.

Many executives read their own e-mail, which means that it is often possible to contact them directly. Many systems make it easy to send e-mail to everyone at the health-care institution. For this reason, it is important to keep e-mail professional. Remember the "chain of command": always go through the proper channels.

The fact that you have the capability to send e-mail instantly to large groups of people does not necessarily make sending it a good idea. Be careful if you have access to an all-company mailing list. It is easy to send e-mail throughout the system without intending this to happen. Consider the following example:

A respiratory therapist and a department administrator at a large health-care institution were engaged in a relationship. They started sending each other personal notes over the company e-mail system. One day, one of them accidentally sent one of these notes to all the employees at the health-care institution. Both were fired. The moral of this story is simple: Don't send anything via e-mail that you would not want published on the front page of a national newspaper or hear on your favorite radio station tomorrow morning.

Although voice tone cannot be "heard" in e-mail, the use of certain words and writing styles indicate emotion. A rude tone in an e-mail message may provoke extreme reactions. Follow the "rules of netiquette" (Shea, 2000) when communicating through e-mail. Some of these rules are listed in Box 6-3.

BOX 6-3
Rules of Netiquette

1. If you were face-to-face, would you say this?
2. Follow the same rules of behavior online that you follow when dealing with individuals in the real world.
3. Send copies of information only to those individuals who need the information.
4. Avoid flaming; that is, sending remarks intended to cause a negative reaction.
5. Do not write in all capital letters; this suggests anger.
6. Respect other people's privacy.
7. Do not abuse the power of your position.
8. Proofread your e-mail before sending it.

Adapted from Shea, V. (2000). *Netiquette*. San Rafael, CA: Albion.

REPORTING CLIENT INFORMATION

Change-of-Shift Report

It is important to understand exactly how your day at work will begin. Regardless of which shift an individual works, some things never change. Nurses traditionally give one another a "report." The change-of-shift report has become the accepted method of communicating client care needs from one nurse to another. In the report, pertinent information related to events that occurred is given to the individuals responsible for providing continuity of care (Box 6-4). Although historically the report has been given face to face, there are newer ways to share information. Many health-care institutions use audiotape and computer printouts as mechanisms for sharing information. These mechanisms allow the nurses from the previous shift to complete their tasks and those coming on duty to make inquiries for clarification as necessary.

The report should be organized, concise, and complete, with relevant details. Not every unit uses the same system for giving a change-of-shift report. The system is easily modified according to the pattern of nursing care delivery and the types of clients serviced. For example, many intensive care units, because of their small size and the more acute needs of their clients, use walking rounds as a means for giving the report. This system allows nurses to

---

BOX 6-4

Information for Change-of-Shift Report

◆ Identify the client, including the room and bed numbers.
◆ Include the client diagnosis.
◆ Account for the presence of the client on the unit. If the client has left the unit for a diagnostic test, surgery, or just to wander, it is important for the oncoming staff members to know the client is off the unit.
◆ Provide the treatment plan that specifies the goals of treatment. Note the goals and the critical pathway steps either achieved or in progress. Personalized approaches can be developed during this time and client readiness for those approaches evaluated. It is helpful to mention the client's primary care physician. Include new orders and medications and treatments currently prescribed.

◆ Document client responses to current treatments. Is the treatment plan working? Present evidence for or against this. Include pertinent laboratory values as well as any untoward reactions to medications or treatments. Note any comments the client has made regarding the hospitalization or treatment plan that the oncoming staff members need to address.
◆ Omit personal opinions and value judgments about clients as well as personal/confidential information not pertinent to providing client care. If you are using computerized information systems, make sure you know how to present the material accurately and concisely.

---

discuss the current client status and to set goals for care for the next several hours. Together, the nurses gather objective data as one nurse ends a shift and the other begins. This way, there is no confusion as to the client's status at shift change. This same system is often used in emergency departments and labor and delivery units. Larger client care units may find the "walking report" time-consuming and an inefficient use of resources.

It is helpful to take notes or create a worksheet while listening to the report. A worksheet helps organize the work for the day (Fig. 6-1). As specific tasks are mentioned, the nurse coming on duty makes a note of the activity in the appropriate time slot. Medications and treatments can also be added. Any changes from the previous day are noted, particularly when the nurse is familiar with the client. Recording changes counteracts the tendency to remember what was done the day before and repeat it, often without checking for new orders. During the day, the worksheet acts as a reminder of the tasks that have been completed and those that still need to be done.

Reporting skills improve with practice. When presenting information in a report, certain details must be included. Begin the report by identifying the client and the admitting as well as current diagnoses. Include the expected treatment plan and the client's responses to the treatment. For example, if the client has had multiple antibiotics and a reaction occurred, this information is important to relay

to the next nurse. Value judgments and personal opinions about the client are inappropriate (Fig. 6-2).

Team Conferences

Members of a team also share information through verbal and written communication in an interdisciplinary team conference. The team conference begins by stating the client's name, age, and diagnoses. Each member of an interdisciplinary team then explains the goal of his or her discipline, the interventions, and the outcome. Effectiveness of treatment, development of new interventions, and setting of new goals are then discussed. The key to a successful interdisciplinary conference is presenting the information in a clear, concise manner and ensuring input from all disciplines and levels of care providers from unlicensed assistive personnel to physicians.

Communicating With Other Disciplines

In many settings, nurses are the client care managers. Integration, coordination, and communication among all disciplines delivering care to a specific client ultimately are the responsibility of the nurse care manager. Nurses are usually in a particularly advantageous position to observe the client's responses to treatments. For example:

Name_____ **Room #**_____ **Allergies** _____

0700	0800	0900	1000	1100	1200	1300	1400	1500	1600	1700	1800

Name_____ **Room #**_____ **Allergies** _____

0700	0800	0900	1000	1100	1200	1300	1400	1500	1600	1700	1800

Name_____ **Room #**_____ **Allergies** _____

0700	0800	0900	1000	1100	1200	1300	1400	1500	1600	1700	1800

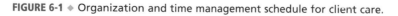

FIGURE 6-1 ◆ Organization and time management schedule for client care.

Mr. Richards is a 75-year-old man who was in a motor vehicle accident with closed head trauma. He had right-sided weakness and dysphagia. The speech therapy, physical therapy, and social services departments were called in to see Mr. Richards. A speech therapist was working with Mr. Richards to assist him with swallowing. He was to receive pureed foods for the second day. The RN assigned an LPN to feed Mr. Richards. The LPN reported that although Mr. Richards had done well the previous day, he had difficulty swallowing today. The RN immediately notified

Room # _____   Patient Name _____   Diagnoses _____

Diet _____   Acitivity_____

1900	0100
2000	0200
2100	0300
2200	0400
2300	0500
2400	0600

FIGURE 6-2 ◆ Client information report.

the speech therapist, and a new treatment plan was developed.

The function of professional nurses in relation to their clients' physicians is to communicate changes in the client's condition, share other pertinent information, discuss modifications of the treatment plan, and clarify physician orders. This can be stressful for a new graduate who still has some role insecurity. Using good communication skills and having the necessary information at hand are helpful when discussing client needs.

Before calling a physician, make sure that all the information you need is available. The physician may want more clarification. If you are calling to report a drop in a client's blood pressure, be sure to have at hand the list of the client's medications, laboratory results, vital signs, and blood pressure trends, together with a general assessment of the client's present status.

Sometimes when a nurse calls a physician, the physician does not return the call. It is important to document all physician contacts in the patient's record. Many units keep physician calling logs. In the log, enter the physician's name, the date, the time, the reason for the call, and the time the physician returns the call.

Professional nurses are responsible for accepting, transcribing, and implementing physicians' orders. The two main types of orders are *written* and *verbal*. *Written orders* are dated and placed on the appropriate institutional form. *Verbal orders* are given from the physician directly to the nurse, either by telephone or in person. A verbal order needs to be written on the appropriate institutional form, the time and date noted, and the form signed as a verbal order by the nurse. Most institutions require the physician to cosign the order within 24 hours. When receiving a verbal order, repeat it back to the physician for confirmation. If the physician is speaking too rapidly, ask him or her to speak more slowly. Then repeat the information for confirmation.

Professionalism and a courteous attitude by all parties are necessary to maintain collegial relationships with physicians and other health-care professionals. Here's how one nurse explained their importance:

RN satisfaction simply is not about money. A major factor is how well nurses feel supported in their work. Do people listen to us—our managers, upper management, human resources? Being able to communicate with each other—to be able to speak directly with your peers, physicians, or managers in a way that is nonconfrontational—is really important to having good working relationships and to providing good care. You need to have mutual respect. (Quoted by Trossman, 2005, p. 1.)

Communicating With Clients and Their Families

Communicating with clients and their families occupies a major portion of the nurse's day. Nurses teach clients and their families about medications and the client's condition, clarify the treatment plan, and explain procedures. To do this effectively, nurses need to use communication skills and recognize the barriers to communication.

The health-care consumer may enter the setting in a highly emotional state. Nurses need to recognize the signs of an anxious or angry client and promptly intervene to defuse the situation before it escalates. Practicing good listening skills and showing interest in the client often helps.

Short-term stays and early morning admissions on the day of surgery make client teaching a challenge. The nurse must complete the admission requirements, surgical checklists, and preoperative teaching within a short time. Time for postoperative teaching is also shortened. It is important for the nurse to communicate clearly and concisely what will be done and what is expected of the client. Allow time for questions and clarifications. For many clients, a written preoperative and/or postoperative teaching guide helps to clarify the instructions.

◼ FEEDBACK

Why Do People Need Feedback?

In good weather, Herbert usually played basketball with his kids after dinner. Yesterday, however, he told them he was too tired. This evening, he said the same thing. When they urged him to play anyway, he snapped at them and told them to leave him alone.

"Herbert!" his wife exclaimed, "Why did you do that?"

"I don't know," he responded. "I'm just so tense these days. My annual review was supposed to be today, but my nurse manager was out sick. I have no idea what she is going to say. I can't think about anything else."

If Herbert's nurse manager had been providing informal feedback to staff on a regular basis, Herbert would have known where he stood. He would have had a good idea about what his strengths and weaknesses were and would not be afraid of an unpleasant surprise during the review. He would also be looking forward to the opportunity to review his accomplishments and make plans with his manager for further developing his skills. He still would have been disappointed that she was unavailable, but he would not have been as distressed by it.

The process of giving and receiving evaluative feedback is an essential leadership responsibility. Done well, it is very helpful, promoting growth and increasing employee satisfaction. Done poorly, as in Herbert's case, it can be stressful, even injurious. This section considers the do's and don'ts of giving and receiving feedback, how to share positive and negative evaluative comments with coworkers, and how people can respond constructively when they are on the receiving end of such comments.

We all need feedback because it is difficult for us to see ourselves as others see us. Curiously, competent people generally underestimate their ability and focus on their shortcomings, and incompetent people generally fail to recognize their incompetence (Channer & Hope, 2001). The following are just a few of the reasons that evaluative feedback is so important:

◆ **Reinforces constructive behavior.** Positive feedback lets people know which behaviors are the most productive and encourages continuation of those behaviors.

◆ **Discourages unproductive behavior.** Correction of inappropriate behavior begins with provision of negative feedback.

◆ **Provides recognition.** The power of praise (positive feedback) to motivate people is underestimated.

◆ **Develops employee skills.** Feedback helps people identify their strengths and weaknesses and guides them in seeking opportunities to further develop their strengths and manage their weaknesses (Rosen, 1996).

Guidelines for Providing Feedback

Done well, evaluative feedback can reinforce motivation, strengthen teamwork, and improve the quality of care given. When done poorly, evaluation can reinforce poor work habits, increase insecurity, and destroy motivation and morale (Table 6-2).

Evaluation involves making judgments and communicating these judgments to others. People make judgments all the time about all types of things. Unfortunately, these judgments are often based on opinions, preferences, and inaccurate or partial information.

Subjective, biased judgment offered as objective feedback has given evaluation a bad

---

TABLE 6-2
Do's and Don'ts of Providing Feedback

Do	Don't
Include positive comments.	Focus only on the negative.
Be objective.	Let personalities intrude.
Be specific when correcting someone.	Be vague.
Treat everyone the same.	Play favorites.
Correct people in private.	Correct people in front of others

Adapted from Gabor, D. (1994). *Speaking Your Mind in 101 Difficult Situations.* New York: Stonesong Press (Simon & Schuster).

---

name. Poorly communicated feedback has an equally negative effect. Many people who are uncomfortable with evaluation have been recipients of subjective, biased, or poorly communicated evaluations.

Evaluative feedback is most effective when given immediately, frequently, and privately. To be constructive, it must be objective, based on observed behavior, and skillfully communicated. The feedback message should include the reasons that a behavior has been judged satisfactory or unsatisfactory. If the message is negative, it should include both suggestions and support for change and improvement (Box 6-5).

Provide Both Positive and Negative Feedback

Leaders and managers often neglect to provide positive feedback. If questioned about this, they often say, "If I don't say anything, that means everything is okay." They do not realize that some people assume that everything is *not* okay when they receive no feedback. Others

---

BOX 6-5

Tips for Providing Helpful Feedback

◆ Provide both positive and negative feedback.
◆ Give feedback immediately.
◆ Provide feedback frequently.
◆ Give negative feedback privately.
◆ Base feedback on observable behavior.
◆ Communicate effectively.
◆ Include suggestions for change.

assume that no one is aware of how much effort they have made unless it is acknowledged with positive feedback.

Most people want to do their work well. They also want to know that their efforts are recognized and appreciated. Kron (1981) called positive feedback a "psychological paycheck." She pointed out that it is almost as important to people as their actual paychecks. It is a real pleasure, not only for staff members but also for their leaders and managers, to be able to share the satisfaction of a job well done with someone else. Leaders and managers should do everything they can to reward and retain their best staff members (Bowers & Lapziger, 2001). In fact, some claim that the very best managers focus on people's strengths and work around their weaknesses (DiMichele & Gaffney, 2005).

Providing negative feedback is just as necessary but probably more difficult to do well. Too often, negative feedback is critical rather than helpful. Simply telling someone that something has gone wrong or could have been done better is inadequate. Instead, make feedback a learning experience by suggesting ways to make changes or by working together to develop a strategy for improvement. It is easier to make broad, critical comments (e.g., "You're too slow") than to describe the specific behavior that needs improvement (e.g., "Waiting in Mr. D.'s room while he cleans his dentures takes up too much of your time.") and then add a suggestion for change (e.g., "You could get your bath supplies together while he finishes.").

Unsatisfactory work must be acknowledged and discussed with the people involved. Too many managers avoid it, not wanting to hurt people's feelings (Watson & Harris, 1999). Tolerating poor work encourages its continuation.

Give Immediate Feedback

The most helpful feedback is given as soon as possible after the behavior has occurred. There are several reasons for this. Immediate feedback is more meaningful to the person receiving it. Address inappropriate behavior when it occurs, whether it is low productivity, tardiness, or other problems. Problems that are ignored often get worse. Ignoring them puts stress on others and reduces morale. Resolving them boosts productivity, lowers stress, increases retention of good staff, and ultimately results in higher-quality care (Briles, 2005).

Provide Frequent Feedback

Frequent feedback keeps motivation high. It also becomes easier with practice. If giving and receiving feedback are frequent, integral parts of team functioning, they will be easier to accomplish and will be less threatening. It becomes an ordinary, everyday occurrence, one that happens spontaneously and is familiar to everyone on the team.

Give Negative Feedback Privately

Giving negative feedback privately rather than in front of others prevents unnecessary embarrassment. It also avoids the possibility that those who overhear the discussion misunderstand it and draw erroneous conclusions. A good manager praises staffers in public but corrects them in private (Matejka, Ashworth, & Dodd-McCue, 1986).

Be Objective

Being objective can be very difficult. First, evaluate people on the basis of job expectations and the results of their efforts (Fonville, Killian, & Tranberger, 1998). Do not compare them, favorably or unfavorably, with other staff members (Gellerman & Hodgson, 1988).

Another way to increase objectivity is to always give a reason that you have judged a behavior as good or poor. Be sure you consider the effect or outcome of the behavior in forming your conclusion. Give reasons for both positive and negative messages. For example, if you tell a coworker, "That was a good patient interview," you have only told that person that the interview pleased you. However, when you add, "because you asked open-ended questions that encouraged the client to explore personal feelings," you have identified and reinforced this specific behavior that made your evaluation positive.

Finally, use broad and generally accepted standards for making judgments as much as possible, rather than basing evaluation on your personal likes and dislikes. Objectivity can be increased by using standards that reflect the consensus of the team, the organization, the community, or the nursing profession. Formal evaluation is based on agreed-upon, written standards of what is acceptable behavior. Informal evaluation, however, is based on unwritten standards. If these unwritten standards are based on personal preferences, the evaluation will be highly subjective. The following are examples:

◆ A team leader who describes a female social worker as having a professional appearance because she wears muted suits instead of bright dresses to work is using a personal standard to evaluate that social worker.

◆ A supervisor who asks an employee to stop wearing jewelry that could get caught in the equipment used at work is applying a standard for safety in making the evaluative statement.

Base Feedback on Observable Behavior

An evaluative statement should describe observed performance, not your interpretation of another's behavior. For example, saying, "You were impatient with Mrs. G. today" is an interpretive comment. Saying, "You interrupted Mrs. G. before she finished explaining her problem" is based on observable behavior. The second statement is more specific and may be more accurate because the caregiver may have been trying to redirect the conversation to more immediate concerns rather than being impatient. The latter statement is also more likely to evoke an explanation than a defensive response.

Include Suggestions for Change

When you give feedback that indicates that some kind of change in behavior is needed, it is helpful to suggest some alternative behaviors. This is easier to do when the change is a simple one.

When complex change is needed (as with Mr. S. below), you may find that the person is aware of the problem but does not know how to solve it. In such a case, offering to engage in searching for the solution is appropriate. A willingness to listen to the other person's side of the story and assist in finding a solution indicates that your purpose is to help rather than to criticize.

Accept Feedback in Return

An evaluative statement is a form of confrontation. Any message that contains a statement about the behavior of a staff member confronts that staff member with his or her behavior. The leader who gives evaluative feedback needs to be prepared to receive feedback in return and to engage in active listening. Active listening is especially important because the person receiving the evaluation may respond with high emotion. The following is an example of what may happen:

You point out to Mr. S. that his patients need to be monitored more frequently. Mr. S. responds, with some agitation, that he is doing everything possible for the patients and does not have a free moment all day for one extra thing. In fact, Mr. S. tells you, he never even takes a lunch break and goes home exhausted. Active listening and problem solving aimed at relieving his overloaded time schedule are a must in this situation.

When you give negative feedback, allow time for the receiver to express his or her opinions and for problem solving. This is particularly important if the problem has been ignored or has become serious (Box 6-6).

SEEKING EVALUATIVE FEEDBACK

It is equally important to be able to accept constructive criticism (Kelly & Aiken, 1999). The reasons for seeking feedback are the same as

---

BOX 6-6

TACTFUL Guidelines for Providing Negative Feedback

T	=	Think before you speak.
A	=	Apologize quickly if you make a mistake.
C	=	Converse; do not be patronizing or sarcastic.
T	=	Time your comments carefully.
F	=	Focus on behavior, not on personality.
U	=	Uncover hidden feelings.
L	=	Listen for feedback.

Gabor, D. (1994). *Speaking Your Mind in 101 Difficult Situations.* New York: Stonesong Press (Simon & Schuster).

those for giving it to others. The criteria for evaluating the feedback you receive are also the same.

When Is Evaluative Feedback Needed?

You may find yourself in a work situation in which you receive very little feedback, or you may be getting only positive and no negative comments (or vice versa) (Box 6-7).

You also need to look for feedback when you feel uncertain about how well you are doing or whether you have correctly interpreted the expectations of the job. The following are examples of these situations:

◆ You have been told that good client care is the highest priority but you feel totally frustrated by never having enough staff members to give good care.

◆ You thought you were expected to do case finding and health teaching in your community, but you receive the most recognition for the number of home visits made and the completeness of your records.

Another instance in which you should request feedback is when you believe that your needs for recognition and job satisfaction have not been met adequately.

Request feedback in the form of "I" messages. If you have received only negative comments, ask, "In what ways have I done well?" If you receive only positive comments, you can ask, "In what areas do I need to improve?" Or, if you are seeking feedback from a client, you could ask, "How can I be of more help to you?"

Responding to Evaluative Feedback

Sometimes, it is appropriate to critically analyze the feedback you are getting. If the feedback seems totally negative or you feel threatened by receiving it, ask for further explanation. You may have misunderstood what your nurse manager intended to say.

It is hard to avoid responding defensively to negative feedback that is subjective or laced with threats and blame. If you are the recipient of such a poorly done evaluation, however, it may help both you and your supervisor to try to guide the discussion into more constructive areas. You can ask for reasons why the evaluation was negative, on what standard it was based, what the person's expectations were, and what the person suggests as alternative behavior.

When the feedback is positive but nonspecific, you may also want to ask for some clarification so that you can learn what that person's expectations really are. Do not hesitate to seek that psychological paycheck. Tell other people about your successes; most are happy to share the satisfaction of a successful outcome or positive development in a client's care.

PERFORMANCE APPRAISAL

Performance appraisal is the formal evaluation of an employee by a superior, usually a manager or supervisor. To prepare an appraisal, the employee's behavior is compared with his or her job description and the standard describing how the employee is expected to perform (Hayes, 2002). Employees need to know what has to be done, how much has to be done, and when it has to be done. Evaluate actual performance, not good intentions.

Procedure

In the ideal situation, the performance appraisal begins when the employee is hired. Based on the written job description, the employee and manager discuss performance expectations and then write a set of objectives they think the employee can reasonably accomplish within a given time. The objectives should be written at a level of performance that demonstrates that some learning, refinement of skill, or advancement toward some long-range objective will have occurred. The following are examples of objectives a new staff nurse

---

BOX 6-7

Situations in Which to Ask for Feedback

◆ When you do not know how well you are doing.
◆ When you receive only positive comments.
◆ When you receive only negative comments.
◆ When you believe that your accomplishments have not been recognized.

could accomplish in the first 6 months of employment:

- ◆ Complete the staff nurse orientation program successfully.
- ◆ Master the basic skills necessary to function as a staff nurse on the assigned unit.
- ◆ Supervise the unlicensed assistive personnel assigned to his or her patients.

Monthly reviews of progress toward these goals help keep the new staff member on track and provide opportunities to identify needs for further orientation or extended training (Hayes, 2002; Lombardi, 2001). Six months later, the staff nurse and nurse manager sit down again and evaluate the staff nurse's performance in terms of the previously set goals. The evaluation is based on the staff nurse's self-evaluation and the nurse manager's observation of specific behaviors. New objectives for the next 6 months and plans for achieving them may be agreed on at the time of the appraisal or at a separate meeting (Beer, 1981). A copy of the performance appraisal and the new goals must be available to employees so that they can refer to them and check on their progress.

It is important to set aside adequate time for feedback and goal-setting processes. Both the staff nurse and the nurse manager bring data for use at this session. These data include a self-evaluation by the staff nurse and observations by the evaluator of the employee's activities and their outcomes. Data may also be obtained from peers and clients. Some organizations use surveys for getting this information from clients.

Most of the guidelines for providing informal evaluative feedback discussed earlier apply to the conduct of performance appraisals. Although not as frequent or immediate as informal feedback, formal evaluation should be just as objective, private, skillfully communicated, and growth-promoting.

Standards for Evaluation

Unfortunately, many organizations' employee evaluation procedures are far from ideal. Their procedures may be inconsistent, subjective, and even unknown to the employee in some cases. The following is a list of standards for a

fair and objective employee evaluation procedure that you can use to judge your employer's procedures:

- ◆ Standards are clear, objective, and known in advance.
- ◆ Criteria for pay raises and promotions are clearly spelled out and uniformly applied.
- ◆ Conditions under which employment may be terminated are known.
- ◆ Appraisals are part of the employee's permanent record and have space for employee comments.
- ◆ Employees may inspect their own personnel file.
- ◆ Employees may request and be given a reasonable explanation of any rating and may appeal the rating if they do not agree with it.
- ◆ Employees are given a reasonable amount of time to correct any serious deficiencies before other action is taken, unless the safety of self or others is immediately threatened.

In some organizations, collective bargaining agreements are used to enforce adherence to fair and objective performance appraisals. However, collective bargaining agreements may emphasize seniority (length of service) over merit, a situation that does not promote growth or change.

PEER REVIEW

Peer review is the evaluation of an individual's practice by his or her colleagues (peers) who have similar education, experience, and occupational status. Its purpose is to provide the individual with feedback from those who are best acquainted with the requirements and demands of that individual's position: colleagues. Peer review is directed to both *actions* (process) and the *outcomes* of actions. It also encompasses decision-making (critical thinking), technical, and interpersonal skills (Mustard, 2002).

Professionals frequently observe and judge their colleagues' performance. Many feel uncomfortable telling colleagues directly what they think of their performance, however, so they do not indicate their thoughts unless informal feedback is shared regularly or a formal system of peer review is established (Katzenbach & Smith, 2003). Whenever staff members meet to audit records or otherwise evaluate the quality of care they have given, they are engaging in a kind of peer review.

Formal peer review programs are often one of the last formal evaluation procedures to be implemented in a health-care organization. They increase the number of sources of feedback and contribute to a rich, comprehensive evaluation process (Guthrie & King, 2004).

Fundamentals of Peer Review

There are many possible variations of the peer review process. The observations may be shared only with the person being reviewed, with the person's supervisor, or with a review committee. The evaluation report may be written by the reviewer, or it may come from the review committee. The use of a committee defeats the purpose of peer review if the committee members are not truly peers of the individual being reviewed.

A Comprehensive Peer Review System

Peer review systems can simply be informal feedback regularly shared among colleagues, or they may be comprehensive systems that are fully integrated into the formal evaluation structure of a health-care organization. When a peer review system is fully integrated, the evaluative feedback from peers is joined with the performance appraisals by the nurse manager, and both are used to determine pay raises and promotions for individual staff nurses. This is a far more collegial approach than the hierarchical one typically used, in which employees are evaluated only by their manager.

A comprehensive peer review system begins with the development of job descriptions and performance standards for each level within the nursing staff. The job description is a very general statement, whereas the standards are specific behaviors that can be observed and recorded.

In a participative environment, the standards are developed by committees having representatives from different units and from each staff level, from the new staff nurse to top-level management. In some instances, they are very specific, quantifiable criteria, but others are likely to require professional judgment as to the quality of the care provided (Chang, et al., 2002).

In some organizations, the standards may be considered the minimal qualifications for each level. In this case, additional activities and professional development are expected before promotion to the next level. The candidate for promotion to an advanced-level position prepares a promotion portfolio for review (Schultz, 1993). The promotion portfolio may include a self-assessment, peer reviews, patient surveys, a management performance appraisal, and evidence of professional growth. Such evidence can derive from participating in the quality improvement program, evaluating a new product or procedure, serving as a translator or disaster volunteer, making postdischarge visits to clients from the unit, or taking courses related to nursing.

Writing useful job descriptions and measurable standards of performance is an arduous but rewarding task. It requires clarification and explication of the work nurses actually do and goes beyond the usual generalizations about what nursing is and what nurses do. Under effective group leadership and with strong administrative support for this process, it can be a challenging and stimulating experience. Without administrative support and guidance, however, the committee work can be frustrating when the group gets bogged down in details and disagreements.

When the job descriptions and performance standards for each level have been developed and agreed on, a procedure for their use must also be worked out. This can be done in several ways. In some organizations, an evaluation form that lists the performance standards can be completed by one or two colleagues selected by the individual staff member. In some organizations, the information from these forms is used along with the nurse manager's evaluation to determine pay raises and promotions. In others, the evaluation from one's peers is used for counseling purposes only and is not taken into consideration in determining pay raises or promotions. This second approach provides useful feedback but weakens the impact of peer review.

A different approach is the use of a professional practice committee. The committee, consisting of colleagues selected by the nursing staff, reviews the peer evaluation forms and makes its recommendations to the director of nursing or vice president for client care services, who then makes the final decision regarding the appropriate rewards (raises, promotions, commendations) or penalties (demotion, transfer, termination of employment).

CONCLUSION

The responsibility for delivering and coordinating client care is an important part of the role of the professional nurse. To accomplish this, nurses need good communication skills. Being assertive without being aggressive and conducting interactions in a professional manner enhance the relationships nurses develop with colleagues, physicians, and other members of the interdisciplinary team.

A comprehensive evaluation system can be an effective mechanism both for improving staff skills and morale and for reducing costs by increasing staff productivity. Constructive feedback demands objectivity and fairness in dealing with each other and leadership of both staff members and management. Done well, feedback can provide many opportunities for increased professionalism and learning as well as ensure appropriate rewards for high performance levels and professionalism on the job.

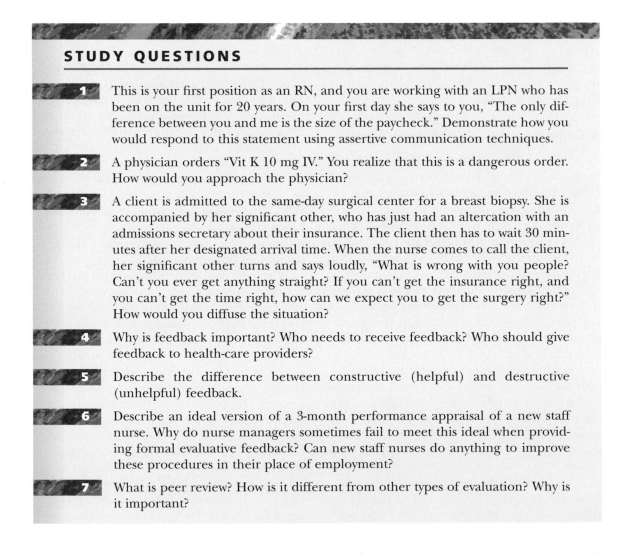

STUDY QUESTIONS

1. This is your first position as an RN, and you are working with an LPN who has been on the unit for 20 years. On your first day she says to you, "The only difference between you and me is the size of the paycheck." Demonstrate how you would respond to this statement using assertive communication techniques.

2. A physician orders "Vit K 10 mg IV." You realize that this is a dangerous order. How would you approach the physician?

3. A client is admitted to the same-day surgical center for a breast biopsy. She is accompanied by her significant other, who has just had an altercation with an admissions secretary about their insurance. The client then has to wait 30 minutes after her designated arrival time. When the nurse comes to call the client, her significant other turns and says loudly, "What is wrong with you people? Can't you ever get anything straight? If you can't get the insurance right, and you can't get the time right, how can we expect you to get the surgery right?" How would you diffuse the situation?

4. Why is feedback important? Who needs to receive feedback? Who should give feedback to health-care providers?

5. Describe the difference between constructive (helpful) and destructive (unhelpful) feedback.

6. Describe an ideal version of a 3-month performance appraisal of a new staff nurse. Why do nurse managers sometimes fail to meet this ideal when providing formal evaluative feedback? Can new staff nurses do anything to improve these procedures in their place of employment?

7. What is peer review? How is it different from other types of evaluation? Why is it important?

CRITICAL THINKING EXERCISE

Tyrell Jones is a new unlicensed assistant who has been assigned to your acute rehabilitation unit. Tyrell is a hard worker; he comes in early and often stays late to finish his work. But Tyrell is gruff with the clients, especially with the male clients. If a client is reluctant to get out of bed, Tyrell often challenges him, saying, "C'mon, man. Don't be such a wimp. Move your big butt." Today, you overheard Tyrell telling a female client who said she didn't feel well, "You're just a phony. You like being waited on, but that's not why you're here." The woman started to cry.

1. You are the newest staff nurse on this unit. How would you handle this situation? What would happen if you ignored it?

2. If you decided that you should not ignore it, with whom should you speak? Why? What would you say?

3. Why do you think Tyrell speaks to clients this way?

REFERENCES

Arnold, J., & Pearson, G. (eds.). (1992). *Computer Applications in Nursing Education and Practice.* New York: National League for Nursing.

Beer, M. (1981, Winter). Performance appraisal: Dilemmas and possibilities. *Organizational Dynamics,* 24.

Blais, K.B., Hayes, J.S., Kozier, B., & Erb, G. (2002). *Professional Nursing Practice: Concepts and Perspectives,* 4th ed. Upper Saddle River, NJ: Prentice-Hall.

Bowers, B., & Lapziger D. (2001). *The New York Times Management Reader.* New York: Times Books.

Briles, J. (2005). Steer your solution in the right direction. *Nursing Management,* 36:5, 68.

Chang, B.L., Lee, J.L., Pearson, M.L., Kahn, K.L., Elliott, M.N., & Rubenstein, L.L. (July/August 2002). Evaluating quality of nursing care. *Journal of Nursing Administration,* 32 (7/8), 405–415.

Channer, P., & Hope, T. (2001). *Emotional Impact: Passionate Leaders and Corporate Transformation.* Hampshire, UK: Palgrave.

Dee, C. (2005). Making the most of nursing's electronic resources. *American Journal of Nursing,* 105:9, 79–85.

DiMichele, C. & Gaffney, L. (2005). Proactive teams yield exceptional care. *Nursing Management,* 36:5, 61.

Fontaine, K.L., & Fletcher, J.S. (2002). *Mental Health Nursing,* 5th ed. Redwood City, CA: Prentice-Hall.

Fonville, A.M., Killian, E.R., & Tranberger, R.E. (1998). Developing new nurse leaders. Nurse Economics, 16, 83–87.

Gabor, D. (1994). *Speaking Your Mind in 101 Difficult Situations.* New York: Stonesong Press (Simon & Schuster).

Gellerman, S.W., & Hodgson, W.G. (1988). Cyanamid's new take on performance appraisal. *Harvard Business Review,* 88(3), 36–41.

Guthrie, V.A., & King, S.N. (2004). Feedback-Intensive Program. In McCauly, C.D., & Van Velsor, E. (eds.). *The Center for Creative Leadership Handbook of Leadership Development.* San Francisco: Jossey-Bass.

Hayes, H. (Winter 2002). Employee training and job descriptions. *Maryland Medicine,* 3(1), 39–41.

Hebda, T., Czar, P., & Mascara, C. (1998). *Handbook of Informatics for Nurses and Health Care Professionals.* Menlo Park, CA: Addison-Wesley.

Katzenbach, J.R., & Smith, D.K. (2003). *The Wisdom of Teams.* New York: Harper Collins.

Kron, T. (1981). *The Management of Patient Care: Putting Leadership Skills to Work.* Philadelphia: WB Saunders.

Lombardi, D.N. (2001). *Handbook for the New Health Care Manager.* San Francisco: Jossey-Bass.

Matejka, J.K., Ashworth, D.N., & Dodd-McCue, D. (1986). Discipline without guilt. *Supervisory Management,* 31(5), 34–36.

Mustard, L.W. (2002). Caring and competency. *JONA's Healthcare Law, Ethics and Regulation,* 4(2), 36–43.

Rees, F. (2005). *25 Activities for Developing Team Leaders.* San Francisco: Pfeiffer.

Rosen, R.H. (1996). *Leading People: Transforming Business From the Inside Out.* New York: Viking Penguin.

Schultz, A.W. (1993). Evaluation for clinical advancement systems. *Journal of Nursing Administration,* 23(2), 13–19.

Shea, V. (2000). *Netiquette.* San Rafael, CA: Albion.

Tappen, R.M. (2001). *Nursing Leadership and Management: Concepts and Practice,* 4th ed. Philadelphia: FA Davis.

Trossman, S. (2005). Who you work with matters. *American Nurse,* 37:4, 1, 8. American Nurses Association.

Watson, T., & Harris, P. (1999). *The Emergent Manager.* London: Sage Publications.

Dealing With Problems and Conflicts

OBJECTIVES

After reading this chapter, the student should be able to:

◆ Identify common sources of conflict in the workplace.

◆ Guide an individual or small group through the process of problem resolution.

◆ Participate in informal negotiations.

◆ Discuss the purposes of collective bargaining.

OUTLINE

CHAPTER 7 SELF-ASSESSMENT
How Do You Respond to Conflict?

Answer the following questions honestly:

1. When someone disagrees with you, do you usually
   a. Avoid the subject
   b. Try to find the basis for the disagreement
   c. Argue with the person

2. If you walked in on an argument between two nursing aides in the utility room, would you
   a. Turn around and leave
   b. Ask what the problem might be
   c. Tell them to stop arguing

3. If your paycheck were $100 less than you expected it to be, would you
   a. Wait to see if the shortfall was made up in the next pay period
   b. Call the payroll department to find out why it was short
   c. Tell payroll you want a check for the missing $100 immediately

4. If a patient told you he was going to sue the hospital after he was sent home, would you
   a. Try to be especially nice to him for the rest of his stay
   b. Find out how the hospital usually handles threats to sue
   c. Explain to him that lawsuits are one of the reasons health care is so expensive

5. If your team leader spends her day at the desk or in meetings and does not conduct patient rounds, would you
   a. Request reassignment to a better team leader
   b. Discuss the problem with the nurse manager
   c. Tell the team leader she's not setting a good example for the rest of the team

ASSESS YOUR STYLE

Problem Avoidance: If you selected **a** for most of your answers.

Negotiation and Resolution: If you selected **b** for most of your answers.

Direct Confrontation: If you selected **c** for most of your answers.

Each of us brings different experiences, beliefs, values, and habits to work. These differences are a natural part of our being unique individuals and members of different segments of our society. Various pressures and demands in the workplace generate problems and conflicts among people at work. Any or all of these can interfere with the ability to work together. Consider Case 1, which is the first of three in this chapter that will be used to illustrate how to deal with problems and conflicts.

CONFLICT

There are no conflict-free work groups (Van de Vliert & Janssen, 2001). Small or large, conflicts are a daily occurrence in the life of nurses (McElhaney, 1996), and they can

Case 1

Team A and Team B

Team A has stopped talking to Team B. If several members of Team A are out sick, no one on Team B will help Team A with their work. Likewise, Team A members will not take telephone messages for anyone on Team B. Instead, they ask the person to call back later. When members of the two teams pass each other in the hall, they either glare at each other or turn away to avoid eye contact. Arguments erupt when members of the two teams need the same computer terminal or another piece of equipment at the same time.

When a Team A nurse reached for a pulse oximeter at the same moment as a Team B nurse did, the second nurse said, "You've been using that all morning."

"I've got a lot of patients to monitor," was the response.

"Oh, you think you're the only one with work to do?"

"We take good care of our patients."

"Are you saying we don't?"

The nurses fell silent when the nurse manager entered the room.

"Is something the matter?" she asked. Both nurses shook their heads and left quickly.

"I'm not sure what's going on here," the nurse manager thought to herself, "but something's wrong, and I need to find out what it is right away."

We will return to this case later as we discuss workplace problems and conflicts, their sources, and how to resolve them.

---

interfere with getting work done, as shown in Case 1.

Serious conflicts can be very stressful for the people involved. Stress symptoms, such as difficulty concentrating, anxiety, sleep disorders, and withdrawal, or other interpersonal relationship problems can occur. Bitterness, anger, and even violence can erupt in the workplace if conflicts are not handled well.

Conflict also has a positive side, however. For example, in the process of learning how to manage conflict, people can develop more open, cooperative ways of working together (Tjosvold & Tjosvold, 1995). They can begin to see each other as people with similar needs, concerns, and dreams instead of as competitors or blocks in the way of progress. Being involved in successful conflict resolution can be an empowering experience (Horton-Deutsch & Wellman, 2002).

The goal in dealing with conflict is to create an environment in which conflicts are dealt with in as cooperative and constructive a manner as possible rather than in a competitive and destructive manner.

SOURCES OF CONFLICT

Why do conflicts occur? Health care brings people of different ages, genders, income levels, ethnic groups, educational levels, lifestyles, and professions together for the purpose of restoring or maintaining people's health. Differences of opinion over how to best accomplish this goal are a normal part of working with people of various skill levels and backgrounds (Wenckus, 1995). In addition, the workplace itself can be a generator of conflict (Box 7-1). Following are some of the most common reasons why conflict occurs in the workplace.

Competition Between Groups

Disagreements over professional "territory" can occur in any setting. For example, nurse practitioners and physicians may disagree over limitations on nurse practitioner independence. Physician dominance and the expectation of self-sacrifice and giving beyond reasonable limits from nurses may need rene-

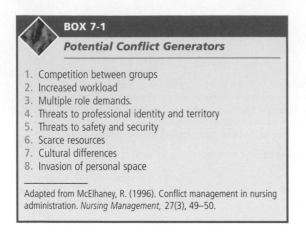

Adapted from McElhaney, R. (1996). Conflict management in nursing administration. *Nursing Management, 27*(3), 49–50.

gotiaton in some settings (Block, 2004). Union-management conflicts regularly occur in some workplaces. Gender-based conflicts, including equal pay for women and sexual harassment issues, are other examples (Ehrlich, 1995).

Increased Workload

Emphasis on cost reductions has resulted in increased pressure to get as much work as possible out of each employee, sometimes more work than a person can reasonably do in a day (Trossman, 1999). This leaves many health-care workers believing that their employers are taking advantage of them (Ketter, 1994) and causes conflict if these workers believe others are not working as hard as they are.

Multiple Role Demands

Inappropriate task assignments (e.g., asking nurses to mop floors as well as nurse their clients), often the result of cost control efforts, can lead to disagreements about who does what task and who is responsible for the outcome.

Threats to Professional Identity and Territory

When role boundaries are blurred (sometimes even erased), professional identities are threatened, and people may react in defense of them. Who, for example, is supposed to teach the discharged client about taking medication at home: the pharmacist, physician, nurse, or all three? If all three do this, who does what part of the teaching?

Threats to Safety and Security

When roles are blurred, cost saving is emphasized, and staff members face layoffs. People's economic security is threatened. This can be a source of considerable stress and tension (Qureshi, 1996; Rondeau & Wagar, 2002).

Scarce Resources

Inadequate money for pay raises, equipment, supplies, or additional help can increase competition between or among departments and individuals as they scramble to grab their share of the little there is to distribute.

Cultural Differences

Different beliefs about how hard a person should work, what constitutes productivity, and even what it means to arrive at work "on time" can lead to problems if they are not reconciled.

Invasion of Personal Space

Crowded conditions and the constant interactions that occur at a busy nurses' station can increase interpersonal tension and lead to battles over scarce work space (McElhaney, 1996).

WHEN CONFLICT OCCURS

Conflicts can occur at any level and involve any number of people, including your boss, subordinates, peers, or patients (Sanon-Rollins, 2000). On the individual level, they can occur between two people on a team, between two people in different departments, or between a staff member and a client or family member (Box 7-2). On the group level, conflict can occur between two teams (as in Case 1), two departments, or two different professional groups (e.g., nurses and social workers, over who is responsible for discharge planning). On the organizational level, conflicts can occur between two organizations (e.g., when two home health agencies compete for a contract with a large hospital). The focus in this chapter is primarily on the first two levels, between or

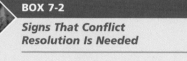

BOX 7-2

Signs That Conflict Resolution Is Needed

◆ You feel very uncomfortable in a situation.
◆ Members of your team are having trouble working together.
◆ Team members stop talking with each other, are withdrawing from conversation.
◆ Team members begin "losing their cool," are attacking each other verbally.

Adapted from Patterson, K., Grenny, J., McMillan, R., & Surtzler, A. (18 March 2003). Crucial conversations: Making a difference between being healed and being seriously hurt. *Vital Signs,* 13(5), 14–15.

among individuals and groups of people within a health-care organization.

RESOLVING PROBLEMS AND CONFLICTS

Win, Lose, or Draw?

Some people think about problems and conflicts that occur at work in the same way they think about a football game or tennis match: unless the score is tied at the end of the game, someone has won, and someone has lost. There are some problems in this comparison with sports competition. First, the aim is to work together more effectively, not to defeat the other party. Second, the people who lose are likely to feel bad about losing. As a result, they may spend their time and energy preparing to win the next round rather than on their work. Third, a tie (neither side wins or loses) may be just a stalemate; no one has won or lost, but the problem still exists.

So the answer to the question "Win, lose, or draw?" is "none of the above." Instead, a win-win result in which both sides gain some benefit is the best resolution (Haslan, 2001).

Other Conflict Resolution Myths

Many people think of what can be "won" as a fixed amount: "I get half, and you get half." The problem is that if one side gets three-quarters or everything, the other side gets only one-quarter or nothing. This is the *fixed pie*

myth of conflict resolution (Thompson & Fox, 2001). Another erroneous assumption is called the *devaluation reaction*: "If the other side is getting what they want, that is, if what we've agreed to is good for them, then it has to be bad for us." These erroneous beliefs can be serious barriers to achievement of a mutually beneficial (win-win) resolution of a conflict.

When differences and disagreements first arise, *problem solving* may be sufficient. If the situation has already developed into a full conflict, however, *negotiation,* either informal or formal, of a settlement may be necessary.

Problem Resolution

The use of the problem-solving process in patient care should be familiar. The same approach can be used when staff problems occur. The goal is to find a solution to a given problem that satisfies everyone involved. The process itself, illustrated in Figure 7-1, includes identifying the issue, generating solutions, evaluating the suggested solutions, choosing what appears to be the best solution, implementing that solution, evaluating the extent to which the problem has been resolved, and, finally, concluding either that the problem is resolved or that it will be necessary to repeat the process to find a better solution.

Identify the Problem or Issue

Ask participants in the conflict what they want (Sportsman, 2005). If the issue is not a highly charged, highly political one, they may be able to give a direct answer. At other times, however, some discussion and exploration of the issues are necessary before the real problem emerges. "It would be nice," wrote Browne and Kelley, "if what other people were really saying was always obvious, if all their essential thoughts were clearly labeled for us ... and if all knowledgeable people agreed about answers to important questions" (1994, p. 5). Of course, this is not what usually happens. People are often vague about what their real concern is; sometimes they are genuinely uncertain about what the real problem is. Emotional involvement may further cloud the issue. All of this needs to be sorted out so that the problem is identified clearly and a solution can be sought.

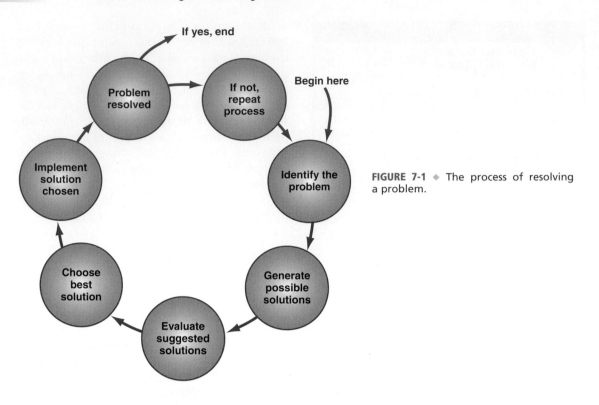

FIGURE 7-1 ◆ The process of resolving a problem.

Generate Possible Solutions

Here, creativity is especially important. If you are guiding people through this process, try to discourage them from using old solutions for new problems. It is natural for people to try to repeat something that has already worked well, but previously successful solutions may not work in the future (Walsh, 1996). Instead, encourage people to spend some time searching for innovative solutions (Smialek, 2001).

When an innovative solution is needed, suggest that the group take some time to *brainstorm*. Ask everyone to write down (or call out and you write on a flip chart or board) as many solutions as he or she can come up with (Rees, 2005). Then give everyone a chance to consider each suggestion on its own merits.

Evaluate Suggested Solutions

An open-minded evaluation of each suggestion is needed, but accomplishing this is not always easy. Some groups are "stuck in a rut," unable to "think outside the box." Other times, groups find it difficult to separate the suggestion from its source. On an interdisciplinary team, for example, the status of the person who made the suggestion may influence whether the suggestion is judged to be useful. Whose solution is most likely to be the best one: the physician's or the unlicensed assistant's? That depends. Judge the suggestion on its merits, not its source.

Choose the Best Solution

Which of the suggested solutions is most likely to work? A combination of suggestions is often the best solution.

Implement the Solution Chosen

The true test of any suggested solution is how well it actually works. Once a solution has been implemented, it is important to give it time to work. Impatience sometimes leads to premature abandonment of a good solution.

Is the Problem Resolved?

Not every problem is resolved successfully on the first attempt. If the problem has not been resolved, the process needs to be resumed with even greater attention to what the real problem is and how it can be successfully resolved.

Consider the following situation in which problem solving was helpful (Case 2).

Case 2

The Vacation

Francine Deloitte has been a unit secretary for 10 years. She is prompt, efficient, accurate, courteous, flexible, and productive—everything a nurse manager could ask for in a unit secretary. When nursing staff members are very busy, she distributes afternoon snacks or sits with a family for a few minutes until a nurse is available. There is only one issue on which Ms. Deloitte is insistent and stubborn: taking her 2-week vacation over the Christmas and New Year holidays. This is forbidden by hospital policy, but every nurse manager has allowed her to do this because it is the only special request she ever makes and because it is the only time she visits her family during the year.

A recent reorganization of the administrative structure had eliminated several layers of nursing managers and supervisors. Each remaining nurse manager was given responsibility for two or three units. The new nurse manager for Ms. Deloitte's unit refused to grant her request for vacation time at the end of December. "I can't show favoritism," she explained. "No one else is allowed to take vacation time at the end of December." Assuming that she could have the time off as usual, Francine had already purchased a nonrefundable ticket for her visit home. When her request was denied, she threatened to quit. On hearing this, one of the nurses on Francine's unit confronted the new nurse manager saying, "You can't do this. We are going to lose the best unit secretary we've ever had if you do."

The nurse manager asked Ms. Deloitte to meet with her to discuss the problem. The following is a summary of their problem solving:

◆ **The Issue.** Ms. Deloitte wanted to take her vacation from the end of December through early January. Assuming this was all right, she had purchased nonrefundable tickets. The policy forbids vacations from December 20 to January 2. The former nurse manager had not enforced this policy with Ms. Deloitte, but the new nurse manager thought it fair to enforce the policy with everyone, including Ms. Deloitte.

◆ **Possible Solutions**
1. Ms. Deloitte resigns.
2. Ms. Deloitte is fired.
3. Allow Ms. Deloitte to take her vacation as planned.
4. Allow everyone to take vacations between December 20 and January 5 as requested.
5. Allow no one to take a vacation between December 20 and January 5.

◆ **Evaluate Suggested Solutions.** Ms. Deloitte preferred solutions 3 and 4. The new nurse manager preferred 5. Neither wanted 1 or 2. They could agree only that none of the solutions satisfied both of them, so they decided to try again.

◆ **Second List of Possible Solutions**
1. Reimburse Ms. Deloitte for the cost of the tickets.
2. Allow Ms. Deloitte to take one last vacation between December 20 and January 5.
3. Allow Ms. Deloitte to take her vacation during Thanksgiving instead.
4. Allow Ms. Deloitte to begin her vacation on December 26 so that she would work on Christmas Day but not on New Year's Day.
5. Allow Ms. Deloitte to begin her vacation earlier in December so that she could return in time to work on New Year's Day.

◆ **Choose the Best Solution.** As they discussed the alternatives, Ms. Deloitte said she could change the day of her flight without a penalty. The nurse manager said she would allow solution 5 on the second list if Ms. Deloitte understood that she could not take vacation time between December 20 and January 5 in the future. Ms. Deloitte agreed to this.

◆ **Implement the Solution.** Ms. Deloitte returned on December 30 and worked both New Year's Eve and New Year's Day.

◆ **Evaluate the Solution.** The rest of the staff members had been watching the situation very closely. Most believed that the solution finally agreed on had been fair to them as well as to Ms. Deloitte. Ms. Deloitte thought she had been treated honestly and fairly. The nurse manager believed both parties had found a solution that was fair to Ms. Deloitte but still reinforced the manager's determination to enforce the vacation policy.

◆ **Resolved, or Resume Problem Solving?** Ms. Deloitte, staff members, and the nurse manager all thought the problem had been solved satisfactorily.

Negotiating an Agreement Informally

When a problem has become too big, too complex, or too heated, a more elaborate process may be required to resolve it. On evaluating Case 1, the nurse manager decided that the tensions between Team A and Team B had become so great that negotiation would be necessary.

The process of negotiation is a complex one that requires much careful thought beforehand and considerable skill in its implementation. Box 7-3 is an outline of the most essential aspects of negotiation. Case 1 is used to illustrate how it can be done.

Scope the Situation

To be successful, it is important that the entire situation be understood thoroughly. Walker

---

BOX 7-3

The Informal Negotiation Process

◆ Scope the situation. Ask yourself:
   What am I trying to achieve?
   What is the environment in which I am operating?
   What problems am I likely to encounter?
   What does the other side want?
◆ Set the stage.
◆ Conduct the negotiation.
◆ Set the ground rules.
◆ Clarify the problem.
◆ Make your opening move.
◆ Continue with offers and counteroffers.
◆ Agree on the resolution of the conflict.

---

and Harris (1995) suggested asking three questions:

1. What am I trying to achieve? The nurse manager in Case 1 is concerned about the tensions between Team A and Team B. She wants the members of these two teams to be able to work together in a cooperative manner, which they are not doing at the present time.
2. What is the environment in which I am operating? The members of Teams A and B were openly hostile to each other. The overall climate of the organization, however, was benign. The nurse manager knew that teamwork was encouraged and that her actions to resolve the conflict would be supported by administration.
3. What problems am I likely to encounter? The nurse manager knew that she had allowed the problem to go on too long. Even physicians, social workers, and visitors to the unit were getting caught up in the conflict. Team members were actively encouraging other staff to take sides, making clear they thought that "if you're not with us, you're against us." This made people from other departments very uncomfortable because they had to work with both teams. The nurse manager knew that resolution of the conflict would be a relief to many people.

It is important to ask one additional question in preparation for negotiations:

4. What does the other side want? In this situation, the nurse manager was not certain what either team really wanted. She realized that she needed this information before she could begin to negotiate.

Set the Stage

When a conflict such as the one between Teams A and B has gone on for some time, the opposing sides are often unwilling to meet to discuss the problem. If this occurs, it may be necessary to confront them with direct statements designed to open communications between the two sides and challenge them to seek resolution of the situation. At the same time, it is important to avoid any implication of blame because this provokes defensiveness rather than willingness to change.

To confront Teams A and B with their behavior toward one another, the nurse manager called them together at the end of the day shift. "I am very concerned about what I have been observing lately," she told them. "It appears to me that instead of working together, our two teams are working against each other." She continued with some examples of what she had observed, taking care not to mention individual names and not blaming anyone for the problem. She was also prepared to take responsibility for having allowed the situation to deteriorate before taking this much-needed action.

Conduct the Negotiation

As indicated earlier, conducting a negotiation requires a great deal of skill.

1. **Manage the emotions.** When staff members are very emotional, they have trouble thinking clearly. Acknowledging these emotions is essential to negotiating effectively (Fiumano, 2005). When faced with a highly charged situation, do not respond with even more emotion. Take time out if you need to get your own feelings under control. Then find out why emotions are high (watch both verbal and nonverbal cues carefully) (Hart & Waisman, 2005), and refocus the discussion on the issues (Shapiro & Jankowski, 1998). Without effective leadership to prevent emotional outbursts and personal attacks, a mishandled negotiation can worsen a situation. With effective leadership, the conflict may be resolved (Box 7-4).

2. **Set ground rules.** Members of Teams A and B began flinging accusations at each other as soon as the nurse manager made her statement. The nurse manager stopped this quickly and said, "First, we need to set some ground rules for this discussion. Everyone will get a chance to speak, but not all at once. Please speak for yourself, not for others. And please do not make personal remarks or criticize your coworkers. We are here to

> ### BOX 7-4
> #### *Tips for Leading the Discussion*
>
> - Create a climate of comfort.
> - Let others know the purpose is to resolve a problem or conflict.
> - Freely admit your own contribution to the problem.
> - Begin with the presentation of facts.
> - Recognize your own emotional response to the situation.
> - Set ground rules.
> - Do not make personal remarks.
> - Avoid placing blame.
> - Allow each person an opportunity to speak.
> - Do speak for yourself but not for others.
> - Focus on solutions.
> - Keep an open mind.
>
> Adapted from Patterson, K., Grenny, J., McMillan, R., & Surtzler, A. (18 March 2003). Crucial conversations: Making a difference between being healed and being seriously hurt. *Vital Signs,* 13(5), 14–15.

resolve this problem, not to make it worse." She had to remind the group of these ground rules several times during the meeting. Teaching others how to negotiate can create a more collaborative environment in which the negotiation will take place (Schwartz & Pogge, 2000).

3. **Clarification of the problem.** The nurse manager wrote a list of problems raised by team members on a chalkboard. As the list grew longer, she asked the group, "What do you see here? What is the real problem?" The group remained silent. Finally, someone in the back of the room said, "We don't have enough people, equipment, or supplies to get the work done." The rest of the group nodded in agreement.

4. **Opening move.** Once the problem is clarified, it is time to obtain everyone's agreement to seek a way to resolve the conflict. In more formal negotiations, you may make a statement about what you wish to achieve. For example, if you are negotiating a salary increase, you might begin by saying, "I am requesting a 10% increase for the following reasons . . . ." Of course, your employer will probably make a counteroffer, such as, "The best I can do

is 3%." These are the opening moves of a negotiation.

5. **Continue the negotiations.** The discussion should continue in an open, non-hostile manner. Each side's concerns may be further explained and elaborated. Additional offers and counteroffers are common. As the discussion continues, it is usually helpful to emphasize areas of agreement as well as disagreement so that both parties are encouraged to continue the negotiations (Tappen, 2001).

Agree on a Resolution of the Conflict

After much testing for agreement, elaboration of each side's positions and concerns, and making of offers and counteroffers, the people involved should finally reach an agreement.

The nurse manager of Teams A and B led them through a discussion of their concerns related to working with severely limited resources. The teams soon realized that they had a common concern and that they might be able to help rather than compete with each other. The nurse manager agreed to become more proactive in seeking resources for the unit. "We can simultaneously seek new resources and develop creative ways to use the resources we already have," she told the teams. Relationships between members of Team A and Team B improved remarkably after this meeting. They learned that they could accomplish more by working together than they had ever achieved separately.

Formal Negotiation: Collective Bargaining

There are many varieties of formal negotiations, from real estate transactions to international peace treaty negotiations. A formal negotiation process of special interest to nurses is collective bargaining, which is highly formalized because it is governed by law and contracts called *collective bargaining agreements.*

Collective bargaining involves a formal procedure governed by labor laws, such as the National Labor Relations Act. Nonprofit health-care organizations were added to the

organizations covered by these laws in 1974. Once a union or professional organization has been designated as the official bargaining agent for a group of nurses, a contract defining such important matters as salary increases, benefits, time off, unfair treatment, and promotion of professional practice is drawn up. This contract then governs employee-management relations within the organization.

Case 3 is an example of how collective bargaining agreements can influence the outcome of a conflict between management and staff in a health-care organization.

A collective bargaining contract is a legal document that governs the relationship between management and staff represented by the union (which, for nurses, may be the nurses' association or another health-care workers' union). The contract may cover some or all of the following:

◆ **Economic issues.** Salaries, shift differentials, length of the workday, overtime, holidays, sick leave, breaks, health insurance, pensions, severance pay.

◆ **Management issues.** Promotions, layoffs, transfers, reprimands, grievance procedures, hiring and firing procedures.

◆ **Practice issues.** Adequate staffing, standards of care, code of ethics, other quality-of-care issues, staff development opportunities.

Concerns over issues such as restructuring and lower levels of RN staffing have increased interest in unionization (Murray, 1999).

The Pros and Cons of Collective Bargaining

Some nurses think that it is unprofessional to belong to a union. Others point out that physicians and teachers are union members and that the protections offered by a union outweigh the downside. There is no easy answer to this question.

Probably the greatest advantages of collective bargaining are protection of the right to fair treatment and the availability of a written grievance procedure that specifies both the

Case 3

Collective Bargaining

The chief executive officer (CEO) of a large home health agency in a southwestern resort area called a general staff meeting. She reported that the agency had grown rapidly and was now the largest in the area. "Much of our success is due to the professionalism and commitment of our staff members," she said. "With growth come some problems, however. The most serious problem is the fluctuation in patient census. Our census peaks in the winter months when seasonal residents are here and troughs in the summer. In the past, when we were a small agency, we all took our vacations during the slow season. This made it possible to continue to pay everyone his or her full salary all year. However, given pressures to reduce costs and the large number of staff members we now have, we cannot continue to do this. We are very concerned about maintaining the high quality of patient care currently provided, but we have calculated that we need to reduce staff by 30 percent over the summer in order to survive financially."

The CEO then invited comments from the staff members. The majority of the nurses said they wanted and needed to work full-time all year. Most supported families and had to have a steady income all year. "My rent does not go down in the summer," said one. "Neither does my mortgage payment or the grocery bill," said another. A small number said that they would be happy to work part-time in the summer if they could be guaranteed full-time employment from October through May. "We have friends who would love this work schedule," they added.

"That's not fair," protested the nurses who needed to work full-time all year. "You can't replace us with part-time staff." The discussion grew louder and the participants more agitated. The meeting ended without a solution to the problem. Although the CEO promised to consider all points of view before making a decision, the nurses left the meeting feeling very confused and concerned about the security of their future income. Some grumbled that they probably should begin looking for new positions "before the ax falls."

The next day the CEO received a telephone call from the nurses' union representative. "If what I heard about the meeting yesterday is correct," said the representative, "your plan is in violation of our collective bargaining contract." The CEO reviewed the contract and found that the representative was correct. A new solution to the financial problems caused by the seasonal fluctuations in patient census would have to be found.

---

employee's and the employer's rights and responsibilities if an issue or complaint arises that cannot be settled between employee and manager informally (Forman & Merrick, 2003).

The greatest disadvantage of using collective bargaining as a way to deal with conflict is that it clearly separates management-level people from staff-level people. Any nurses who make staffing decisions may be classified as supervisors and, therefore, may be ineligible to join the union, separating them from the rest of their colleagues (Martin, 2001). The result is that "management" and "staff" are treated as opposing parties rather than as people who are trying to work together to provide essential services to their clients. The collective bargaining contract also adds another layer of rules and regulations between staff members and their supervisors. Because management of such employee-related rules and regulations can take almost one-quarter of a manager's time (Drucker, 2002), this can become a drain on a nurse manager's time and energy.

CONCLUSION

Conflict is inevitable within any large, diverse group of people who are trying to work together over an extended period. However, it does not have to be destructive, nor does it have to be a negative experience if it is handled skillfully by everyone involved. In fact, conflict can stimulate people to learn more about each other and how to work together in more effective ways. Resolution of a conflict, when it is done well, can lead to improved working relationships, more creative methods of operation, and higher productivity.

STUDY QUESTIONS

1 Debate the question of whether conflict is constructive or destructive. How can good leadership affect the outcome of a conflict?

2 Give an example of how each of the eight sources of conflict listed in this chapter can lead to a serious problem or conflict. Then discuss ways to prevent the occurrence of conflict from each of the eight sources.

3 What is the difference between problem resolution and negotiation? Under what circumstances would you use one or the other?

4 Identify a conflict (or potential conflict) in your clinical area, and explain how either problem resolution or negotiation could be used to resolve it.

CRITICAL THINKING EXERCISE

A not-for-profit hospice center in a small community received a generous gift from the grateful family of a client who had died recently. The family asked only that the money be "put to the best use possible."

Everyone in this small facility had an opinion about the best use for the money. The administrator wanted to renovate their old, run-down headquarters. The financial officer wanted to put the money in the bank "for a rainy day." The chaplain wanted to add a small chapel to the building. The nurses wanted to create a food bank to help the poorest of their clients. The social workers wanted to buy a van to transport clients to health-care providers. The staff agreed that all the ideas had merit, that all of the needs identified were important ones. Unfortunately, there was enough money to meet only one of them.

The more the staff members discussed how to use this gift, the more insistent each group became that their idea was best. At their last meeting, it was evident that some were becoming frustrated and that others were becoming angry. It was rumored that a shouting match between the administrator and the financial officer had occurred.

1. In your analysis of this situation, identify the sources of the conflict that are developing within this facility.

2. What kind of leadership actions are needed to prevent the escalation of this conflict?

3. If the conflict does escalate, how could it be resolved?

4. Which idea do you think has the most merit? Why did you select the one you did?

5. Try role-playing a negotiation among the administrator, the financial officer, the chaplain, a representative of the nursing staff, and a representative of the social work staff. Can you suggest a creative solution?

REFERENCES

Block, P. (2004). A time to heal. *Reflections.* Fourth Quarter, 20, 22.

Browne, M.M., & Kelley, S.M. (1994). *Asking the Right Questions: A Guide to Critical Thinking.* Englewood Cliffs, NJ: Prentice-Hall.

Drucker, P.F. (2002). They're not employees, they're people. *Harvard Business Review,* 80(2), 70–77, 128.

Ehrlich, H.J. (1995). Prejudice and ethnoviolence on campus. *Higher Education Extension Service Review,* 6(2), 1–3.

Fiumano, J. (2005). Navigate through conflict, not around it. *Nursing Management,* 36(8), 14, 18.

Forman, H., & Merrick, F. (2003). Grievances and complaints: Valuable tools for management and for staff. *Journal of Nursing Administration,* 33(3), 136–138.

Hart, L.B., & Waisman, C.S. (2005). *The Leadership Training Activity Book.* New York: AMACOM.

Haslan, S.A. (2001). *Psychology in Organizations.* Thousand Oaks, CA: Sage.

Horton-Deutsch, S.L., & Wellman, D.S. (2002). Christman's principles for effective management. *Journal of Nursing Administration,* 32, 596–601.

Ketter, J. (1994). Protecting RNs with the Fair Labor Standards Act. *American Nurse,* 26(9), 1–2.

Martin, R.H. (June 2001). Ruling may limit ability to unionize. *Advance for Nurses,* 9.

McElhaney, R. *(1996).* Conflict management in nursing administration. *Nursing Management,* 27(3), 49–50.

Murray, M.K. (1999). Is healthcare reengineering resulting in union organizing of registered nurses? *Journal of Nursing Administration,* 29(10), 4–7.

Patterson, K., Grenny, J., McMillan, R., & Surtzler, A. (18 March 2003). Crucial conversations: Making a difference between being healed and being seriously hurt. *Vital Signs,* 13(5), 14–15.

Qureshi, P. (1996). The effects of threat appraisal. *Nursing Management,* 27(3), 31–32.

Rees, F. (2005). *25 Activities for Developing Team Leaders.* San Francisco: Pfeiffer.

Rondeau, K.V., & Wagar, T.H. (2002). Reducing the hospital workforce: What is the role of human resource management practices? *Hospital Topics,* 89(1), 12–18.

Sanon-Rollins, G. (2000). Surviving conflict on the job. *Nursing Spectrum Career Fitness Guide* (pp. 6767–6868). Barrington, IL: Gannett.

Schwartz, R.W., & Pogge, C. (2000). Physician leadership: Essential skills in a changing environment. *American Journal of Surgery,* 180(3), 187–192.

Shapiro, R.M., & Jankowski, M.A. (1998). *The Power of Nice.* New York: John Wiley & Sons.

Smialek, M.A. (2001). *Team Strategies for Success.* Lanham, MD: The Scarecrow Press.

Sportsman, S. (2005). Build a framework for conflict assessment. *Nursing Management,* 36(4), 32–40.

Tappen, R.M. (2001). *Nursing Leadership and Management: Concept and Practice.* Philadelphia: FA Davis.

Thompson, L., & Fox, C.R. (2001). Negotiation within and between groups in organizations: Levels of analysis. In Turner, M.E. (ed.). *Groups at Work* (pp. 221–266). Mahwah, NJ: Laurence Erlbaum.

Tjosvold, D., & Tjosvold, M.M. (1995). *Psychology for Leaders: Using Motivation, Conflict, and Power to Manage More Effectively.* New York: John Wiley & Sons.

Trossman, S. (1999). Stress! It's everywhere! And it can be managed. *American Nurse,* 31(4), 1–2.

Van de Vliert, E., & Janssen, O. (2001). Description, explanation and prescription of intragroup conflict behaviors. In Turner, M.E. (ed.). *Groups at Work* (pp. 267–297). Mahwah, NJ: Laurence Erlbaum.

Walker, M.A., & Harris, G.L. (1995). *Negotiations: Six Steps to Success.* Upper Saddle River, NJ: Prentice-Hall.

Walsh, B. (3 June 1996). When past perfect isn't. *Forbes ASAP,* p. 18.

Wenckus, E. (21 February 1995). Working with an interdisciplinary team. *Nursing Spectrum,* 5, 12–14.

People and the Process of Change

OBJECTIVES

After reading this chapter, the student should be able to:

◆ Describe the process of change.

◆ Recognize resistance to change and identify its sources.

◆ Suggest strategies to reduce resistance to change.

◆ Assume a leadership role in implementing change.

CHAPTER 8 SELF-ASSESSMENT
Do You Know How to Play the Change Game?

Following is a list of "rules" for leading change. Mark each one either as a useful rule to *keep* or a rule to *delete*.

Rule 1. Squelch all dissent immediately—eliminate anyone who opposes the change.
Keep _____ Delete _____

Rule 2. Keep the pace of change high at all times.
Keep _____ Delete _____

Rule 3. Make sure everyone understands what changes will be made and why.
Keep _____ Delete _____

Rule 4. Keep everyone informed as the change progresses.
Keep _____ Delete _____

Rule 5. Don't allow any modifications once the change process is under way.
Keep _____ Delete _____

Rule 6. Demonstrate clearly why the change is a beneficial one.
Keep _____ Delete _____

Rule 7. Show people that the "old" way of doing things was not as good as the "new" way.
Keep _____ Delete _____

Keep: Rules 3, 4, 6, & 7

Delete: Rules 1, 2, & 5

When asked the theme of a recent nursing management conference, a top nursing executive replied, "Change, change, and more change." Whether we call it innovation, turbulence, or change, this theme seems to be a constant in the workplace today. Mismanaging change was the primary reason chief exective officers (CEOs) were fired, according to one survey of over a thousand CEOs (Hempel, 2005). This chapter discusses the process of change, how people respond to change, and how you can influence change and help people cope with it when it becomes difficult.

learn something new. We grow up, leave home, graduate from college, and begin a career, perhaps a family as well. Some of these changes are milestones in our lives, ones we have prepared for and anticipated for some time. Some are within our control, others are not (Hart & Waisman, 2005). Others are entirely unexpected, sometimes welcome and sometimes not. Many are exciting, leading to new opportunities and challenges. When change occurs too rapidly or demands too much, it can make people uncomfortable (Bilchik, 2002), even anxious or stressed.

CHANGE

A Natural Phenomenon

Change is a naturally occurring phenomenon: it is a part of everyone's lives. Every day, we have new experiences, meet new people, and

Macro and Micro Change

The "ever-whirling wheel of change" (Dent, 1995, p. 287) in health care seems to spin faster every year. Managed care alone profoundly changed the way health care is delivered in the United States (Trinh & O'Connor, 2002).

Medicare and Medicaid cuts, restructuring, downsizing, and staff shortages are major concerns. These changes sweeping through the health-care system affect clients and caregivers alike. They are the *macro-level* (large scale) changes that affect virtually every health-care facility.

Change anywhere in a system creates "ripples throughout the system" (Parker & Gadbois, 2000, p. 472). Every change that occurs at this macro-level filters down to the *micro-level* (small scale), to teams and to people as individuals. Nurses, colleagues in other disciplines, and clients are participants in these changes. This micro-level of change is the primary focus of this chapter.

THE PROCESS OF CHANGE

The Comfort Zone

The basic stages of the change process are *unfreezing, change,* and *refreezing* (Lewin, 1951; Mander, Gomes, & Castle, 2002). Assume that a work situation is basically stable before change is introduced. Although some changes occur naturally, people are generally accustomed to each other, have a routine for doing their work, and believe they know what to expect and how to deal with whatever problems may arise in the course of a day. In other words, they are operating within their "comfort zone" (Farrell & Broude, 1987; Lapp, 2002). A change of any magnitude is likely to move people out of this comfort zone into discomfort. This first stage in the change process is called *unfreezing* (Fig. 8-1).

Many health-care institutions offer nurses the choice of weekday or weekend work or 12-hour shifts. Given these choices, nurses with school-age children are likely to find their comfort zone on weekday shifts. Imagine the discomfort they would experience if confronted with a transfer to weekends. Such a change would rapidly unfreeze their usual routine and move them into the discomfort zone. They might have to find a new babysitter or begin a search for a new child care center that is open on weekends. An alternative would be the establishment of a child care center where they work. Another alternative would be to find a position that offers better working hours.

Whatever alternative they chose, the nurses would be challenged to find a solution that enabled them to move into a new comfort zone. To do this, they would have to find a consistent, dependable source of child care suited to their new schedule and to the needs of their children and *refreeze* their situation. If they did not find a satisfactory alternative, they could remain in an unsettled state, in a *dis*comfort zone, caught in a conflict between their professional and personal responsibilities.

As this example illustrates, even what seems to be a small change can disturb the people involved in it. In the next section, the many reasons that change can be unsettling and how they provoke resistance are considered.

RESISTANCE TO CHANGE

People resist change for a variety of reasons that can vary from person to person and situation to situation. For example, one client care technician is delighted with an increase in responsibility while another is upset about it. Some people are ready to risk change; others prefer the status quo (Hansten & Washburn, 1999). One change in routine provokes a storm of protest, whereas another change is hardly noticed. Let's see why this happens.

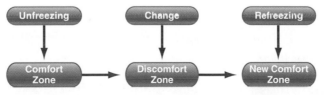

FIGURE 8-1 ◆ The change process. (Based on Farrell, K., & Broude, C. [1987]. *Winning the Change Game: How to Implement Information Systems with Fewer Headaches and Bigger Paybacks.* Los Angeles: Breakthrough Enterprises; and Lewis, K. [1951]. *Field Theory in Social Science: Selected Theoretical Papers.* New York: Harper & Row.)

Sources of Resistance

Resistance to change comes from three major sources: technical concerns, psychosocial needs, and threats to a person's position and power (Araujo Group).

Technical Concerns

Some resistance to change is based on concerns about whether the proposed change is a good idea. In some cases, these concerns are justified:

The Professional Practice Committee of a small hospital suggested, in order to save money, replacing a commercial mouthwash with a mixture of hydrogen peroxide and water. A staff nurse objected to this proposed change, saying that she had read a research study several years ago that found peroxide solutions to be an irritant to the oral mucosa (Tombes & Gallucci, 1993). Fortunately, the chairperson of the Professional Practice Committee recognized that this objection was based on technical concerns and requested that a more thorough study of the research literature be done before instituting the change. "It's important," she reminded the staff committee, "to investigate the evidence supporting a proposed change thoroughly before recommending it."

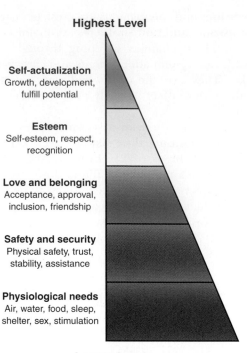

FIGURE 8-2 ◆ Maslow's hierarchy of needs. (Based on Maslow, A.H. [1970]. *Motivation and Personality.* New York: Harper & Row.)

The change itself may have design flaws. For example, if the bar codes on patients' armbands are difficult to scan, nurses may develop a way to work around this safety feature by taping a duplicate armband to the bed or a clipboard (Englebright & Franklin, 2005), thus defeating the purpose of instituting electronic medication administration in the first place.

Psychosocial Needs

According to Maslow (1970), human beings have a hierarchy of needs, from the basic physiological needs for oxygen, fluids, and nutrients to the higher-order needs for belonging, self-esteem, and self-actualization (Fig. 8-2). Maslow observed that the more basic needs (those lower on the hierarchy) must be at least partially met before a person is motivated to seek fulfillment of the higher-order needs.

Change may make it more difficult for a person to meet any or all of his or her needs. In other words, change may threaten these powerful safety and security needs that Maslow discussed (Hunter, 2004). For example, if a massive downsizing occurs and a person's job is

eliminated, fulfillment of all of these levels of needs may be threatened, from having enough money to pay for food and shelter to opportunities to fulfill one's career potential.

In other cases, the threat is subtler and may be harder for the leader or manager to anticipate. For example, an institution-wide reevaluation of the effectiveness of the advanced practice role would be a great concern to a staff nurse who is working toward accomplishing a lifelong dream of becoming an advanced practice nurse in oncology. In contrast, it would have little effect on unlicensed assistive personnel (UAPs) unless an actual change in staffing occurred. A staff reorganization that involves UAPs to different units, however, would threaten the belonging needs of one who has very close friends on his or her unit but few friends outside work.

Position and Power

Status, power, and influence, once gained within an organization, are hard to give up.

This applies to people anywhere in the organization, not just those at the top. For example:

A clerk in the surgical suite had been preparing the operating room schedule for many years. Although his supervisor really had the authority to revise the schedule, she rarely did so because the clerk was skillful in preparing realistic schedules that balanced the needs and desires of various parties, including some very demanding surgeons. When the operating room supervisor was transferred to another facility, her replacement decided that she had to review the schedules before they were posted because they were ultimately her responsibility. The clerk became defensive. He tried to avoid the supervisor and posted the schedules without her approval. This surprised the new supervisor. She had heard how skillful the clerk was and did not think that her review of the schedules would be threatening. She had not realized the importance of this task to the clerk. The opportunity to tell others when and where they could perform surgery had given this clerk a feeling of power and importance. The supervisor's insistence on reviewing his work reduced the importance of his position. What seemed to the new supervisor to be a very small change in routine had provoked surprisingly strong resistance because it threatened the clerk's position and power within the organization.

As you learned in Chapter 5 on power and organizations, empowerment is a source of motivation and satisfaction for most people. Although some changes empower people, others threaten their sense of empowerment, especially when they believe the change was imposed on them.

Recognizing Resistance

It is easy to recognize resistance to a change when the resistance is expressed directly. When a person says to you, "That's not a very good idea," "I'll quit if you schedule me for the night shift," or "There's no way I'm going to do that," there is no doubt that you are encountering resistance. When resistance is less direct, however, it can be difficult to recognize unless you know what to look for.

Resistance may be *active* or *passive* (Heller, 1998). Active resistance can take the form of outright refusal to comply, such as the statements in the previous paragraph, writing "killer" memos that destroy the idea or the person who suggested it, quoting existing rules that make the change difficult to implement, or encouraging others to resist. Passive approaches use avoidance: canceling appointments to discuss implementation of the change, being too busy to make the change, refusing to commit to changing or agreeing to it but doing nothing to change, and simply

TABLE 8-1
Resistance to Change

Active	Passive
Attacking the idea	Avoiding discussion
Refusing to change	Ignoring the change
Arguing against the change	Refusing to commit to the change
Organizing resistance of other people	Agreeing but not acting

ignoring the entire process as much as possible (Table 8-1). Once resistance has been recognized, action can be taken to lower or even eliminate it.

Lowering Resistance

A great deal can be done to lower people's resistance to change. Strategies fall into four categories: sharing information, disconfirming currently held beliefs, providing psychological safety, and dictating change (Tappen, 2001).

Sharing Information

Much resistance is simply the result of misunderstanding about a proposed change. Sharing information about the proposed change can be done on a one-to-one basis, in group meetings, or through written materials distributed to everyone involved via print or electronic means.

Disconfirming Currently Held Beliefs

Leaders can provide the catalyst for change (Lichiello & Madden, 1996). For example, disconfirming current beliefs is often persuasive enough to lower resistance to change. When this happens, providing evidence that what people are currently doing or believing is inadequate, incorrect, or inefficient can increase their willingness to change. For example:

Jolene was a little nervous when it was her turn to present information on a new enteral feeding procedure to the Clinical Practice Committee. Committee members were very demanding: they wanted clear, research-based information presented in a concise manner. Opinions, generalities, and vague references ("Somebody told me....") were not acceptable. She had prepared thoroughly and even

◆ Is the change necessary?

◆ Is the change technically correct?

◆ Will this change work?

◆ Is there a better way to do this?

This is a good time to use creativity and innovation (Handy, 2002). Encourage people to talk about the changes planned, to express their doubts, and to provide their input (Fullan, 2001). Those who do are usually enthusiastic supporters later in the process.

Planning

The next step is to prepare a careful plan to implement the change. All the information presented previously about sources of resistance and ways to overcome that resistance should be taken into consideration when deciding how to implement a change.

You are likely to find supporters, fence-sitters, and resisters within your group (McCarthy, 2005). The supporters will help you lead people on the path to change, but be sure to include those who are neutral (the fence-sitters) and opposed (the resisters) in the process and to analyze why they might be resistant. Ask yourself:

◆ Why might people resist this change?

◆ Is their resistance justified?

◆ What can be done to prevent or overcome this resistance?

The context in which the change will take place is another factor to consider when assessing resistance to change (Lichiello & Madden, 1996). This includes the amount of change occurring at the same time, the organizational climate, and the environment surrounding the organization. For example, there may be external pressure to change because of the competitive nature of the health-care market in the community. In other situations, government regulations may make it difficult to bring about a desired change.

Almost everything you have learned about effective leadership is useful in planning the implementation of change: setting the vision, motivating people, involving people in decisions that affect them, dealing with conflict, eliciting cooperation, providing coordination, and fostering teamwork. Remember, you have to move people out of their comfort zone to unfreeze the situation and get them ready to change (Flower & Guillaume, 2002). Consider all of these things when formulating a plan to implement a proposed change, then act on them in the next step: implementing the change.

Implementing the Change

Now you are ready to make the change that has been carefully planned. In addition to the strategies to lower resistance, increase motivation, and help people work well together, consider the following factors:

◆ What is the magnitude of this change? Is this a major change that affects almost everything people do, or is it a minor one with little effect on what people do every day?

◆ What is the complexity of this change? Is this a difficult change to make? Does it require much new knowledge or skill, or both? How much time will people need to acquire the necessary knowledge and skill?

◆ What is the pace of the change? How urgent is this change? Can it be done gradually, or must it be implemented all at once?

◆ What is the current stress level of the people involved in this change? Is this the only change that is taking place, or is it just one of many changes taking place? How stressful are these changes? How can I help people keep their stress levels low?

A simple change such as introducing a new thermometer may be planned, implemented, and integrated into everyone's work routine easily. But a complex change, such as introducing a medication error reduction system, may require experimentation with the new system, feedback on what works and what does not, and revising the plan several times before the system really works.

As indicated earlier, some discomfort is likely to occur with almost any change, but it is important to keep the discomfort within tolerable limits. Exert pressure to make people pay attention to the change process but not so much that they are overstressed by it. In other words, you want to raise the heat enough to get them moving but not so much that they boil over (Heifetz & Linsky, 2002).

Integrating the Change

Finally, after the change has been made, make sure that everyone has moved into a new comfort zone. Ask yourself:

◆ Is the change well integrated into everyday operations?

◆ Are people comfortable with it now?

◆ Is it well accepted? If not, why not? What can be done to increase acceptance? Is there any residual resistance that could still undermine full integration of the change? If there is, how can this resistance be overcome?

It usually takes some time before a change is fully accepted and integrated into everyday routines (Hunter, 2004). As Kotter noted, change "sticks" when, instead of being the new way to do something, it has become "the way we always do things around here" (1999, p. 18).

Personal Change

The focus of this chapter is on leading others through the process of change. However, choosing to change is also an important part of your own development as a leader. Hart and Waisman (2005) compare personal change with the story of the caterpillar and the butterfly:

Caterpillars cannot fly. They have to crawl or climb to find their food. Butterflies, on the other hand, can soar above an obstacle. They also have a different perspective on their world because they can fly. It is not easy to change from a caterpillar to a butterfly. Indeed, the transition (metamorphosis) may be quite uncomfortable and involves some risk. Are you ready to become a butterfly?

The process of personal change is similar to the process described throughout this chapter: first recognize the need for change, then learn how to do things differently, then become comfortable with the "new you" (Guthrie & King, 2004). A more detailed step-by-step process is given in Box 8-1. You might, for example, decide that you need to stop interrupting people when they speak with you. Or you might want to change your leadership style from laissez-faire to participative.

Will the small change in communication style be easier to accomplish than the radical change in your leadership? Perhaps not. Deutschman (2005) reports research that indicates radical change might be easier to accomplish because the benefits are evident much more quickly. Changing behavior, your own or others', is a challenge. An extreme example: many people could avoid a second coronary bypass or angioplasty by changing their lifestyle, yet 90% do not do so or do not do so long enough after their first bypass to make a difference. Deutschman compares the usual advice to exercise, stop smoking, and eat healthier meals to Dean Ornish's radical vegetarian diet with only 10% of calories from fat. After 3 years, 77% of the patients who went through this extreme change had continued these lifestyle changes. Why? Ornish suggests several reasons: 1) after several weeks, people felt a change—they could walk or have sex without pain 2) information alone is not enough—the emotional aspect is dealt with in support groups and through meditation, relaxation, yoga, and aerobic exercise, 3) the motivation to pursue this change is redefined—instead of focusing on fear of death, which many find too frightening, Ornish focuses on the joy of living, feeling better, and being active without pain.

The traditional approach to change is turned on its head in this approach. Deutschman lists five commonly accepted myths about change that have been refuted by new insights from research (Box 8-2).

It remains to be seen whether these new insights on changing behavior will be useful in the workplace as well.

CONCLUSION

Change is an inevitable part of living and working. How people respond to change, the amount of stress it causes, and the amount of resistance it provokes can be influenced by leadership. Handled well, most changes can become opportunities for professional growth and development rather than just additional stressors with which nurses and their clients have to cope.

BOX 8-1

Which Stage of Change Are You In?

While studying how smokers quit the habit, Dr. James Prochaska, a psychologist at the University of Rhode Island, developed a widely influential model of the "stages of change." What state are you in? See if any of the following statements sound familiar.

TYPICAL STATEMENT	STAGE	RISKS
"As far as I'm concerned, I don't have any problems that need changing." "I guess I have faults, but there's nothing that I really need to change."	1 Precontemplation ("Never")	You're in denial, dude. You proabably feel coerced by other people who are trying to make you change. But they're not going to shame you into it. Their meddling will backfire.
"I've been thinking that I wanted to change something about myself." "I wish I had more ideas on how to solve my problems."	2 Contemplation ("Someday")	Feeling righteous because of your good intentions, you could stay in this stage for years. But you might respond to the emotional persuasion of a compelling leader.
"I have decided to make changes in the next 2 weeks." "I am committed to join a fitness club by the end of the month."	3 Preparation ("Soon")	This "rehearsal" can become your reality. Some 85% of people who need to change their behavior for health reasons never get to this stage or progress beyond it.
"Anyone can talk about changing. I'm actually doing something about it." "I am doing okay, but I wish I was more consistent."	4 Action ("New")	It's an emotional struggle. It's important to change quickly enough to feel the short-term benefits that give a psychic lift and make it easier to stick with the change.
"I may need a boost right now to help me maintain the changes I've already made." "This has become part of my day and I feel it when I don't follow through."	5 Maintenance ("Forever")	Relapse. Even though you've created a new mental pathway, the old pathway is still there in your brain, and when you're under a lot of stress, you might fall back on it.

Adapted from Deutschman's Which Stage of Change Are You In?: "typical statements" adapted from *Stages of Change: Theory and Practice* by Michael Samuelson, executive director of the National Center for Health Promotion.

BOX 8-2

Five Myths About Changing Behavior

MYTH	REALITY
1. Crisis is a powerful impetus for change.	Ninety percent of patients who have had coronary bypasses do not sustain changes in the unhealthy lifestyles, which worsens their severe heart disease and greatly threatens their lives.
2. Change is motivated by fear.	It is too easy for people to go into denial of the bad things that might happen to them. Compelling positive visions of the future are a much stronger inspiration for change.
3. The facts will set us free.	Our thinking is guided by narratives, not facts. When a fact does not fit our conceptual "frames"—the metaphors we use to make sense of the world—we reject it. Also, change is inspired best by emotional appeals rather than factual statements.
4. Small, gradual changes are always easier to make and sustain.	Radical, sweeping changes are often easier because they yield benefits quickly.
5. We cannot change because our brains become "hardwired" early in life.	Our brains have extraordinary "plasticity," meaning that we can continue learning complex new things throughout our lives—assuming we remain truly active and engaged.

Adapted from Deutschman's *Five Myths About Changing Behavior.* Deutschman, A. (2005/May). Why is it so darn hard to change our ways? Fast Company, 53-62.

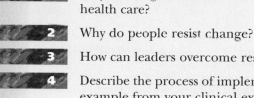

STUDY QUESTIONS

1 Why is change inevitable? What would happen if no change at all occurred in health care?

2 Why do people resist change?

3 How can leaders overcome resistance to change?

4 Describe the process of implementing a change from beginning to end. Use an example from your clinical experience to illustrate this process.

CRITICAL THINKING EXERCISE

A large health-care corporation recently purchased a small (50-bed) rural nursing home. A new director of nursing was brought in to replace the former one, who had retired after 30 years at this facility. The new director addressed the staff members at the reception held to welcome him. "My philosophy is that you cannot manage anything that you haven't measured. Everyone tells me that you have all been doing an excellent job here. With my measurement approach, we will be able to analyze everything you do and become more efficient than ever." The nursing staff members soon found out what the new director meant by his measurement approach. Every bath, episode of incontinence care, feeding of a resident, or trip off the unit had to be counted, and the amount of time each activity required had to be recorded. Nurse managers were required to review these data with staff members every week, questioning any time that was not accounted for. Time spent talking with families or consulting with other staff members was considered time wasted unless the staff member could justify the "interruption" in his or her work. No one complained openly about the change, but absenteeism rates increased rapidly. Personal day and vacation time requests soared. Staff members nearing retirement crowded the tiny personnel office, overwhelming the single staff member with their requests to "tell me how soon I can retire on full benefits." The director of nursing found that shortage of staff was becoming a serious problem and that no new applications were coming in, despite the fact that this rural area offered few good job opportunities.

1. What evidence of resistance to change can you find in this case study?

2. What kind of resistance to change did the staff members exhibit?

3. If you were a staff nurse at this facility, how do you think you would have reacted to this change in administration?

4. Why did staff members resist this change?

5. What could the director of nursing do to increase acceptance of this change? What could the nurse managers and staff nurses do?

REFERENCES

Araujo Group. A Compilation of Opinions of Experts in the Field of the Management of Change. Unpublished report.

Bilchik, G.S. (May 2002). Are you the problem? *Hospitals and Health Networks Magazine*, 38–42.

Conger, J., Spreitzer, G., & Lawler, E.E. (1999). *The Leader's Change Handbook*. San Francisco: Jossey-Bass.

Dent, H.S. (1995). *Job Shock: Four New Principles Transforming Our Work and Business*. New York: St. Martin's Press.

Deutschman, A. (2005). *Making Change*. Fast Company, 94, 52–62.

Englebright, J.D. & Franklin, M. (2005). Managing a new medication administrative process. *Journal of Nursing Administration*, 35(9), 410–413.

Farrell, K., & Broude, C. (1987). *Winning the Change Game: How to Implement Information Systems With Fewer Headaches and Bigger Paybacks*. Los Angeles: Breakthrough Enterprises.

Flower, J., & Guillaume, P. (March/April 2002). Surfing the edge of chaos. *Health Forum Journal*, 17–20.

Fullan, M. (2001). *Leading in a Culture of Change*. San Francisco: Jossey-Bass.

Guthrie, V.A. & King, S.N. (2004). Feedback-Intensive Programs. In McCauley, C.D., & Van Velson, E. (eds.). *The Center for Creative Leadership Handbook of Leadership Development*. San Francisco: Jossey-Bass.

Handy, C. (June 2002). The elephant and the flea: Looking backward to the future. *Times Literary Supplement*, (5157), 30.

Hansten, R.I., & Washburn, M.J. (1999). Individual and organizational accountability for development of critical thinking. *Journal of Nursing Administration*, 29(11), 39–45.

Hart, L.B. & Waisman, C.S. (2005). *The Leadership Training Activity Book*. New York: AMACOM.

Heifetz, R.A., & Linsky, M. (June 2002). A survival guide for leaders. *Harvard Business Review*, 65–74.

Heller, R. (1998). *Managing Change*. New York: DK Publishing.

Hempel, J. (2005). Why the boss really had to say goodbye. *Business Week*, July 4, p. 10.

Holland, L.E. (2002). *Change Is the Rule: Practical Actions for Change: On Target, On Time, On Budget*. Chicago: Dearborn.

Hunter, J.C. (2004). *The World's Most Powerful Leadership Principle: How to Become a Servant Leader*. New York: Crown Business.

Kotter, J.P. (1999). Leading change: The eight steps to transformation. In Conger, J.A., Spreitzer, G.M., & Lawler, E.E. (eds.). *The Leader's Change Handbook*. San Francisco: Jossey-Bass.

Lapp, J. (May 2002). Thriving on change. *Caring Magazine*, 40–43.

Lewin, K. (1951). *Field Theory in Social Science: Selected Theoretical Papers*. New York: Harper & Row.

Lichiello, P., & Madden, C.W. (1996). Context and catalysts for change in health care markets. *Health Affairs*, 15(2), 121–129.

Mander, A., Gomes, A., & Castle, D. (2002). The management of change in a community mental health team. *Australian Health Review*, 25(2), 115–121.

Maslow, A.H. (1970). *Motivation and Personality*. New York: Harper & Row.

McCarthy, J.E. (2005). Five Concepts for Creating Change. *Nursing Management*, 36(5), 20–22.

Parker, M., & Gadbois, S. (2000). Building community in healthcare workplace. Part 3: Belonging and satisfaction at work. *Journal of Nursing Administration*, 30, 466–473.

Pearcey, P., & Draper, P. (1996). Using the diffusion of innovation model to influence practice: A case study. *Journal of Advanced Nursing*, 23, 724–726.

Porter-O'Grady, T. (1996). The seven basic rules for successful redesign. *Journal of Nursing Administration*, 26(1), 46–53.

Porter-O'Grady, T. (2003). A different age for leadership: Part 1. *Journal of Nursing Administration*, 33(2), 105–110.

Tappen, R.M. (2001). *Nursing Leadership and Management: Concepts and Practice*. Philadelphia: FA Davis.

Tombes, M.B., & Gallucci, B. (1993). The effects of hydrogen peroxide rinses on the normal oral mucosa. *Nursing Research*, 42, 332–337.

Trinh, H.Q., & O'Connor, S.J. (2002). Helpful or harmful? The impact of strategic change on the performance of U.S. urban hospitals. *Health Services Research*, 37(1), 145–171.

chapter 9

Delegation of Client Care

OBJECTIVES

After reading this chapter, the student should be able to:

- Define the term *delegation*.

- Define the term *unlicensed assistive personnel*.

- Understand the legal implications of making assignments to other health-care personnel.

- Recognize barriers to successful delegation.

- Make appropriate assignments to team members.

OUTLINE

CHAPTER 9 SELF-ASSESSMENT
Delegation

1. Are you able to ask others to help you?

2. Do you need to do every task yourself?

3. If you ask someone to do something, do you check to see if the job was completed?

4. Do you take responsibility for your own behaviors?

Linda is a new graduate and has just finished her orientation. She works the 7 p.m. to 7 a.m. shift on a busy, monitored neuroscience unit. The client census is 48, making this a full unit. Although there is an associate nurse manager for the shift, Linda is charge nurse for the shift. Her responsibilities include receiving and transcribing orders, contacting physicians with any information or requests, accessing laboratory reports from the computer, reviewing them and giving them to the appropriate staff members, checking any new medication orders and placing them in the appropriate medication administration records, relieving the monitor technician for dinner and breaks, and assigning staff to dinner and breaks. When Linda comes to work, she discovers that one registered nurse (RN) called in sick. She has two RNs and three unlicensed assistive personnel (UAP) for staff and a full census. She panics and wants to refuse to take report. After a discussion with the charge nurse from the previous shift, she realizes that this is not an option. She sits down to evaluate the acuity of the clients and the capabilities of her staff.

INTRODUCTION TO DELEGATION

Delegation is not a new concept. In the *Old Testament,* Moses was instructed to identify 70 elders "so they will share with you the burden of this nation and you will no longer have to carry it by yourself" (Numbers 11:16-17). In her *Notes on Nursing,* Florence Nightingale (1859) clearly stated: Don't imagine that if you, who are in charge, don't look to all these things yourself, those under you will be more careful than you are…." She continued by directing, "But then again to look to all these things yourself does not mean to do them yourself. If you do it, it is by so much the better certainly than if it were not done at all. But can you not insure that it is done when not done by yourself? Can

you insure that it is not undone when your back is turned? This is what being in charge means. And a very important meaning it is, too. The former only implies that just what you can do with your own hands is done. The latter that what ought to be done is always done. Head in charge must see to house hygiene, not do it herself" (p. 17).

Definition of Delegation

By definition, delegation is the reassigning of responsibility for the performance of a job from one person to another (American Nurses Association [ANA], 1996). RNs maintain accountability for supervising those to whom tasks are delegated (ANA, 2005). Although the responsibility for the task is transferred, the accountability for the process or outcome of the task remains with the delegator, or the person delegating the activity. Nightingale referred to this delegation responsibility when she inferred that the "Head in charge" does not necessarily carry out the task but still sees that it is completed.

According to the ANA, specific overlying principles remain firm regarding delegation. These include the following:

◆ The nursing profession delineates the scope of nursing practice.

◆ The nursing profession identifies and supervises the necessary education, training, and use for ancillary roles concerned with the delivery of direct client care.

◆ The RN assumes responsibility and

acountability for the provision of nursing practice.

◆ The RN directs care and determines the appropriate uitilization of any ancillary personnel involved in providing direct client care.

◆ The RN accepts assistance from ancillary nursing personnel in delivering nursing care for the client (ANA, 2005, p. 6).

Nurse-related principles are also designated by the ANA. These are important when considering what tasks may be delegated and to whom they may be assigned. These principles are:

◆ The RN may delegate aspects of care but does not delegate the nursing process itself.

◆ The RN has a duty to be accountable for personal actions related to the nursing process.

◆ The RN considers the knowledge and skills of any ancillary personnel to whom aspects of care are delegated.

◆ The decision to delegate or assign is based on the RN's judgment regarding the following:

　◆ The condition of the client.

　◆ The competence of the members of the nursing team.

　◆ The amount of supervision that will be required of the RN if a task is delegated.

◆ The RN uses critical thinking and professional judgment when following the Five Rights of Delegation delineated by the National Council of State Boards of Nursing (NCSBN) (Box 9-1).

◆ The RN recognizes that a relational aspect exists between delegation and communication. Communication needs to be culturally appropriate, and the individual receiving the communication should be treated with respect.

◆ Chief nursing officers are responsible for creating systems to assess, monitor, verify, and communicate continuous competence requirements in areas related to delegation.

◆ RNs monitor organizational policies, procedures, and job descriptions to ensure they are in compliance with the nurse practice act, consulting with the state board of nursing as needed (ANA, 2005, p. 6).

Delegation may be direct or indirect. *Direct delegation* is usually "verbal direction by the RN delegator regarding an activity or task in a specific nursing care situation" (ANA, 1996, p. 15). In this case, the RN decides which staff member is capable of performing the specific task or activity at this time. *Indirect delegation is* "an approved listing of activities or tasks that have been established in policies and procedures of the health care institution or facility" (ANA, 1996, p. 15). The ANA also differentiated the delegation of a task from the assignment of a task. Although the terms are often used interchangeably, according to the ANA (1997), assignment is the "downward or lateral transfer of both the responsibility and the accountability of an activity from one person to another." When one RN "delegates" to another RN, that RN, based on knowledge and skill, may be responsible and accountable. UAP may also be assigned, rather than "delegated," a task. For example, UAP have the knowledge and skills required for some routine tasks (Ellis & Hartley, 2004).

The recent changes occurring in the health-care environment continue to modify the scope of nursing practice and the activities delegated to UAP. A main concern in almost all health-care settings is that UAP are inappropriately performing functions that belong within the legal realm of nursing (ANA, 2002).

Permitted tasks vary from institution to institution. For example, a certified nursing assistant (CNA) performs specific activities designated by the job description approved by the particular health-care institution. Although

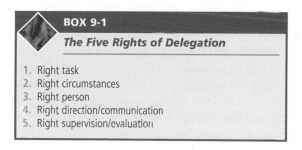

BOX 9-1

The Five Rights of Delegation

1. Right task
2. Right circumstances
3. Right person
4. Right direction/communication
5. Right supervision/evaluation

the institution delineates tasks and activities in the job description, this does not mean that the RN cannot decide to assign other personnel in specific situations. Take the following example:

Ms. Ross was admitted to the neurological unit from the neuroscience intensive care unit. She suffered a grade II subarachnoid hemorrhage 2 weeks ago and has a left hemiparesis. She has difficulty with swallowing and receives tube feedings through a percutaneous endoscopic gastrostomy (PEG) tube; however, she has been advanced to a pureed diet. She needs assistance with personal care, toileting, and feeding. Although a physical therapist comes twice a day to get her up for gait training, the physician wants her in a chair as much as possible.

Assessing this situation, the RN might consider assigning a licensed practical nurse (LPN) to this client. The swallowing problems place the client at risk for aspiration, which means that feeding may present a problem. There is a potential for injury. The LPN is capable of managing the PEG tube feeding. While assisting with bathing, the LPN can perform range-of-motion exercises to all the client's extremities and assess her skin for breakdown. The LPN also knows the appropriate way to assist the client in transferring from the bed to the chair. The RN may not assign an individual to perform a task or activity not specified in his or her job description or within the scope of practice, such as allowing a nursing assistant to administer medications or perform certain types of dressing changes.

Supervision

Do not confuse delegation with supervision. Supervision is more direct and requires directly overseeing the work or performance of others. Supervision includes checking with individuals throughout the day to see what activities have been completed and what may still need to be finished. For example, a nursing assistant has been assigned to take all the vital signs on the unit and give the morning baths to eight clients. Three hours into the morning, she is far behind. At this point, it is important that the RN discover why. Perhaps one of the clients required more care than expected or the nursing assistant needed to run an errand off the floor. Reevaluation of the

assignment may be necessary. When one RN works with another, supervision is not needed. This is a collaborative relationship and includes consulting and giving advice when needed.

Individuals who supervise others also delegate tasks and activities. Chief nursing officers often delegate tasks to associate directors. This may include record reviews, unit reports, client acuities, and other tasks. The chief nursing officer remains accountable for ensuring the activities are completed.

Supervision sometimes entails more direct evaluation of performance. For example, a nurse manager both supervises and delegates. Certain administrative tasks, such as staff scheduling, may be delegated to another staff member such as an associate manager. However, performance evaluations and discussions regarding individual interactions with clients and other staff members remain supervisory duties.

Regardless of where you work, you cannot assume that only those in the higher levels of the organization delegate work to other people. You, too, will be responsible at times to delegate some of your work to other nurses, to technical personnel, or to another department. Decisions associated with this responsibility often cause some difficulty for new nurses. Knowing each person's capabilities and job description can help you decide which personnel can assist with a task.

THE NURSING PROCESS AND DELEGATION

As nurses, we understand the nursing process. The same concept can be applied to delegation. Before deciding who should care for a particular client, the nurse must assess each client's particular needs, set client-specific goals, and match the skills of the person assigned with the tasks that need to be accomplished *(assessment)*. Thinking this through before delegating helps prevent problems later *(plan)*. Next, the nurse assigns the tasks to the appropriate person *(implementation)*. The nurse must then oversee the care and determine whether client care needs have been met *(evaluation)*. It is also important for the nurse to allow time for feedback during the day. This enables all personnel to see where they are and where they want to go.

Often, the nurse must first coordinate care for groups of clients before being able to delegate tasks to other personnel. By looking at the needs of each client, the nurse makes an educated decision about which staff members have the appropriate education and skill to deliver safe, quality care (Ellis & Hartley, 2004). The nurse also needs to consider his or her responsibilities. This includes assisting other staff members with setting priorities, communicating clearly, clarifying instructions, and reassessing the situation.

The NCSBN in 1995 published a paper addressing the issue of delegation. The NCSBN developed a concept called the Five Rights of Delegation, similar to the five rights regarding medication administration. These five rights are listed in Box 9-1. Before being able to delegate tasks and activities to other individuals, however, the nurse must understand the needs of each client.

Coordinating Assignments

One of the most difficult tasks for new nurses to master is coordinating daily activities. Often, you not only have a group of clients for whom you are expected to provide direct care but also must supervise the work of others, such as non-nurse caregivers, LPNs, or vocational nurses. Although care plans, critical (or clinical) pathways, concept maps, and computer information sheets are available to help identify client needs, these items do not provide a mechanism for coordinating the delivery of care. To do this, personalized worksheets can be developed that prioritize tasks to perform for each client. Using the worksheets helps the nurse identify tasks that require the knowledge and skill of an RN and those that can be carried out by UAP.

On the worksheet, tasks are prioritized on the basis of client need, not nursing convenience. For example, an order states that a client is to receive continuous tube feedings. Although it may be convenient for the nurse

to fill the feeding container with enough supplement to last 6 hours, it is not good practice and not safe for the client. Instead, the nurse should plan to check the tube feeding every 2 hours.

As for Linda at the beginning of the chapter, a worksheet can help her determine who can do what. First, she needs to decide what particular tasks she must do. These include receiving and transcribing orders; contacting physicians with information or requests; accessing laboratory reports from the computer, reviewing them, and giving them to the appropriate staff members; and checking any new medication orders and placing them in the medication administration records. Another RN may be able to relieve the monitor technician for dinner and breaks, and a second RN may be able to assign staff to dinner and breaks. Next, Linda needs to look at the needs of each client on the unit and prioritize them. She is now ready to delegate to her staff effectively.

Some activities must be done at a certain time, and their timing may be out of one's control. Examples include medication administration and clients who need special preparation for a scheduled procedure. The following are some tips for organizing work on personalized worksheets to help establish client priorities (Tappen, Weiss, & Whitehead, 2004):

◆ Plan your time around these activities.

◆ Do high-priority activities first.

◆ Determine which activities are best done in a cluster.

◆ Remember that you are still responsible for activities delegated to others.

◆ Consider your peak energy time when scheduling optional activities.

This list acts as a guideline for coordinating client care. The nurse needs to use critical thinking skills in the decision-making process. Rember that this is one of the ANA nurse-related principles of delegation (ANA, 2005). For example, activities that are usually clustered include bathing, changing linen, and parts of the physical assessment. Some clients may not be able to tolerate too much activity at one time. Take special situations into consideration when coordinating client care and deciding who should carry out some of the activities. Remember, however, even when you delegate, you remain accountable.

Figure 9-1 is an example of a personalized worksheet. (See Chapter 11 on time management for a complete discussion.)

THE NEED FOR DELEGATION

The 1990s brought rapid change to the healthcare environment. Several forces coming together at one time contributed to these changes, including the nursing shortage,

---

Nurse/Team _____DNR 8607/Code 99

Patient Room # _____ Name _____ Age _____

Allergies_____

Diagnosis_____

Diet _____Fluids: PO _____IV_____ Type _____

Restrictions: BR _____ BRP _____OOB/Chair_____ Ambulate with assist_____

Activity _____

Assessment_____

Treatments

1. _____

2. _____

3. _____

4. _____

5. _____

Monitor

1. Vital signs: Temp _____ Pulse_____AHR_____ BP _____Parameters _____

2. Cardiac Monitor: Rhythm_____ Rate _____ __

3. Neurologic Status _____

4. CMS: _____ Traction:_____

FIGURE 9-1 ◆ Personalized patient worksheet.

health-care reform, an increased need for nursing services, and demographic trends. These changes continue to have an impact on the delivery of nursing care, requiring institutions to hire other personnel to assist nurses with client care (Zimmerman, 1996).

Health-care institutions often use UAP to perform certain client care tasks (Habel, 2001; Hansten & Jackson, 2004; Huber, Blegan, & McCloskey, 1994). As the nursing shortage becomes more critical, there is a greater need for institutions to recruit the services of UAPs (ANA, 2002). A survey conducted by the American Hospital Association revealed that 97% of hospitals currently employ some form of UAP. Due to the continuing nursing shortage, this trend has continued. Because a high percentage of institutions employ these personnel, many nurses believe they know how to work with and safely delegate tasks to them. This is not the case. Therefore, many nursing organizations have developed definitions for UAP and criteria regarding their responsibilities. The ANA defines UAP as follows:

Unlicensed assistive personnel are individuals who are trained to function in an assistive role to the registered nurse in the provision of patient/client care activities as delegated by and under the supervision of the registered professional nurse. Although some of these people may be certified (e.g., certified nursing assistant [CNA]), it is important to remember that certification differs from licensure. When a task is delegated to an unlicensed person, the professional nurse remains personally responsible for the outcomes of these activities (ANA, 2005).

As the work on the UAP issue is ongoing, the ANA has recently updated its position statements to define direct and indirect patient care activities that may be performed by UAP in the health-care setting. Included in these updates are specific definitions regarding UAP and technicians and acceptable tasks.

Use of the RN to provide all the care a client needs may not be the most efficient or cost-effective use of professional time. More hospitals are moving away from hiring LPNs and utilizing all RN staffing with UAP. For this reason, the nursing focus is directed at diagnosing client care needs and carrying out complex interventions.

The ANA cautions against delegating nursing activities that include the foundation of the nursing process and that require specialized knowledge, judgment, or skill (ANA, 1996, 2002, 2005). Non-nursing functions, such as performing clerical or receptionist duties, taking trips or running errands off the unit, cleaning floors, making beds, collecting trays, and ordering supplies, should not be carried out by the highest paid and most educated member of the team. These tasks are easily delegated to other personnel.

SAFE DELEGATION

In 1990, the NCSBN adopted a definition of delegation, stating that delegation is "transferring to a competent individual the authority to perform a selected nursing task in a selected situation" (p. 1). In its publication *Issues* (1995), the NCSBN again presented this definition. Accordingly, the ANA Code for Nurses (1985) stated, "The nurse exercises informed judgment and uses individual competence and qualifications as criteria in seeking consultation, accepting responsibilities, and delegating nursing activities to others" (p. 1). In 2005, the ANA defined delegation as "The transfer of responsibility for the performance of an activity from one individual to another while retaining accountability for the outcome" (p. 4). It is important to remember that delegation still includes accountability. To delegate tasks safely, nurses must delegate appropriately and supervise adequately.

In 1997, the NCSBN developed a Delegation Decision-Making Grid. This grid is a tool to help nurses delegate appropriately. It provides a scoring instrument for seven categories that the nurse should consider when making delegation decisions. The categories for the grid are listed in Box 9-2.

Scoring the components helps the nurse evaluate the situations, the client needs, and the health-care personnel available to meet the needs. A low score on the grid indicates that the activity may be safely delegated to person-

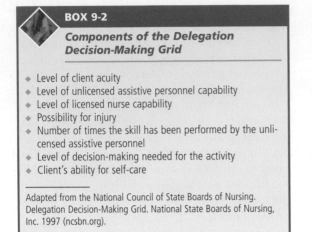

nel other than the RN, and a high score indicates that delegation may not be advisable. Figure 9-2 shows the Delegation Decision-Making Grid. The grid is also available on the NCSBN Web site at ncsbn.com.

Nurses who delegate tasks to UAP should evaluate the activities being considered for delegation (Keeney, Hasson, & McKenna, 2005). The American Association of Critical Care Nurses (AACN) (1990) recommended considering five factors, which are listed in Box 9-3, in making a decision to delegate.

It is the responsibility of the RN to be well acquainted with the state's nurse practice act and regulations issued by the state board of nursing regarding UAP (ANA, 2005). State laws and regulations supersede any publications or opinions set forth by professional organizations. As stated earlier, the NCSBN provides criteria to assist nurses with delegation.

LPNs are trained to perform specific tasks, such as basic medication administration, dressing changes, and personal hygiene tasks. In some states, the LPN, with additional training, may start and monitor intravenous (IV) infusions and administer certain medications.

CRITERIA FOR DELEGATION

The purpose of delegation is not to assign tasks to others that you do not want to do yourself. When you delegate to others effectively, you should have more time to perform the tasks that only a professional nurse is permitted to do.

In delegating, the nurse must consider both the *ability* of the person to whom the task is delegated and the *fairness* of the task to the individual and the team (Tappen, Weiss, & Whitehead, 2004). In other words, both the *task aspects* of delegation (Is this a complex task? Is it a professional responsibility? Can this person do it safely?) and the *interpersonal aspects* (Does the person have time to do this? Is the work evenly distributed?) must be considered.

The ANA (2005) has specified tasks that RNs may not delegate because they are specific to the discipline of professional nursing. These activities include (Boysen & Fischer, 2000):

◆ Initial nursing assessment and follow-up assessments if nursing judgment is indicated.

◆ Decisions and judgments about client outcomes.

◆ Determination and approval of a client plan of care.

◆ Interventions that require professional nursing knowledge, decisions, or skills.

◆ Decisions and judgments necessary for the evaluation of client care.

TASK-RELATED CONCERNS

The primary task-related concern in delegating work is whether the person assigned to do the task has the ability to complete it. Team priorities and efficiency are also important considerations.

Abilities

To make appropriate assignments, the nurse needs to know the knowledge and skill level, legal definitions, role expectations, and job description for each member of the team. It is equally important to be aware of the different skill levels of caregivers within each discipline because ability differs with each level of education. Additionally, individuals within each level

Elements for Review		Client A	Client B	Client C	Client D
Activity/task	Describe activity/task:				
Level of Client Stability	Score the client's level of stability: 0. Client condition is chronic/stable/predictable 1. Client condition has minimal potential for change 2. Client condition has moderate potential for change 3. Client condition is unstable/acute/strong potential for change				
Level of UAP Competence	Score the UAP competence in completing delegated nursing care activities in the defined client population: 0. UAP - expert in activities to be delegated, in defined population 1. UAP - experienced in activities to be delegated, in defined population 2. UAP - experienced in activities, but not in defined population 3. UAP - novice in performing activities and in defined population				
Level of Licensed Nurse Competence	Score the licensed nurse's competence in relation to both knowledge of providing nursing care to a defined population and competence in implementation of the delegation process: 0. Expert in the knowledge of nursing needs/activities of defined client population and expert in the delegation process 1. Either expert in knowledge of needs/activities of defined client population and competent in delegation or experienced in the needs/ activities of defined client population and expert in the delegation process 2. Experienced in the knowledge of needs/activities of defined client population and competent in the delegation process 3. Either experienced in the knowledge of needs/activities of defined client population or competent in the delegation process 4. Novice in knowledge of defined population and novice in delegation				
Potential for Harm	Score the potential level of risk the nursing care activity has for the client (risk is probability of suffering harm): 0. None 1. Low 2. Medium 3. High				
Frequency	Score based on how often the UAP has performed the specific nursing care activity: 0. Performed at least daily 1. Performed at least weekly 2. Performed at least monthly 3. Performed less than monthly 4. Never performed				
Level of Decision Making	Score the decision making needed, related to the specific nursing care activity, client (both cognitive and physical status), and client situation: 0. Does not require decision making 1. Minimal level of decision making 2. Moderate level of decision making 3. High level of decision making				
Ability for Self-Care	Score the client's level of assistance needed for self-care activities: 0. No assistance 1. Limited assistance 2. Extensive assistance 3. Total care or constant attendance				
	Total Score				

FIGURE 9-2 ✦ Delegation decision-making grid.

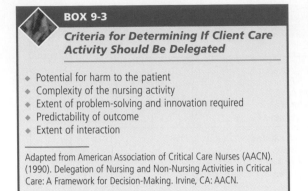

BOX 9-3

Criteria for Determining If Client Care Activity Should Be Delegated

- Potential for harm to the patient
- Complexity of the nursing activity
- Extent of problem-solving and innovation required
- Predictability of outcome
- Extent of interaction

Adapted from American Association of Critical Care Nurses (AACN). (1990). Delegation of Nursing and Non-Nursing Activities in Critical Care: A Framework for Decision-Making. Irvine, CA: AACN.

of skill possess their own strengths and weaknesses. Prior assessment of the strengths of each member of the team will assist in providing safe and efficient care to clients. Figure 9-3 outlines the skills of various health-care personnel.

People should not be assigned a task they are not skilled in or knowledgeable to perform, regardless of their professional level. People are often reluctant to admit they cannot do something. Instead of seeking help or saying they are not comfortable with a task, they may avoid doing it, delay starting it, do only part of it, or even bluff their way through it, a risky choice in health care.

Regardless of the length of time individuals have been in a position, employees need orientation when assigned a new task. Those who seek assistance and advice are showing concern for the team and the welfare of their clients. Requests for assistance or additional explanations should not be ignored, and the person should be praised, not criticized, for seeking guidance (Tappen, Weiss, & Whitehead, 2004).

Priorities

The work of a busy unit rarely ends up going as expected. Dealing with sick people, their families, physicians, and other team members all at the same time is a difficult task. Setting priorities for the day should be based on client needs, team needs, and organizational and community demands. The values of each may be very different, even opposed. These differences should be discussed with team members so that decisions can be made based on team priorities.

One way to determine patient priorities is to base decisions on Maslow's hierarchy of needs. Maslow's hierarchy is frequently used in nursing to provide a framework for prioritizing care to meet client needs. The basic physiological needs come first because they are necessary for survival. Oxygen and medication administration, IV fluids, and enteral feedings are included in this group.

Identifying priorities and deciding the needs to be met first help in organizing care and in deciding which other team members can meet client needs. For example, nursing assistants can meet many hygiene needs, allowing licensed personnel to administer medications and enteral feedings in a timely manner.

Efficiency

Efficiency means that all members of the team know their jobs and responsibilities and work

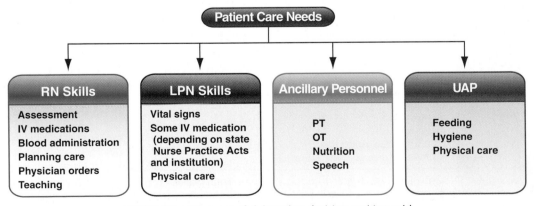

FIGURE 9-3 ◆ Diagram of delegation decision-making grid.

together like gears in a well-built clock. They mesh together and keep perfect time.

The current health-care delivery environment demands efficient, cost-effective care. Delegating appropriately can increase efficiency and save money. Likewise, incorrect delegation can decrease efficiency and cost money in the end. When delegating tasks to individuals who cannot perform the job, the RN must often go back to perform the task.

Although institutions often need to"float" staff to other units, maintaining continuity, if at all possible, is important. Keeping the same staff members on the unit all the time, for example, allows them to develop familiarity with the physical setting and routines of the unit as well as the types of clients the unit services. Time is lost when staff members are reassigned frequently to different units. Although physical layouts may be the same, client needs, unit routines, and use of space are often different, as is the availability of supplies. Time spent to orient reassigned staff members takes time away from delivery of client care. However, when staff members are reassigned, it is important for them to indicate their skill level and comfort in the new setting. It is just as important for the staff members who are familiar with the setting to identify the strengths of the reassigned person and build on them.

Appropriateness

Appropriateness is another task-related concern. Nothing can be more counterproductive than, for example, floating a coronary care nurse to labor and delivery. More time will be spent teaching the necessary skills than on safe mother-baby care. Assigning an educated, licensed staff member to perform non-nursing functions to protect safety is also poor use of personnel.

RELATIONSHIP-ORIENTED CONCERNS

Relationship-oriented concerns include fairness, learning opportunities, health concerns, compatibility, and staff preferences. Each of these is discussed next.

Fairness

Fairness means distributing the workload evenly in terms of both the physical requirements and the emotional investment in providing health care. The nurse who is caring for a dying client may have less physical work to do than another team member, but in terms of emotional care to the client and family, he or she may be doing double the work of another staff member.

Fairness also means considering equally all requests for special consideration. The quickest way to alienate members of a team is to be unfair. It is important to discuss with team members any decisions that have been made that may appear unfair to them. Allow the team members to participate in making decisions regarding assignments. Their participation will decrease resentment and increase cooperation. In some health-care institutions, team members make such decisions as a group.

Learning Opportunities

Including assignments that stimulate motivation, learning, and assisting team members to learn new tasks and take on new challenges is part of the role of the RN.

Health

Some aspects of caregiving jobs are more stressful than others. Rotating team members through the more difficult jobs may decrease stress and allow empathy to increase among the members. Special health needs, such as family emergencies or special physical problems of team members, also need to be addressed. If some team members have difficulty accepting the needs of others, the situation should be discussed with the team, bearing in mind the employee's right to privacy when discussing sensitive issues.

Compatibility

No matter how hard you may strive to get your team to work together, it just may not happen. Some people work together better than others. Helping people develop better working relationships is part of team building. Creating opportunities for people to share and learn from each other increases the overall effectiveness of the team.

As the leader, you may be forced to intervene in team member disputes. Many individuals find it difficult to work with others they do not like personally. It sometimes becomes necessary to explain that liking another person is a plus but not a necessity in the work setting and that personal problems have no place in the work environment. Take the example of Laura:

Laura had been a labor and delivery room supervisor in a large metropolitan hospital for 5 years before she moved to another city. Because a position similar to the one she left was not available, she became a staff nurse at a small local hospital. The hospital had just opened its new birthing center. The first day on the job went well. The other staff members seemed cordial enough. As the weeks went by, however, Laura began to have problems getting other staff to help her. No one would offer to relieve her for meals or a break. She noticed that certain groups of staff members always went to lunch together but that she was never invited to join them. She attempted to speak to some of the more approachable coworkers, but she did not get much information. Disturbed by the situation, Laura went to the nurse manager. The nurse manager listened quietly while Laura related her experiences. She then asked Laura to reflect on some of the events of the past weeks, particularly the last staff meeting. Laura realized that she had alienated the staff during that encounter because she had monopolized the meeting and kept saying that in "her hospital" things were done in a particular way. Laura also realized that, instead of asking for help, she was in the habit of demanding it. Laura and the nurse manager discussed the difficulties of her changing positions, moving to a new place, and trying to develop both professional and social ties. Together, they came up with several solutions to Laura's problem.

Staff Preferences

Considering the preferences of individual team members is important but should not supersede the other criteria for delegating responsibly. Allowing team members to always select what they want to do may cause the less assertive members' needs to be unmet.

It is important to explain the rationale for decisions made regarding delegation so that all team members may understand the needs of the unit or organization. Box 9-4 outlines basic rights for professional health-care team members. Although written originally for women,

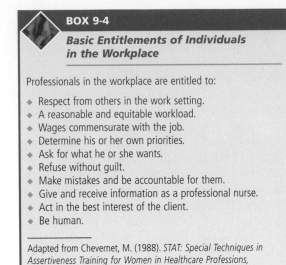

BOX 9-4

Basic Entitlements of Individuals in the Workplace

Professionals in the workplace are entitled to:

◆ Respect from others in the work setting.
◆ A reasonable and equitable workload.
◆ Wages commensurate with the job.
◆ Determine his or her own priorities.
◆ Ask for what he or she wants.
◆ Refuse without guilt.
◆ Make mistakes and be accountable for them.
◆ Give and receive information as a professional nurse.
◆ Act in the best interest of the client.
◆ Be human.

Adapted from Chevernet, M. (1988). *STAT: Special Techniques in Assertiveness Training for Women in Healthcare Professions*, 2nd ed. St. Louis, MO: Mosby.

the concepts are applicable to all professional health-care providers.

BARRIERS TO DELEGATION

Many nurses, particularly new ones, have difficulty delegating. The reasons for this include experience issues, licensure issues, and quality-of-care issues.

Experience Issues

Many nurses received their education during the 1980s, when primary care was the major delivery system. These nurses lacked the education and skill needed for delegation (Mahlmeister, 1999). Nurses educated before the 1970s worked in settings with LPNs and nursing assistants, where they routinely delegated tasks. However, client acuity was lower and the care less complex. Older nurses have considerable delegation experience and can be a resource for younger nurses.

The added responsibility of delegation creates some discomfort for nurses. Many believe that they are unprepared to assume this responsibility, especially when it comes to deciding the competency of another person. To decrease this discomfort, nurses need to participate in establishing the guidelines for

TABLE 9-1 DIRECT AND INDIRECT CLIENT CARE ACTIVITIES	
Direct Client Care Activities	**Indirect Client Care Activities**
Assisting with feeding and drinking	Providing a clean environment
Assisting with ambulation	Providing a safe environment
Assisting with grooming	Providing companion care
Assisting with toileting	Providing transportation for non-critical clients
Assisting with dressing	Assisting with stocking nursing units
Assisting with socializing	Providing messenger and delivery services

Adapted from American Nurses Association. (2002). Position Statement on Utilization of Unlicensed Assistive Personnel. Washington, DC: American Nurses Association.

UAP within the institution. The ANA Position Statements on Unlicensed Assistive Personnel address this. Table 9-1 lists the direct and indirect client care activities that may be performed by UAP.

Licensure Issues

Today's health-care environment requires nurses to delegate. Many nurses voice concerns about the personal risk regarding their licensure if they delegate inappropriately. The courts have usually ruled that nurses are not liable for the negligence of other individuals, provided that the nurse delegated appropriately. Delegation is within the scope of nursing practice. The art and skill of delegation are acquired with practice.

There may be legal implications if a client is injured as a result of inappropriate delegation. Take the following case:

In *Hicks v. New York State Department of Health,* a nurse was found guilty of patient neglect because of her failure to appropriately train and supervise the UAP working under her. In this particular situation, a security guard discovered an elderly nursing home client in a totally dark room undressed and covered with urine and fecal material. The client was partially in his bed and partially restrained in an overturned wheelchair. The court found the nurse guilty on the following: the nurse failed to assess whether the UAP had delivered proper care to the client, and this subsequently led to the inadequate delivery of care (1991).

Quality-of-Care Issues

Nurses have expressed concern over the quality of client care when tasks and activities are delegated to others. Remember Nightingale's words earlier in the chapter, "Don't imagine that if you, who are in charge, don't look to all these things yourself, those under you will be more careful than you are." She added that you do not need to do everything yourself to see that it is done correctly. When you delegate, you control the delegation. You decide to whom you will delegate the task. Remember that there are levels of acceptable performance and that not every task needs to be done perfectly.

Assigning Work to Others

This is difficult for several reasons:

1. Some nurses think they must do everything themselves.
2. Some nurses distrust subordinates to do things correctly.
3. Some nurses think that if they delegate all the technical tasks, they will not reinforce their own learning.
4. Some nurses are more comfortable with the technical aspects of client care than with the more complex issues of client teaching and discharge planning.

Families and clients do not always see professional activities. They see direct client care (Keeney, Hasson, McKenna, & Gillen, 2005). Nurses believe that when they do not participate directly in client care, they do not accomplish anything for the client. The professional aspects of nursing, such as planning care, teaching, and discharge planning, help to promote positive outcomes for clients and their families. When working with LPNs, knowing their scope of practice helps in making delegation decisions.

CONCLUSION

The concept of delegation is not new. The delegation role is essential to the RN-LPN and RN-UAP relationship. Personal organizational skills are a prerequisite to delegation. Before the nurse can delegate tasks to others, he or she needs to understand individual client needs. Using worksheets and Maslow's hierarchy helps the nurse understand these individual client needs, set priorities, and identify which tasks can be delegated to others. Using the Delegation Decision-Making Grid helps the nurse delegate safely and appropriately.

It is also importat the the nurse be aware of the capabilities of each staff member, the tasks that may be delegated, and the tasks that the RN needs to perform. When delegating, the RN uses professional judgment in making decisions. Professional judgment is directed by the state nurse practice act and national standards of nursing. Institutions develop their own job descriptions for UAP and other health-care professionals, but institutional policies cannot contradict the state nurse practice act. Although the nurse delegates the task or activity, he or she remains accountable for the delegation decision.

Understanding the concept of delegation helps the new nurse organize and prioritize client care. Knowing the staff and their capabilities simplifies delegation. Utilizing staff members' capabilities creates a pleasant and productive working environment for everyone involved.

STUDY QUESTIONS

1 What are the responsibilities of the professional nurse when delegating tasks to an LPN or UAP?

2 What factors need to be considered when delegating tasks?

3 What is the difference between the delegation and the assignment of a task?

4 What are the nurse manager's legal responsibilities in supervising UAP?

5 If you were the nurse manager, how would you have handled Laura's situation?

6 How would you have handled the situation if you were Linda?

7 Bring the client census from your assigned clinical unit to class. Using the Delegation Decision-Making Grid, decide which clients you would assign to the personnel on the unit. Give reasons for your decision.

CRITICAL THINKING EXERCISE

Julio works at a large teaching hospital in a major metropolitan area. This institution services the entire geographical region, including indigent clients, and because of its renowned reputation also administers care to international clients and individuals who reside in other states. Like all health-care institutions, this one has been attempting to cut costs by using more UAP. Nurses are often floated to other units. Lately, the number of indigent and foreign clients on Julio's unit has increased. The acuity of these clients has been quite high, requiring a great deal of time from the nursing staff.

Julio arrived at work at 6:30 a.m., his usual time. He looked at the census board and discovered that the unit was filled, and bed control was calling all night to have clients discharged or transferred to make room for several clients who had been in the emergency department since the previous evening. He also discovered that the other RN assigned to his team called in sick. His team consists of himself, two UAP, and an LPN who is shared by two teams. He has eight clients on his team: two need to be readied for surgery, including preoperative and postoperative teaching, one of whom is a 35-year-old woman scheduled for a modified radical mastectomy for the treatment of breast cancer; three are second-day postoperative clients, two of whom require extensive dressing changes, are receiving IV antibiotics, and need to be ambulated; one postoperative client is required to remain on total bedrest, has a nasogastric tube to suction as well as a chest tube, is on TPN and lipids, needs a central venous catheter line dressing change, has an IV, is taking multiple IV medications, and has a Foley catheter; one client is ready for discharge and needs discharge instruction; and one client needs to be transferred to a subacute unit, and a report must be given to the RN of that unit. Once the latter client is transferred and the other one is discharged, the emergency department will be sending two clients to the unit for admission.

1. How should Julio organize his day? Set up an hourly schedule.

2. What type of client management approach should Julio consider in assigning staff appropriately?

3. If you were Julio, which clients and/or tasks would you assign to your staff? List all of them, and explain your rationale.

4. Using the Delegation Decision-Making Grid, make staff and client assignments.

REFERENCES

American Nurses Association (ANA). (1985). Code for Nurses. Washington, DC: ANA.

American Association of Critical Care Nurses (AACN). (1990). Delegation of Nursing and Non-Nursing Activities in Critical Care: A Framework for Decision Making. Irvine, CA: AACN.

American Nurses Association (ANA). (1996). Registered Professional Nurses and Unlicensed Assistive Personnel. Washington, DC: ANA.

American Nurses Association (ANA). (2002). Position Statements on Registered Nurse Utilization of Unlicensed Assistive Personnel. Washington, DC: ANA.

American Nurses Association (ANA). (2005). Principles for Delegation. Washington, DC: ANA.

Boysen, R., & Fischer, C. (2000). Delegation/Practice Boundaries. South Dakota State University College of Nursing. Retrieved on July 29, 2002 from learn.sdstate.edu/nursing/DelegationModule2

Chevernet, M. (1988). STAT: Special Techniques in Assertiveness Training for Women in Healthcare Professions, 2nd ed. St. Louis, MO: Mosby.

Ellis, J.R., & Hartley, C.L. (2004). Nursing in Today's World. Philadelphia: Lippincott, Williams & Wilkins.

Habel, M. (Winter 2001). Delegating nursing care to unlicensed assistive personnel. Continuing Education for Florida Nurses, 39–54.

Hansten, R.I., & Jackson, M. (2004). Clinical Delegation Skills: A Handbook for Professional Practice. Sudbury, MA: Jones & Bartlett Publishers.

Hicks v. New York State Department of Health. (1991). 570 N.Y.S. 2d 395 (A.D. 3 Dept).

Huber, D., Blegan, M., & McCloskey, J. (1994). Use of nursing assistants: Staff nurse opinions. Nursing Management, 25(5), 64–68.

Keeney, S., Hasson, F., McKenna, H., & Gillen, P. (2005). Health care assistants: The view of managers of health care agencies on training and employment. Journal of Nursing Management, 13(1), 83–92.

Keeney, S., Hasson, F., & McKenna, H. (2005). Nurses', midwives', and patients' perceptions of trained health care assistants. Journal of Advanced Nursing, 50(4), 345–355.

Mahlmeister, L. (1999). Professional accountability and legal liability for the team leader and charge nurse.

Journal of Obstetric, Gynecologic, and Neonatal Nursing, 28, 300–309.

National Council of State Boards of Nursing. (1990). Concept Paper on Delegation. Chicago: National Council of State Boards of Nursing.

National Council of State Boards of Nursing. (1995). Delegation: Concepts and decision-making process. Issues (December), 1–2.

National Council of State Boards of Nursing. (1997). Delegation Decision-Making Grid. Chicago: National Council of State Boards of Nursing.

Nightingale, F. (1859). *Notes on Nursing: What It Is and What It Is Not.* London: Harrison and Sons. (Reprint 1992. Philadelphia: JB Lippincott.)

Tappen, R., Weiss, S.A., & Whitehead, D.K. (2004). *Essentials of Leadership and Management.* Philadelphia: FA Davis.

Zimmerman, P.G. (1996). Delegating to assistive personnel. *Journal of Emergency Nursing,* 22, 206–212.

chapter **10**

Managing Client Care

1. Describe the nursing care delivery system on the unit of your current clinical site.

2. Based on your observations, how well does the model promote client and staff satisfaction?

3. What suggestions do you have for improvement?

Risk Management

Identify how you will decrease your risk in the following common areas of risk to nurses.

1. Medication errors

2. Documentation errors and/or omissions

3. Failure to correctly perform nursing care or treatments

4. Errors in patient safety that result in falls

5. Failure to communicate significant data to clients and other providers

All the results of good nursing, as detailed in these notes, may be spoiled or utterly negated by one defect, viz.: in petty management, or in other words, by not knowing how to manage.... How few men, or even women, understand, either in great or in little things....know how to carry out a "charge." To be "in charge" is certainly not only to carry out the proper measure yourself but to see that every one else does so too; to see that no one either willfully or ignorantly thwarts or prevents such measures. It is neither to do everything yourself nor to appoint a number of people to each duty, but to ensure that each does that duty to which he is appointed (Nightingale & Barnum, 1992, pp. 20, 24).

Although Florence Nightingale wrote these words in the 1800s, they are still true. Major changes in our health-care system are occurring as administrators in all types of agencies try to find the correct balance between "lean and mean" efficiency and high-quality care (Sharp, 1994, p. 32). These efforts affect the way nursing care is delivered. The search for ways to provide safe, effective health care without spending too much money has led to the creation of new models for managing nursing care.

This chapter will help you understand and develop your role in the management of client care. The chapter begins by considering the economic context in which health care is provided. A review of the past, present, and future models for managing nursing care is presented next. This includes the traditional models of total care, primary care, functional care, and team care. The contemporary use of case management, the multidisciplinary team approach, product line management, and differentiated practice complete this section. This is followed by a discussion of the ways in which the quality of the care given is monitored and evaluated.

THE ECONOMIC CLIMATE IN THE HEALTH-CARE SYSTEM

For many years, decisions about care were based primarily on providing the best quality care, whatever the cost. As the economic support for health care is challenged, however, health-care providers are pressured to seek methods of care delivery that achieve quality outcomes at lower cost.

Economic Perspective

The economic perspective is rooted in three fundamental observations:

1. **Resources are scarce.** Due to scarce resources, three choices result:
   ◆ The amount to be spent on health-care services and the composition of those services.
   ◆ The methods for producing those services.
   ◆ The method of distribution of health care, which influences the equity of these services to various people within the population; note that health-care needs are not met for more than 40 million uninsured individuals in America.
2. **Resources have alternative uses.** As a result of this scarcity, the choice to expend resources in one area eliminates the use of those same resources in another area. If more nursing homes are going to be built, for example, then there will be fewer hospitals, less housing, less education, or other uses of those same resources.
3. **Individuals want different services or have different preferences.** Some people choose alternative treatment modalities such as acupuncture, herbal therapy, or massage therapy rather than traditional health care. The assumption exists that preferences for products and services can be influenced, which explains the extensive marketing of health-care services.

During the past three decades, federal and state governments have attempted a variety of cost-containment programs to restrain the cost of health care. Some were carried out through broad federal programs, whereas others targeted specific issues or industries. Among them were:

1. **Economic Stabilization Program (ESP).** A broad-based federal government program, the ESP was initiated by Richard Nixon in 1971. This program froze wages and prices of all goods and services, including health care, for 90 days. Less stringent restrictions followed, and the program ended in 1974.
2. **Voluntary Effort (VE).** The VE program, proposed by Jimmy Carter in 1977, urged hospitals to reduce their costs voluntarily. The proposal was defeated by Congress in 1979.
3. **Certificate of Need (CON).** The CON program aims at regulating hospital expenditures for new beds, equipment, and facility construction. The rationale is that excessive hospital growth is the root cause of hospital inflation due to empty beds and underutilized facilities that must be maintained.
4. **Medicare Prospective Payment System (PPS).** In 1983 the federal government changed its method of paying hospitals for treating Medicare clients. Instead of paying for actual costs, the PPS pays hospitals a fixed, predetermined sum for a particular admission. If a hospital can provide the service at a cost below the fixed amount, it pockets the difference. If more resources and money are used than the predetermined amount, the hospital incurs a loss.
5. **Diagnostic Related Groups (DRGs).** Tied to the PPS, DRGs are the patient classification systems by which the Medicare PPS determines payment. Each of the 495 DRGs represents a particular case type.
6. **Managed Care.** Managed care is a system of health care that combines the financing and delivery of health services into a single entity. Currently, more than 75% of the enrolled population in the private sector is in a managed care plan of some form. Managed care plans are seen as cost-saving alternatives to traditional fee-for-service delivery systems. Through provider networks and selective provider contracting, they attempt to control

Factors Increasing Costs

- Expansion of national economy
- General inflation
- Aging population
- Growth of third-party payments
- Employer-provided health insurance
- Tax deduction for medical expenses
- Increased costs of labor and equipment
- Expansion of medical technology and products
- Malpractice insurance and litigation

Factors Containing Costs

- Federal economic stabilization program
- Voluntary effort hospital regulation program
- State-level health-care payment programs
- Medicare prospective payment system (PPS) with payments of fixed amount per admission
- Diagnostic related groups (DRGs) for hospital payments
- Resource-based relative value scale (RBRVS) for physician payments
- Managed care plans

FIGURE 10-1 ◆ Factors affecting the cost of health care. (From Chang, C.F., Price, S.A., & Pfoutz, S.K. [2001]. *Economics and Nursing: Critical Professional Issues.* Philadelphia: FA Davis, p. 79.)

resource use and health-care costs (Chang, Price, & Pfoutz, 2001). Figure 10-1 depicts the current factors increasing and containing health-care costs.

The season of change continues in nursing and health care. Three important drivers are cultural diversity, the aging population, and new services and technologies (Wakefield, 2003).

1. **Cultural diversity.** Health-care environments are acknowledging the complex cultural diversity across the country. The need for health-care providers to provide culturally sensitive and competent care continues to grow.
2. **Aging population.** The growth of the aging population is causing health-care

providers to recognize the differences in providing chronic versus acute care and the need to provide services that will help clients and families manage their health care over years and even decades.

3. **New services and technologies**. As Medicare and Medicaid programs cut back on their funding, resource consumption grows. New services and new technologies, especially in biotechnology and pharmacology, are causing change at a rapid rate. Time and distance are continuing to become irrelevant through telehealth technologies.

Nursing Labor Market

Registered nurses (RNs) comprise 77% of the nurse workforce, and almost 60% of them are employed in hospitals. The nationwide unemployment rate for RNs is only 1%. Even with this low rate, vacancy rates nationwide are reported at anywhere from 13% to 20% and are rising. A serious nursing shortage is here, and it will continue at least until 2020. The demand for nurses is expected to increase even more dramatically as the baby boomers reach their 60s, 70s, and beyond. From now until 2030, the population age 65 years and older will double. What has caused the nursing shortage?

◆ **Nursing shortage.** In the previous edition of this book (2004), enrollments in associate degree nursing programs had declined 11% in the past 2 years, and enrollment in bachelor of science in nursing (BSN) programs had declined 19% in the same period (Heinrich, 2001). Research in 2004 by Dr. Peter Buerhaus and colleagues found that "despite the increase in employment of nearly 185,000 hospital RNs since 2001, there is no empirical evidence that the nursing shortage has ended. To the contrary, national surveys of RNs and physicians conducted in 2004 found that a clear majority of RNs (82%) and doctors (81%) perceived shortages where they worked." (aacn.nche. edu/Media/shortageresource.htm#about) In 2002 over 100,000 new RNs were hired; the majority were foreign-born nurses and

nurses over age 50 returning to the workforce in tough economic times. Though the new hires and a sharp increase in RN salaries are positive, the current nursing shortage is far from over. According to projections from the Bureau of Labor Statistics (BLS), there will be more than one million vacant positions for registered nurses (RNs) by 2010 (aacn.nche.edu/Publications/WhitePapers/FacultyShortages.htm)

◆ **High acuity of clients in hospitals.** Medically complex clients require skilled nursing care.

◆ **Increased demand for nurses.** As health care moves to a variety of community settings, only the most acute clients remain in the hospital. The transfer of less acute clients to nursing homes and community settings creates additional job opportunities and increased demand for nurses.

◆ **Aging nursing workforce.** In 2000, fewer than one in three RNs was younger than 40 years of age. The percentage of nurses age 40 to 49 years is currently more than 35%.

◆ **Job dissatisfaction.** Staffing levels, heavy workloads, increased use of overtime, lack of sufficient support staff, and salary discrepancies between nurses and other health-care professionals have contributed to growing dissatisfaction and retention of nurses. Many facilities are now using workplace issues and incentives as a retention strategy.

◆ **Reduction in nursing faculty.** As retirements for faculty continue, the shortage of faculty continues to affect the number of students admitted to nursing programs. The need to control spiraling health-care costs along with the issues of supply and demand for nursing services will continue well into this century. According to the American Nurses Association (ANA), more than 40% of nurses initially graduate from associate degree nursing programs. You, personally, will not only be affected by trends in health-care delivery but also can be a major voice in decision making (Nelson, 2002). As in the past, cost control and demand for nursing services will most likely involve changing nurse staffing, the model of care, and professional nursing practice (Ritter-Teitel, 2002).

MODELS OF CARE DELIVERY

Nursing care delivery systems provide the structure that allows nurses to plan and deliver nursing care to groups of clients. Even today, there is no one right way to structure and deliver nursing care. The institution size, staff availability, environment, budget, and organizational goals all affect the model of nursing care delivery. The current acute nursing shortage continues to fuel the frenzy of work redesign in acute care hospitals across the nation. Regardless of the model, a delivery system focuses on four organizing principles (Manthey, 2001, p. 425):

1. **Decision making.** Who is responsible for making what decisions?
2. **Care allocation.** Who gives what care to the client?
3. **Communication.** Who tells what to whom?
4. **Management.** Who is overseeing the process?

Traditional Models

Although the following models are categorized as traditional, this does not imply that they are old or outdated. Many models are still used, and all of them have historical significance in the development of the more contemporary models.

Total Care

The total care, or case, method is one of the earliest models of nursing care delivery. One nurse assumes total responsibility for the planning and delivery of care to a particular client or group of clients. This method may be used in community health nursing, in private duty, in intensive care and isolation units, and in making assignments for students in nursing school. The client may have different nurses within a 24-hour period, but each nurse provides all of the care needed for the period assigned. The case method is considered a precursor of primary nursing. Although the

method has the advantage of being extremely client-focused, it is not considered the most efficient use of staff and is not used in the majority of health-care settings.

Functional

The functional method of care delivery grew out of the 1950s' emphasis on an assembly-line style of management that focused on division of labor and tasks that need to be completed. The nurse manager is responsible for making work assignments. Roles such as those of the medication nurse and treatment nurse are part of the functional delivery approach. Job descriptions, procedures, policies, and lines of communication are clearly defined. The functional model is generally considered efficient, economical, and productive. The disadvantage is that this model leads to fragmentation of care because the client receives care from several different types of nursing personnel. In addition, the emotional needs of both the staff members and the client are overlooked in the interest of time management and task completion (Loveridge & Cummings, 1996).

Team

In the later 1950s and into the 1960s, the emphasis moved from a task focus to group dynamics and promotion of job satisfaction. In response to the fragmentation of the functional method and the continued scarcity of RNs after World War II, the team method was developed. Each team consists of a mix of staff members, such as an RN, a licensed practical nurse (LPN), and a nursing assistant. The team is responsible for providing care to a group of assigned clients during the shift. The team leader, usually the RN, makes assignments for the team based on members' abilities and client needs. Compared with the functional method, the team method emphasizes holistic care and increases client and employee satisfaction.

Modular Nursing

A more current version of team nursing is modular nursing. Modular nursing takes into account the actual structure of the unit, allowing nurses to be located nearer the clients, with a wider range of responsibility delegated to them. Modular nursing is often used when primary nursing is not an option. Each RN, assisted by paraprofessional team members, delivers care to a group of clients. The grouping of one 50-bed unit into three modular substations may allow staff to even further emphasize efficiency in this era of RN scarcity (Huber, 2000; Loveridge & Cummings, 1996).

Primary Nursing

Primary nursing became popular in the 1960s and 1970s as nurses voiced concern over the fragmentation of care provided to their clients. In this model, an RN is assigned care of a client for 24 hours a day for the client's entire hospital stay, including discharge planning. This RN is responsible for developing the care plan and managing the associate nurses and other staff members who provide additional care for the client. Primary nursing decreases the number of persons who have contact with each client and usually increases accountability and client satisfaction. However, primary nursing severely limits the number of clients each nurse can serve and can place the client in jeopardy if the primary nurse is not capable of meeting the client's needs. As the pressures for cost containment and restructuring increased in the late 1980s and early 1990s, the primary care concept was almost totally eliminated in acute care settings (Huber, 2000; Loveridge & Cummings, 1996).

Contemporary Models

Health-care administrators continue to seek delivery models that will ensure quality, promote client and staff satisfaction, and contain costs. Several of these models are case management, client-focused care with cross-training, product line management, and differentiated practice.

Case Management

The term *case management* is used to describe a variety of health-care delivery systems in acute, long-term, and community settings. Case management is not a new concept. Public health programs have used case management to provide care since the early 1900s. In 1970 insurance companies began case management in an attempt to control long-term, expensive cases. When mental health services moved out of institutions into the community in the 1960s, case management programs became important to psychiatric–mental health nursing as well (Lyon, 1993). These examples of "external" case management were models for the "internal" case management that began in the 1980s within the acute care setting.

The Case Management Society of America defines case management as a collaborative process that assesses, plans, implements, coordinates, monitors, and evalutes the options and services required to meet an individual's health needs, using communication and available resources to promote quality, cost-effective outcomes (Harrison, Nolin, & Suero, 2004). The process of case management is easily placed within the framework of the nursing process (Table 10-1).

According to Newell (1996), the primary functions of case managers include:

◆ **Negotiation services and/or treatments.** Obtain maximum quality services at an acceptable cost (e.g., negotiate RN hourly rates for home care services, obtain prices for equipment such as a wheelchair).

TABLE 10-1
Comparison of Nursing Process and Nursing Case Management Process

Assessment/Diagnosis	Planning	Intervention	Evaluation
Determine physical, emotional, psychological needs	Determine resources	Link clients to services	Ensure needs are met
Reassess and begin process again	Develop care plans, critical pathways	Act as a "broker" and advocate	Monitor and document cost effectiveness and client progress

Adapted from Mass, S., & Johnson, B. (November 1998). Case management and clinical guidelines. *Journal of Care Management,* 18.

◆ **Communication.** Communicate with service providers, clients, families, and information systems.

◆ **Coordination of care.** Oversee services and resources to avoid duplication and breakdowns in quality.

◆ **Clinical expertise.** Acquire technical knowledge of disease processes and interventions to assess, plan, and evaluate client services.

◆ **Holistic approach.** Be able to understand human beings' biological, social, and behavioral needs.

◆ **Ethics with caring.** Maintain a focus on advocacy, honesty, and understanding in dealing with clients.

◆ **Coaching.** This important skill affects all of the preceding functions; be successful in working with clients, families, staff, and physicians.

Nursing care management is designed to decrease fragmentation of care, use of hospitalization, and cost through better coordination and monitoring of client care. Effective nursing case management can improve the quality of services, the quality of life for clients, and the functioning of the interdisciplinary team.

Case management systems must act like human beings who are functioning well: they are focused on the task at hand, interact without duplicity, learn and respond to new situations and information, and are honest and forthright in communicating with all parties. Well-functioning case managers and case management systems may not always do everything right, but they strive to do the right thing, thus affecting others in the system to also act with integrity (Newell, 1996).

Nursing care management is a system for delivering nursing care that is based on the philosophy of case management. The goals of nursing care management follow (Girard, 1994):

◆ **Outcomes based on standards of care.** Evaluation of the quality of nursing practice is based on desired measurable outcomes and accepted practices of the nursing profession.

◆ **Well-coordinated continuity of care**

through collaborative practice. All providers of services work together to plan services and meet client needs. Effective collaboration requires that providers also work together to meet each other's needs.

◆ **Efficient use of resources to reduce wasted time, energy, and materials.** Continued monitoring of material and personnel resources can eliminate duplication of steps and services, resulting in increased efficiency and job satisfaction.

◆ **Timely discharge within prospective payment guidelines.** Grouping of medical conditions into categories that have allowable lengths of stay and payment schedules designated by Medicare has been in effect since the 1980s. Enabling clients to be discharged safely within the designated length of stay is an ongoing challenge for the nursing care manager.

◆ **Professional development and satisfaction.** Through coordination of services and collaboration with providers, family, and clients, the case management model can enhance clients' quality of life (Christensen & Bender, 1994).

Although many different health-care personnel claim to have in-depth knowledge of client and family care needs and understanding of organizational and financial services and community resources, the RN is ideally suited to serve as care manager. "In an era of decreasing reimbursements and increasing accreditation requirements, hospital administrators view nurse case managers as one answer to balancing cost and quality" (Wayman, 1999, p. 236).

Nursing has traditionally considered the client from a total-systems perspective of person, environment, and health, with a focus on the multidisciplinary efforts needed to optimize care for the individual. Nurses, accustomed to focusing on a holistic approach to nursing care, are best able to use a whole-system approach to care delivery rather than a parts-oriented approach (Newell, 1996).

The case management system of care helps clients learn to cope with the challenges of their illness. Case management services can be delivered in a variety of settings. *External case management* involves activities that are external to provider organizations. For example, case managers may work with victims of catastrophic motor vehicle accidents, workers' compensation clients, major medical insurance clients, and individual clients with complex chronic conditions. *Internal case managers* provide services within the walls of institutions or provider organizations. Internal case managers work in acute care, subacute care, rehabilitation, long-term care, home care, and managed care organizations (Newell, 1996).

The following is a case management example:

Maria is a 71-year-old Salvadoran-American woman with a history of childhood rheumatic heart disease. She has given birth to four children, the last one when Maria was 41. During that pregnancy, she spent the last trimester on bedrest. She complained of fatigue, shortness of breath, and swelling in her feet and ankles after her last child was born; 4 years after the birth of this child, she had a mitral commissurotomy to open the calcified mitral valve. Since then, she has complained of the same symptoms, and she has been unable to walk up the flight of stairs in her two-story home. Maria and her husband depend on his small pension and Social Security for their living expenses. Their home is paid, and the children are always sending "gifts," but money is limited. The couple joined a Medicare health maintenance organization (HMO) to cover the cost of drugs and to avoid having to carry a supplemental policy to augment traditional Medicare coverage.

As Maria's condition deteriorated, she experienced liver enlargement, sleep apnea, and petechiae on her face. She was very depressed regarding her continued illness. The HMO physician tried to talk Maria into a mitral valve replacement. She stated emphatically, "I will never go through what I did when I had that surgery, so don't even mention it!" The physician asked the nurse case manager to see Maria. The nurse case manager met with Maria and her husband in their home. She observed that, although the house appeared clean, Maria complained that she was unable to keep house like she used to and felt useless as a wife and mother. The case manager helped Maria and her husband evaluate their options for treatment of Maria's illness. She made several visits to their home and, after forming a positive relationship with them, began to discuss the potential benefits of surgery and the possibility of improving Maria's quality of life. Maria finally consented to having a cardiac catheterization, which subsequently showed that both the mitral and tricuspid valves were leaking. She agreed to surgery, which was successful. The case manager continues to call Maria monthly to monitor her progress. Maria said recently, "I owe my new life to my wonderful nurse."

Client-Focused Care

In the client-focused care model, services and staff are organized around client needs rather than the other way around. Traditionally, hospitals have been organized by departments, which the client goes to for services. In the client-focused care model, the services are brought to the client (Greenberg, 1994). Clients with similar needs are placed on the same nursing units, with ancillary and support services present on the unit. The traditional boundaries between disciplines are blurred. Although licensed members of the team retain their professional expertise and function within state and national practice acts and accrediting agency requirements, members of the team share all nonregulated tasks. Members of disciplines such as nursing, physical therapy, respiratory therapy, and pharmacy are unit-based. They receive additional training so they can provide services across disciplinary lines. Their combined functions may range from clinical to managerial responsibilities and may be of higher, lower, or parallel levels when compared with their original functions.

In addition, new all-purpose "client care technicians" or unlicensed assistive personnel (UAP) roles are usually created. These new workers perform such tasks as meal delivery, cleaning and maintenance of rooms, and assisting clients with comfort needs. Under the supervision of licensed personnel, client care technicians may also perform skilled tasks that are not restricted by various practice acts, such as insertion of indwelling urinary catheters or simple dressing changes (Christensen & Bender, 1994; Flarey, 1995).

Response to this model has been mixed. Some nursing administrators say that staff dissatisfaction and stress have increased, whereas others report favorable client experiences and staff satisfaction (Christensen & Bender, 1994). Since its inception in 1989, use of the client-focused care model has increased, but further research on its effectiveness is needed (Clouten & Weber, 1994). The following is a client-focused care example:

Esperanza has been the nurse manager on a 50-bed medical-surgical unit for 5 years. Since the advent of the prospective payment system, reimbursement for care has been limited. Clients come in sicker and go home more quickly. Esperanza just left a management meeting in which the chief executive officer informed them that nursing costs make up over half of the hospital's total budget. To cut costs and maximize effectiveness, the nurse managers must decrease the number of nurses on each shift, making sure that RNs do only those tasks that require an RN. A consultant will be brought in to implement a new system called *client-focused care.*

Each unit formed a committee of management personnel, staff nurses, and nursing assistants to meet with the consultant. In addition, representatives of other services, such as rehabilitation services, respiratory care, pharmacy, and housekeeping, were included. The consultant made clear that the decisions made would be what worked for this organization and were not a blueprint from another organization. The committees met weekly. Specific indirect and direct client-care activities that could be delegated to nonlicensed personnel in accordance with the state nurse practice act were identified. The committees decided that there would be two levels of clinical assistants. Job descriptions and work standards were developed for each level. Training workshops were developed, and a skill competency workshop was required for all new personnel. The hospital worked in conjunction with the local community college to offer certificates for the two clinical assistant levels. By the end of the program, 9.6 full-time RN positions were converted into 15.6 clinical assistant positions. The hospital predicted savings in recruitment, orientation, and training costs as well as increased job satisfaction for all participants. Esperanza thought that only time would tell if the program worked for both staff and clients.

Product Line Management

Product line management is used in business to create a center to plan, manage, and market a specific product within the larger company. In health-care delivery, use of this system results in a new organizational structure in which components of various clinical services or departments are merged to create a distinct "product line," such as drug abuse treatment, women's health care, or pediatric care. For example, the orthopedic product line would include nursing care, therapies, technician services, orthotic and prosthetic devices, and educational programs. In this type of delivery system, a product line manager directs these operations.

Unlike traditional systems in which the RN was the manager, the product line manager may be a member of a discipline other than nursing. In some instances, the manager may not even have a related health-care background (Christensen & Bender, 1994, p. 68). The non-nurse manager may have a substantial business and financial background and make purely business decisions regarding client care. Unfortunately, the non-nurse manager may have difficulty focusing on client and family needs that are incongruent with business decisions.

Differentiated Practice

Differentiated practice is the structuring of nursing roles and functions based on the individual's education, experience, and competence. Differentiated practice was the model for the first associate degree nursing programs. For example, a nurse with an associate degree would care for a client in a hospital under the supervision of a BSN nurse manager, whereas the nurse with a baccalaureate degree would plan the client's care in the home. The reasons for implementing a differentiated practice model focus on organizational and professional benefits (Huber, 2000):

◆ **Organizational benefits.** Decreasing costs and increasing efficiency, this argument describes differentiated practice as a means of better use of nursing resources.

◆ **Professional benefits.** This argument focuses on the need to decide what nursing is and what it is not and on delineating the role of the RN based on education. The most common models of differentiated nursing practice are based on nursing education (AONE, 1994):

◆ *Associate degree nurse.* The associate nurse is responsible for the shift of service, with a strong emphasis on meeting the physiological and comfort needs of the client assigned by the primary nurse. The associate nurse implements nursing care plans developed by the nurse clinician and primary nurse.

◆ *Baccalaureate degree nurse or primary nurse.* The primary nurse's responsibility extends from admission to discharge, focusing on coordination of medical and nursing orders, client education, and a well-planned, timely discharge. The primary nurse must be able to match client needs with staff abilities using an interdisciplinary team approach.

◆ *Master's degree nurse.* This advanced practice role may include the advanced registered nurse practitioner (ARNP), advanced practice nurse (APN), and certified nurse midwife (CNM). The APN is the case manager and client advocate. The ARNP extends beyond acute care into multiple health-care arenas.

Informally, differentiated practice among RNs exists in almost every setting. It occurs each time a nurse manager plans staff assignments according to the knowledge, competence, and licensure of the staff members involved, for example. Other members of the health-care team and even clients develop a "sixth sense" about the abilities of the nurses with whom they interact (McClure, 1991).

The controversy over RN licensure has raged within the profession since 1965, when the ANA endorsed the concept of two levels of educational preparation and licensure. Forty years later, the organization is still fighting the idea that "a nurse is a nurse is a nurse." Regardless of educational preparation or background, nurses are often used interchangeably in the workplace. The result is that they are not used in a cost-effective manner, and many are not challenged to reach their full potential. As the nursing shortage continues, differentiated

practice models are expanding to include LPNs, UAP, and other specially trained nurse extenders.

The rationale for implementing differentiated nursing practice is both professional and economic. Professionally, differentiated practice for the RN may lead to increased satisfaction and improved client care. Used effectively, differentiated practice models also ensure efficient use of nursing resources (Allender, Egan, & Newman, 1995; Koerner, et al., 1995; Ray & Hardin, 1995; Vena & Oldaker, 1994). Table 10-2 outlines the advantages and disadvantages of each model. Regardless of the client care delivery system, the shortage of professional nurses will continue to increase the use of UAP. The ANA defines UAP as "individuals trained to function in an assistive role to the registered professional nurse in the provision of patient/client care activities as delegated by and under the supervision of the registered

TABLE 10-2
Advantages and Disadvantages of Nursing Care Delivery Systems

Delivery System	Major Concept	Advantages	Disadvantages
TOTAL CARE	One RN with total responsibility for care	Continuity of care	Costly; not efficient use of staff
FUNCTIONAL	Division of tasks with clearly defined roles	Efficient, economical, productive	Fragments care
TEAM	RN team leader supervises ancillary staff	More holistic	RN must take time to delegate appropriately
MODULAR NURSING	Derivative of team nursing; takes structure of unit into account	More efficient than team	Substations must be organized on unit
PRIMARY CARE	RN maintains 24-hour responsibility for client(s)	Emphasis on accountability and client satisfaction	Extremely costly; primary nurse must be capable of meeting all client's needs
CASE MANAGEMENT	Management and coordination of care for episode of illness	Focuses on entire episode of illness; goal is achievement of outcomes	Nurse must be knowledgeable in coordinating care throughout illness
CLIENT-FOCUSED CARE	Services and staff organized around client needs	Interdisciplinary team approach	RN must be able to delegate and supervise; ancillary staff must be trained; organization of all services must be present on unit
PRODUCT LINE MANAGEMENT	Components of clinical services and departments organized around a distinct product	Makes distinct services available	Manager may not be a nurse or even have a health-care background
DIFFERENTIATED PRACTICE	Nursing roles and functions based on education, experience, and competence	Recognizes roles and functions of RN	Hard to overcome mentality of "a nurse is a nurse is a nurse"

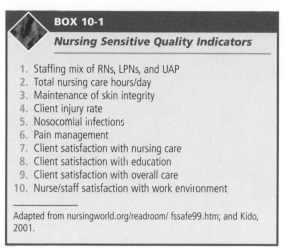

professional nurse" (Kido, 2001, p. 28). State nurse practice acts define the legal scope of nursing in each state and enumerate the nursing activities that cannot be delegated to UAP.

In March 1994, the ANA Board of Directors launched a major multiphase initiative to investigate the effect of health-care restructuring on the safety and quality of client care as well as on nursing. Through a program called Nursing's Safety and Quality Initiative, ANA highlights the strong linkages between nursing actions and client outcomes. In this initiative, many state nurses associations collect data on nursing-sensitive quality indicators. The list of 10 indicators is shown in Box 10-1.

The use of UAP need not affect patient safety or quality care. RNs must be actively involved in the training, educating, monitoring, and supervising of UAPs. Above all, the belief in the nurse-patient relationship as the foundation of professional nursing practice and the value placed on the delivery of direct patient care by the decision maker are central to maintaining positive outcomes for clients and nurses (Scott, Sochalski, & Aiken, 1999).

MONITORING AND EVALUATING THE QUALITY OF CARE

Quality management activities have been part of nursing care since Florence Nightingale

evaluated the care of soldiers during the Crimean War (Nightingale, 1992). Quality monitoring and standard setting occur through many avenues:

1. Professional organizations.
2. Federal and state governments.
3. State licensure.
4. Private accreditation.

Continuous quality improvement in health care is called by many names: quality assurance, total quality management (TQM), and continuous quality improvement (CQI) being the most common. Regardless of the term, TQM/CQI is a structured organizational process for involving personnel in planning and executing a continuous flow of improvements to provide quality health care that meets or exceeds expectations (McLaughlin & Kaluzny, 2006, p. 3).

Although quality improvement may be called by a varity of names, it usually involves common characteristics (McLaughlin & Caluzny, 2006, p 3):

◆ A link to key elements of the organizations' strategic plan.

◆ A quality council made up of the institution's top leadership.

◆ Training programs for all levels of personnel.

◆ Mechanisms for selecting improvement opportunities.

◆ Formation of process improvement teams.

◆ Staff support for process analysis and redesign.

◆ Personnel policies that motivate and support staff participation in process improvement.

Professional Organizations

Joint Commission on Accreditation of Healthcare Organizations

In 1951 the Joint Commission on Accreditation of Healthcare Organizations (JCAHO) was established. The focus of its evaluation at that time was on structural measures of quality, assessment of the physical plant, number of client beds per nurse, credentialing of service providers, and other standards for each department. This system of evaluation has given way to a more process- and outcome-focused model: CQI.

Today, JCAHO accredits more than 19,000 health-care organizations. Evaluation of nursing services is an important part of the accreditation. JCAHO-accredited agencies are measured against national standards set by health-care professionals. Hospitals, health-care networks, long-term care facilities, ambulatory care centers, home health agencies, behavioral health-care facilities, and clinical laboratories are among the organizations seeking JCAHO accreditation. Although accredita-

tion by JCAHO is voluntary, Medicare and Medicaid reimbursement cannot be sought by organizations not accredited by JCAHO.

American Nurses Association

Shortly after the establishment of JCAHO, the ANA began publishing standards related to nursing. Table 10-3 identifies current standards published by the American Nurses Credentialing Center.

Subjectively, most nurses agree that they recognize high-quality care when they see it. Objectively, however, quality in nursing care has been difficult to define. Quality encompasses effectiveness, efficiency, optimality (a balance between cost and effectiveness), acceptability,

---

TABLE 10-3
Certifications Available from the American Nurses Credentialing Center (AACC)

Specialty Certifications Baccalaureate RN, BC	Specialty Certifications Associate/Diploma RN, C	Modular Certification RN, C	Advanced Practice Certification ARNP, BC	Clinical Nurse Specialist
Cardiac/ Vascular Nurse	Cardiac/Vascular Nurse	Nursing Case Management	Acute Care NP	Community/Public Health Nurse
Community/Public Health Nurse	Gerontological Nurse	Ambulatory Nursing	Adult NP	Gerontological Nurse
Nursing Professional Development	Pediatric Nurse	Pain Management	Family NP	
Gerontology Nurse	Psychological/Mental Health Nurse		Gerontological NP	Medical-Surgical Nurse
Informatics Nurse; BSN in Nursing Informatics Nurse; BSN in other relevant field of study	Medical-Surgical Nurse		Pediatric NP	Pediatric Nurse
Medical-Surgical Nurse	Perinatal Nurse		Psychological/Mental Health NP Adult or Family	Adult or Child and Adolescent Psychological/Mental Health Nurse
Nursing Administration RN, CNA, BC			Advanced Diabetes Management NP	Advanced Diabetes Management
Pediatric Nurse				
Perinatal Nurse				
Psychological/Mental Health Nurse				

Adapted from American Nurses Credentialing Center, nursingworld.org/ancc/, accessed on November 26, 2005.

legitimacy (conformance to social norms and ethical principles), and equity (Donabedian quoted in Mark, Salyer, & Geddis, 1997). Should we strive for perfection in health care? Is it good enough to provide just adequate care? Leebov (1991) suggested considering the following before answering these questions:

◆ How many babies is it permissible to drop?

◆ How many medication errors are allowable in a week or a month?

◆ How many rude comments to clients is too many?

◆ How long can a call light be ignored?

JCAHO does not mandate a specific model to perform CQI. It does, however, have a survey of standards that address organizational performance in specific areas. The goal of the survey is to assess both what the organization says it does and what it actually accomplishes. As of 2006, all JCAHO surveys have been unannounced.

Institute of Medicine

Beginning in 1996, the Institute of Medicine (IOM) began publishing its Quality Chasm Series (available at jcaho.com). The series consists of the following publications:

◆ Crossing the Quality Chasm: The IOM Health Care Quality Initiative (1996).

◆ Crossing the Quality Chasm: A New Health System for the 21st Century (2001).

◆ Leadership by Example: Governmental Roles (2003).

◆ Health Professions Education: A Bridge to Quality (2003).

◆ Keeping Patients Safe: Transforming the Work Environment of Nurses (2004).

◆ Academic Health Centers: Leading Change in the 21st Century (2004).

The IOM idenitifed essential competencies necessary for health-care providers to move health care into the 21st century (IOM, 2003):

◆ Provide client-centered care.

◆ Work in interdisciplinary teams.

◆ Employ evidence-based practice (EBP).

◆ Apply quality improvement.

◆ Utilize informatics.

Focusing on medical errors, the IOM found that at least 44,000 and as many as 98,000 people die in hospitals each year from preventable medical errors. The total cost of these errors is estimated to be between $17 billion and $29 billion per year. The impact of medical errors is costly in terms of loss of trust, physical and psychological discomfort, loss of morale, reduced work productivity, reduced school attendance, and lower levels of population health status (IOM, 1999). JCAHO developed the International Center for Patient Safety, which establishes patient safety goals each year. Health-care facilities wishing to be accredited must conform to these patient safety goals. Box 10-2 describes the work of the International Center for Patient Safety.

In May 2005, JCAHO affirmed its "do not use" list of abbreviations. Current information on the "do not us" list, patient safety goals, and other JCAHO information related to patient safety can be found on the JCAHO Web site at jcaho.org. It is your responsibility to be aware of the patient safety guidelines and requirements in your facility. It is also your responsibility to report any information related to a

---

BOX 10-2

Joint Commission International Center for Patient Safety

1. Sets patient safety standards.
2. Implements and oversees sentinel event policy and advisory group.
3. Publishes *Sentinel Event Alert* newsletter and quality check reports.
4. Sets yearly national patient safety goals.
5. Developed the universal protocol related to surgical procedures.
6. Evaluates organizations' monitoring of quality of care issues.
7. Conducts patient safety research.
8. Provides patient safety resources.
9. Supports the Speak Up program.
10. Involved with patient safety coalitions and legistative efforts.

Adapted from Joint Commission on Accreditation of Healthcare Organizations (JCAHO), accessed on November 26, 2005, from jcipatientsafety.org

lack of safety. Most of the time, errors are a result of fauty systems, processes, and conditions, causing people to make mistakes or at least fail to prevent them. The patient safety guidelines are intended to focus facilities systems to design more preventive health-care systems. However, safer systems will never take the place of human vigilance and responsibility. Nursing-caused client errors are generally the result of medication errors, knowledge errors, or procedure errors (Simpson, 2005).

Medication errors. Nurses are responsible for following the rules learned in their fundamental nursing courses about giving medications. However, information systems and health-care delivery processes can be designed to intercept the human errors that inevitably occur. Programmable "smart" pumps and bar codes are tools that can save money and prevent errors.

Knowledge errors. Given the rapid changes and advancements in medicine, it is impossible for nurses to know everything. But nurses can utilize current research evidence (evidence-based medicine), clinical expertise, and client preferences in planning and implementing care. Performing EBP allows nurses to put research-based knowledge into practice.

Procedural errors. Nurses function as a surveillance system for early detection of and intervention against adverse occurrences and as the institutional advocate for patients. Surveillance is influenced by nurse staffing adequacy. Nurses' error rates increase significantly during overtime, after 12 hours per day, and more than 60 hours per week (Rogers, et al., 2004). Clinical decision support systems and point of care computers that automate care management through monitoring can enable nurses to make the best decision in the least amount of time.

CQI

CQI is a process of identifying areas of concern (indicators), continuously collecting data on these indicators, analyzing and evaluating the data, and implementing needed changes. When the indicator is no longer a concern, another indicator is selected. Common indicators include the number of falls, medication errors, and infection rates. Indicators can be identified by the accrediting agency and/or by the facility itself. The purpose of CQI is to continuously improve the capability of everyone involved in providing care, including the organization itself. Early quality programs concentrated mainly on structure and processes; the focus today is on identifying key performance indicators of nursing care and defining the patient outcomes that nurses directly or indirectly influence. These outcomes are measured and attributed to nursing (Long, 2003).

CQI consists of four basic elements (McLaughlin & Kaluzny, 2006):

1. Localized improvement efforts.
2. Organizational learning.
3. Process reengineering.
4. Evidence-based medicine and management.

CQI relies on collecting information and analyzing it. The time frame used in a CQI program can be retrospective (evaluating past performance), concurrent (evaluating current performance), or prospective (future-oriented, collecting data as they come in). The procedures used to collect data depend on the purpose of the program. Data may be by observation, performance appraisals, client satisfaction surveys, statistical analyses of length-of-stay and costs, surveys, peer reviews, and chart audits (Huber, 2000).

In the CQI framework, data collection is everyone's responsibility. You may be asked to brainstorm your ideas with other nurses or members of the interdisciplinary team, complete surveys or check sheets, or keep a time log of your daily activities for a week or longer. Collecting comprehensive, accurate, and representative data is the first step in revisiting the process. How do you actually administer medications to a group of clients? What steps are involved? Are the medications always available at the right time and in the right dose, or do you have to wait for the pharmacy to bring them to the floor? Is the pharmacy technician delayed by emergency orders that must be processed? Looking at the entire process and mapping it out on paper in the form of a flowchart may be part of the CQI process for your organization (Fig. 10-2).

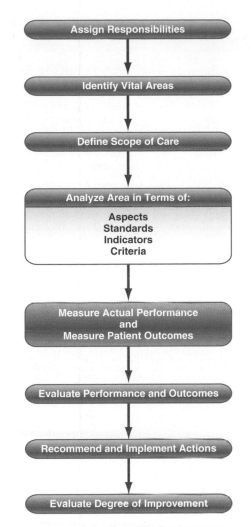

FIGURE 10-2 ◆ Unit level quality improvement process. (Adapted from Hunt, D.V. [1992]. *Quality in America: How to Implement a Competitive Quality Program.* Homewood, IL: Business One Irwin; and Duquette, A.M. [1991]. Approaches to monitoring practice: Getting started. In Schroeder, P. [ed.]. *Monitoring and Evaluation in Nursing.* Gaithersburg, MD: Aspen.)

Aspects of Health Care to Evaluate

Three aspects of health care can be evaluated in a CQI program: the structure within which the care is given, the process of giving care, and the outcome of that care. To be comprehensive, an evaluation program must include all three aspects (Brook, Davis, & Kamberg, 1980; Donabedian, 1969, 1977, 1987). When focused on nursing care, the independent, dependent, and interdependent functions of nurses may be added to the model (Irvine,

1998). Each of these dimensions is described here, and their interrelationship is illustrated in Table 10-4.

Structure

Structure refers to the setting in which the care is given and the resources (human, financial, and material) that are available. It is the easiest of the three aspects to measure and yet is still overlooked in some evaluation procedures. The following is a list of some of the structural aspects of a health-care organization that can be evaluated:

◆ **Facilities.** Comfort, convenience of layout, accessibility of support services, and safety.

◆ **Equipment.** Adequate supplies, state-of-the-art equipment, and staff ability to use equipment.

◆ **Staff.** Credentials, experience, absenteeism, turnover rate, staff-client ratios.

◆ **Finances.** Salaries, adequacy, sources.

Although none of these structural factors alone can guarantee that good care will be given, they can make good care more likely. A higher level of nurses each shift and a higher proportion of RNs in the skill mix are structural factors that are associated with shorter lengths of stay; higher proportions of RNs are also related to fewer adverse patient outcomes (Lichtig, Knauf, & Milholland, 1999; Rogers, et al., 2004).

A common pitfall in evaluating structural factors, however, has been to neglect the other two aspects, process and outcome. The following example illustrates the problems that occur when only structure is evaluated:

A hospital measured the quality of nursing care given in its eight-bed critical care unit by comparing its staffing ratio with the standard ratio of one nurse to two clients. The inadequacy of this structural measure became apparent during a period when the unit had six (out of a total of eight) clients who each required the care of one nurse. Under the standard that was set, only four nurses were on duty, which created a severe staff shortage because seven nurses were actually needed to provide adequate care.

Process

Process refers to the activities carried out by the health-care providers and the decisions

		TABLE 10-4		

TABLE 10-4
Dimensions of Quality Improvement in Nursing: Examples

	Independent Function	Dependent Function	Interdependent Function
STRUCTURE	Pressure ulcer risk assessment form available	High-speed automatic dial-up system puts nurses in touch with physicians rapidly	Nursing case management model of care adopted on rehabilitation unit
PROCESS	Assesses risk for development of pressure ulcer and implements preventive measures	Order to increase dosage of pain medication obtained and processed within 1 hour	Communicates with therapists about need for customized wheelchair
OUTCOME	Skin intact at discharge	Relief from pain	Able to enter narrow doorway to bathroom unassisted

Adapted from Irvine, D. (1998). Finding value in nursing care: A framework for quality improvement and clinical evaluation. *Nursing Economics,* 16(3), 110–118.

made from the time an individual approaches the health-care system through assessment, diagnosis, treatment, and follow-up care (Irvine, 1998). Examples include the following:

◆ Setting an appointment.

◆ Conducting a physical assessment.

◆ Ordering a radiograph and magnetic resonance imaging scan.

◆ Administering a blood transfusion.

◆ Completing a home environment assessment.

◆ Preparing the client for discharge.

◆ Telephoning the client post discharge.

Each of these processes can be evaluated in terms of timeliness, appropriateness, accuracy, and completeness (Irvine, 1998). Process variables include psychosocial interventions, such as teaching and counseling, as well as physical care measures. It can include leadership activities, such as interdisciplinary team conferences. When process data are collected, a set of objectives, procedures, or guidelines is needed to serve as a standard or gauge against which to compare the activities. This set can be highly specific, such as listing all the steps in a catheterization procedure, or it can be a list of objectives, such as: offer information on breastfeeding to all expectant parents or conduct weekly staff meetings.

The ANA Standards of Care are process standards. These standards answer the question: What should the nurse be doing, and

what process should he/she follow to ensure quality care?

Outcome

An outcome is the result of activities in which the health-care providers have been involved. Outcome measures evaluate the effectiveness of these nursing activities by answering such questions as: Did the patient recover? Is the family more independent now? Has team functioning improved? Outcome standards address indicators such as physical and mental health status, social and physical function, health attitudes/knowledge/behavior, utilization of services, and customer satisfaction (Huber, 2000).

These questions are very general and reflect overall goals of health-care providers and the organizations in which they work. The outcome questions asked during an evaluation should be far more specific and should measure observable behavior, such as the following:

Client: Wound healed; blood pressure within normal limits; infection absent.

Family: Increased time between visits to the emergency department; applied for food stamps.

Team: Decisions reached by consensus; attendance at meetings by all team members.

Some of these outcomes, such as blood pressure or time between emergency department visits, are easier to measure than are other, equally important, outcomes, such as increased satisfaction or changes in attitude. Although the latter cannot be measured as precisely, it is still important to include them so that the full spectrum of biological, psychological, and social aspects are represented (Strickland, 1997). For this reason, considerable effort has been put into identifying the client outcomes that are affected by the quality of nursing care. As mentioned earlier, the ANA identified 10 quality indicators in acute care that are likely to relate to the availability and quality of professional nursing services in hospitals. Across the United States, data are being collected from nursing units using these quality indicators.

A major problem in using and interpreting outcome measures in evaluation is that outcomes are influenced by many factors. For example:

The outcome of client teaching done by a nurse on a home visit is affected by the client's interest and ability to learn, the quality of the teaching materials, the presence or absence of family support, information from other caregivers (which may conflict), and the environment in which the teaching is done. If the teaching is successful, can the nurse be given full credit for the success? If it is not successful, who has failed?

It is necessary to evaluate the process as well as the outcome to determine why an intervention such as client teaching succeeds or fails. A comprehensive evaluation includes all three aspects: structure, process, and outcome. However, it is much more difficult to gather and monitor outcome data than to measure structure or process.

In the early 2000s, the IOM put several issues related to health-care quality before the public. In addition to safety, the IOM looked at health-care delivery systems, racial and ethnic disparities, and the 2003 publication Keeping Patients Safe: Transforming the Work Environment of Nurses (IOM, 2004). Interest in quality of care has clearly moved from the professional to the public domain. Who are the interested parties?

QUALITY IMPROVEMENT AND ORGANIZATIONAL AND UNIT LEVEL

Strategic Planning

Leaders and managers are so often preoccupied with immediate issues that they lose sight of their ultimate objectives. Quality cannot be found at the unit level if the organization is not focusing on quality issues. In order to stay on track, an organization needs a strategic plan. A strategic plan is a short, visionary, conceptual document that (planware.org/strategy.htm):

◆ Serves as a framework for decisions or for securing support/approval.

◆ Provides a basis for more detailed planning.

◆ Explains the business to others in order to inform, motivate, and involve.

◆ Assists benchmarking and performance monitoring.

◆ Stimulates change and becomes the building block for the next plan.

During the strategic planning process, the organization develops or reviews its vision, mission statement, and corporate values. The group develops business objectives and key strategies to meet these objectives. In order to do this, a SWOT analysis is done—a review of the organization's Strengths, Weaknesses, Opportunities, and Threats. Key strategies are identified, and action plans developed. The organization's mission, goals, and strategic plan ultimately drive the outcomes and quality improvement plan for that organization. Be proactive, and participate in the process. Ask your nurse manager if there are opportunities for the staff to participate in the planning process.

Issues related to quality improvement may come out of the strategic planning process. More often, they are identified at the unit level. Quality issues are not often apparent to senior managers. The impact of these issues, however, is often felt by staff.

Once a process that needs improvement is identified, a team is organized. The team members need to have knowledge of the identified process; therefore, team members change depending on the issue to be addressed. The suggestion from the IOM that health care have an interdisciplinary team focus is present in quality improvement planning. The team identifies and analyzes problems, discusses solutions, and evaluates changes. The team clarifies the current knowledge of the process. Causes

BOX 10-3

Questions the Team Needs to Ask

1. Who are our customers, stakeholders, markets?
2. What do they expect from us?
3. What are we trying to accomplish?
4. What changes do we think will make an improvement?
5. How and when will we pilot-test our predicted improvement?
6. What do we expect to learn from the pilot test?
7. What will we do with negative results? positive results?
8. How will we implement the change?
9. How will we measure success?
10. What did we learn as a team from this experience?
11. What changes would we make for the future?

Adapted from McLaughlin, C., & Kaluzny, A. (2006). *Continuous Quality Improvement in Health Care: Theory, Implementations, and Applications.* 3rd ed. Massachsetts: Jones & Bartlett.

of variations in the process are identified, and the team works to unify the process.

Box 10-3 identifies questions that team members might ask as they work on the quality improvement plan.

Most agencies have tools for tracking outcomes. These tools are called *structured care methodologies* (SCMs). SCMs are interdisciplinary tools to "identify best practices, facilitate standardization of care, and provide a mechanism for variance tracking, quality enhancement, outcomes measurement, and outcomes research" (Cole & Houston, 1999, p. 53). SCMs include guidelines, protocols, algorithms, standards of care, critical pathways, and order sets.

◆ **Guidelines.** Guidelines first appeared in the 1980s as statements to assist health-care providers and clients in making appropriate health-care decisions. Guidelines are based on current research strategies and are often developed by experts in the field. The use of guidelines is seen as a way to decrease variations in practice.

◆ **Protocols.** Protocols are specific, formal documents that outline how a procedure or intervention should be conducted. Protocols have been used for many years in research and specialty areas but have been introduced into general health care as a way to standardize approaches to achieve

desired outcomes. An example in many facilities is a chest pain protocol.

◆ **Algorithms.** Algorithms are systematic procedures that follow a logical progression based on additional information or client responses to treatment. They were originally developed in mathematics and are frequently seen in emergency medical services. Advanced cardiac life support algorithms are now widely used in health-care agencies.

◆ **Standards of care.** Standards of care are often discipline-related and help to operationalize client care processes and provide a baseline for quality care. Lawyers often refer to a discipline's standards of care in evaluating whether a client has received appropriate services.

◆ **Critical (or clinical) pathways.** Critical pathways were first used in manufacturing during the late 1950s and appeared in health care in the 1980s. A critical pathway is a "multidisciplinary map" that outlines the expected course of treatment for clients with similar diagnoses. The critical pathway should easily orient the nurse to the client outcomes for the day. In some institutions, nursing diagnoses with specific time frames are incorporated into the critical pathway. This standardized map is designed to describe the course of events that lead to successful client outcome within the diagnosis-related group (DRG)–defined time frame. For the client with an uncomplicated myocardial infarction (MI), a proposed course of events leading to successful client outcomes within the 4-day DRG-defined time frame might be as follows (Doenges, Moorhouse, & Geissler, 1997):

◆ Client states that chest pain is relieved.

◆ ST- and T-wave changes resolve, and pulse oximeter reading is greater than 90%; client has clear breath sounds.

◆ Client ambulates in hall without experiencing extreme fatigue or chest pain.

◆ Client verbalizes feelings about having an MI and future fears; client identifies effective coping strategies.

◆ Ventricular dysfunction, dysrhythmia, or crackles resolved.

Critical pathways are clinical protocols involving all disciplines. They are designed for tracking a planned clinical course for clients based on average and expected lengths of stay. Financial outcomes can be evaluated from critical pathways by assessing any variances from the proposed length of stay. The health-care agency can then focus on problems within the system that extend the length of stay or drive up costs because of overutilization or repetition of services. For example:

Mr. J. was admitted to the telemetry unit with a diagnosis of MI. He had no previous history of heart disease and no other complicating factors such as diabetes, hypertension, or elevated cholesterol levels. His DRG-prescribed length of stay was 4 days. He had an uneventful hospitalization for the first 2 days. On the third day, he complained of pain in the left calf. The calf was slightly reddened and warm to the touch. This condition was diagnosed as thrombophlebitis, which increased his length of hospitalization. A review of the events leading up to the complaints of calf pain by the case manager indicated that, although the physician ordered compression stockings for Mr. J., the stockings never arrived, and no one followed through on the order. The variances related to his proposed length of stay were discussed with the team providing care, and measures were instituted to make sure that this oversight would not occur again.

Critical pathways provide a framework for communication and documentation of care. They are also excellent teaching tools through which staff members from various disciplines can learn about the expected care of given client populations and an institution's practice patterns. Critical pathways can be used by an institution to evaluate the cost of care for different client populations (Capuano, 1995; Crummer & Carter, 1993; Flarey, 1995; Lynam, 1994).

Most institutions have adopted a chronological, diagrammatic format for presenting a critical pathway. Time frames may range from daily (day 1, day 2, day 3) to hourly, depending on client needs. Key elements of the critical pathway include discharge planning, client education, consultations, activities, nutrition, medications, diagnostic tests, and treatment (Crummer & Carter, 1993). Table 10-5 is an example of a critical pathway. Although originally developed for use in acute care institutions, critical pathways can be developed for home care and long-term care. The client's nurse is usually responsible for monitoring and recording any deviations from the critical pathway. When deviations occur, the reasons are discussed with all members of the health-care team, and the appropriate changes in care are made. The nurse must identify general trends in client outcomes and develop plans to improve the quality of care to reduce the number of deviations. Through this close monitoring, the health-care team can avoid last-minute surprises that may delay client discharge and can more effectively predict lengths of stay.

SCMs may be used alone or together. A client who is admitted for an MI may have care planned using a critical pathway for his acute MI, a heparin protocol, and a dysrhythmia algorithm. In addition, the nurses may refer to the standards of care in developing a traditional nursing care plan.

SCMs can improve physiological, psychological, and financial outcomes. Services and interventions are sequenced to provide safe and effective outcomes in a designated time and with most effective use of resources. They also give an interdisciplinary perspective that is not found in the traditional nursing care plan. Computer programs allow health-care personnel to track variances (differences from the identified standard) and use these variances in planning quality improvement activities.

The use of SCMs does not take the place of the expert clinical judgment of the RN. The fundamental purpose of the SCM is to assist health-care providers in implementing practices identified with good clinical judgment, research-based interventions, and improved client outcomes. Data from SCMs allow comparisons of outcomes, development of research based decisions, identification of high-risk clients, and identification of issues and problems before they escalate into pending disasters. Do not be afraid to learn and understand the different SCMs.

You may hear nurses talking about root cause analysis. *Root cause analysis* is the process of learning from consequences. The consequences can be desirable, but most root cause analysis deals with adverse consequences. An example of a root cause analysis is a review of a medication error, especially one resulting in a death or severe complications. Principles of root cause analysis include:

ND and Categories of Care	Day 1 _____	Day 2 _____	Day 3 _____	Day 4 _____
Decreased cardiac output R/T decreased myocardial contractility, altered electrical conduction, structural changes	Goals Participate in actions to reduce cardiac workload	Display VS within acceptable limits; dysrhythmias controlled; pulse oximetry within acceptable range → Meet own self-care needs with assist as necessary	Dysrhythmias controlled or absent → Free of signs of respiratory distress Demonstrate measurable increase in activity tolerance	→
Fluid volume: excess R/T compromised regulatory mechanism	Verbalize understanding of fluid/food restrictions	Verbalize understanding of general condition and health-care needs Breath sounds clearing Urinary output adequate Weight loss (reflecting fluid loss)	Plan for lifestyle/ behavior changes Breath sounds clear Balanced I&O Edema resolving	Plan in place to meet postdischarge needs Weight stable (continued loss if edema present)
Referrals	Cardiology Dietitian	Cardiac rehabilitation Occupational therapist (for ADLs) Social services Home care	Community resources	
Diagnostic studies	ECG Echo-Doppler CXR ABGs/pulse oximetry Cardiac enzymes BUN/Cr CBC, electrolytes Mg^{++} PT/aPTT Liver function studies Serum glucose Albumin Uric acid Digoxin level (as indicated)	Echo-Doppler (if not done day 1) or MUGA Cardiac enzymes (if ↑) BUN/Cr Electrolytes PT/aPTT (if on anticoagulants)	CXR BUN/Cr Electrolytes PT/aPTT (as indicated) Repeat digoxin level (if indicated)	

ND and Categories of Care	Day 1 _____	Day 2 _____	Day 3 _____	Day 4 _____
Additional assessments	UA			
	Apical pulse, heart/breath sounds q8h →		→ bid	→
	Cardiac rhythm (telemetry) q4h →		→ D/C	→
	B/P, P.R. q2h until stable, q4h Temp q8h →	q8h	→	→
	I&O q8h →		→	→ D/C
	Weight qAM →		→	→
	Peripheral edema q8h →		→	→ qd
	Peripheral pulses q8h →		→	→ D/C
	Sensorium q8h →		→	→ D/C
	DX check qd →		→	→
	Response to activity →		→	→
	Response to therapeutic interventions →		→	→
Medications Allergies: _____ _____	IV diuretic →	po	→	→
	ACE inhibitor →		→	→
	Digoxin →		→	→
	PO/cutaneous nitrates →		→	→
	Morphine sulfate →		→ D/C	
	Daytime/HS sedation →		→	→ D/C
	PO/low-dose anticoagulant →		→ PO or D/C	→
	IV/PO potassium →		→ D/C	
	Stool softener/ laxative →		→	→
Client education	Orient to unit/room	Cardiac education per protocol	Signs/systems to report to health-care provider	Provide written instructions for home care
	Review advance directives	Review medications: dose, time, route, purpose, side effects	Plan for home care needs	Schedule for follow-up appointments
	Discuss expected outcomes, diagnostic tests/ results	Progressive activity program		
	Fluid/nutritional restrictions/ needs	Skin care		

(Continued on following page)

TABLE 10-5 *(Continued)* **Sample Critical Pathway: Heart Failure, Hospital. ELOS 4 Days Cardiology or Medical Unit**				
ND and Categories of Care	Day 1 _____	Day 2 _____	Day 3 _____	Day 4 _____
Additional nursing actions	Bed/chair rest →	BPR/ambulate as tolerated, cardiac program →	Up ad lib/graded program →	
	Assist with physical care →	→		→ (send home)
	Egg-crate mattress →	→		→
	Dysrhythmia/angina care per protocol →	→	D/C	
	Supplemental O_2 →	→		→
	Cardiac diet →	→		→

CP = critical path; ELOS = estimated length of stay; ND = nursing diagnosis.
Doenges, M.E., Moorhouse, M.F., and Geissler, A.C. (2002). *Nursing Care Plans: Guidelines for Individualizing Patient Care,* ed. 6, pp. 59–60. Philadelphia: FA Davis, with permission.

1. Determine what influenced the consequences, i.e., determine the necessary and sufficient influences that explain the nature and the magnitude of the consequences.

2. Establish tightly linked chains of influence.
3. At every level of analysis, determine the necessary and sufficient influences.
4. Whenever feasible, drill down to root causes.
5. There are always multiple root causes.

A most important part of any quality plan is how success is measured. There is not one specified point in the CQI process where one needs to start measuring. Measurement and analysis should be done on a continuous basis. There are numerous tools and techniques used in organiztions to monitor and improve processes. Table 10-6 identifies some of the measurement tools used in CQI.

TABLE 10-6 **Measurement Tools Used in Quality**	
FLOWCHARTS AND DIAGRAMS	Pictorial representation of how a process works by tracing the steps from start to finish
CAUSE AND EFFECT DIAGRAMS (ISHIKAWA OR FISHBONE DIAGRAMS)	Identify sources of variation once the process has been documented with a flowchart
PARETO DIAGRAMS OR HISTOGRAMS	Bar diagrams to display data
RUN CHARTS	Chart ongoing data to observe trends
REGRESSION ANALYSIS	Statistical analysis of data to support hypotheses
CONTROL CHARTS	Identify if the process is or remains under control

Adapted from McLaughlin, C. & Kaluzny, A. (2006). *Continuous Quality Improvement in Health Care,* 3rd ed. Massachusetts: Jones and Bartlett.

RISK MANAGEMENT

An important part of CQI is risk management. Defined as a process of identifying, analyzing, treating, and evaluating real and potential hazards, *risk management* addresses liability and financial loss. JCAHO recommends the integration of a quality control/risk management program in order to monitor and maintain continuous feedback and communication. In order to plan proactively, an organization must identify real or potential exposures that might threaten it. As you saw from the statistics on medical errors, health care is a high-risk business. As a nurse, it is your responsibility to report adverse incidents to the risk manager. In many states, this duty is written into law.

Risk events are categorized according to severity. Although all untoward events are important, not all carry the same severity of outcomes (Benson-Flynn, 2001).

1. **Service occurrence.** A service occurrence is an unexpected occurrence that does not result in a clinically significant interruption of services and that is without apparent client or employee injury. Examples of a service occurrence include minor property or equipment damage, unsatisfactory provision of service at any level, or inconsequential interruption of service. Most occurrences in this category are addressed within the client complaint process.

2. **Serious incident.** A serious incident results in a clinically significant interruption of therapy or service, minor injury to a client or employee, or significant loss or damage of equipment or property. Minor injuries are usually defined as needing medical intervention outside of hospital admission or physical or psychological damage.

3. **Sentinel events.** A sentinel event is an unexpected occurrence involving death or serious/permanent physical or psychological injury, or the risk thereof. The phrase, "or the risk thereof" includes any process variation for which a recurrence would carry a significant chance of a serious adverse outcome. Such events are called sentinel because they signal the need for immediate investigation and response. When a sentinel event occurs in a health-care organization, it is necessary that appropriate individuals within the organization be made aware of the event, they investigate and understand

the causes that underlie the event, and they make changes in the organization's systems and processes to reduce the probability of such an event in the future (jcaho.org/ptsafety_frm.html).

The subset of sentinel events that is subject to review by JCAHO includes any occurrence that meets any of the following criteria:

◆ The event has resulted in an unanticipated death or major permanent loss of function, not related to the natural course of the client's illness or underlying condition.

◆ The event is one of the following (even if the outcome was not death or major permanent loss of function):

  ◆ Suicide of a client in a setting where the client receives around-the-clock care (e.g., hospital, residential treatment center, crisis stabilization center).

  ◆ Infant abduction or discharge to the wrong family.

  ◆ Rape.

  ◆ Hemolytic transfusion reaction involving administration of blood or blood products having major blood group incompatibilities.

  ◆ Surgery on the wrong client or wrong body part (jcaho.org/ptsafety_frm.html).

Adhering to nursing standards of care as well as the policies and procedures of the institution greatly decreases the nurse's risk. Common areas of risk for nursing include:

◆ Medication errors.

◆ Documentation errors and/or omissions.

◆ Failure to correctly perform nursing care or treatments.

◆ Errors in patient safety that result in falls.

◆ Failure to communicate significant data to clients and other providers (Swansburg & Swansburg, 2002).

Risk management programs also include attention to areas of employee wellness and prevention of injury. Latex allergies, repetitive stress injuries and carpal tunnel syndrome, barrier protection for tuberculosis, back injuries, and the rise of antibiotic-resistant organisms all fall under the attention of risk management (Huber, 2000).

Adhering to standards of care and exercising the amount of care that a reasonable nurse would demonstrate under the same or similar circumstances can protect the nurse from negligent litigation. Understanding what actions to take when something goes wrong is imperative. The main goal is client safety. Reporting and remediation must occur quickly (Huber, 2000).

Once an incident has occurred, an incident report must be completed. The incident report is used to collect and analyze data for future determination of risk. The incident report should be completed in a timely manner. It should be accurate, objective, complete, and factual. If there is future litigation, the plaintiff's attorney can subpoena the report. The incident report should be prepared in only a single copy and never placed in the medical record (Swansburg & Swansburg, 2002). It is kept with internal hospital correspondence.

Nurses have a responsibility to remain educated and informed and to become active participants in understanding and identifying potential risks to their clients and to themselves. Ignorance of the law is no excuse. Maintaining a knowledgeable, professional, and caring nurse-client relationship is the first step in decreasing your own risk.

CONCLUSION

Pressure from JCAHO and health-care consumers, payers, and providers has caused the focus in the health-care system to shift from client care to issues of cost and quality. Experts indicate that quality promotes decreased costs and increased satisfaction. This is an opportunity for nurses to become more professional and empowered to organize and manage client care so that it is safe, efficient, and of the highest quality. Begin early in your career to actively participate in quality improvement initiatives.

Regardless of the care model used or the indicators selected, in patient care delivery focus attention on the following (Hansten, & Washburn, 2001, p. 24D):

1. **Think critically.** Use your creative, intuitive, logical, and analytical processes continually in working with clients.
2. **Plan and report outcomes.** Emphasizing results is a necessary part of managing resources in today's cost-conscious environment. Focusing on the outcomes moves the nurse out of the mindset of just focusing on tasks.
3. **Make introductory rounds.** Begin each shift with the health-care team members introducing themselves, describing their roles, and providing clients updates.
4. **Plan in partnership with the client.** In conjunction with the introductory rounds, spend a few minutes early in the shift with each client discussing shift objectives and long-term goals. This event becomes the center of the nursing process for the shift and ensures that the client and nurse are working toward the same outcomes.
5. **Communicate the plan.** Avoid confusion among members of the team by communicating the intended outcomes and the important role that each member plays in the plan.
6. **Evaluate progress.** Schedule time during the shift to quickly evaluate outcomes and the progress of the plan and to make revisions as necessary.

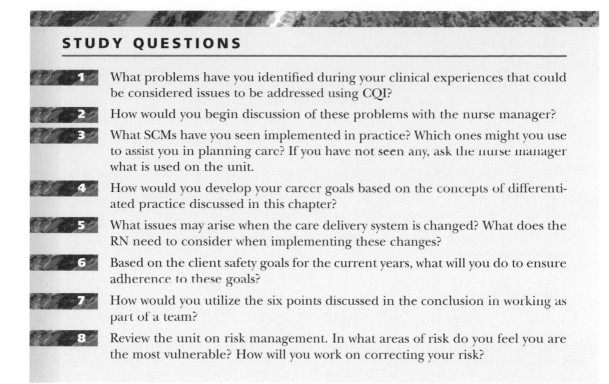

STUDY QUESTIONS

1   What problems have you identified during your clinical experiences that could be considered issues to be addressed using CQI?

2   How would you begin discussion of these problems with the nurse manager?

3   What SCMs have you seen implemented in practice? Which ones might you use to assist you in planning care? If you have not seen any, ask the nurse manager what is used on the unit.

4   How would you develop your career goals based on the concepts of differentiated practice discussed in this chapter?

5   What issues may arise when the care delivery system is changed? What does the RN need to consider when implementing these changes?

6   Based on the client safety goals for the current years, what will you do to ensure adherence to these goals?

7   How would you utilize the six points discussed in the conclusion in working as part of a team?

8   Review the unit on risk management. In what areas of risk do you feel you are the most vulnerable? How will you work on correcting your risk?

CRITICAL THINKING EXERCISE

The director of CQI has called a meeting of all the staff members on your floor. Based on last quarter's statistics, the length of stay of clients with uncontrolled diabetes is 2.6 days longer than that of clients for the first half of the year. She has requested that the staff identify members who wish to be CQI team members looking at this problem. You, the staff nurse, have volunteered to be a member of the team. The team will consist of the diabetes educator, a client-focused care assistant, a pharmacist, and you.

1. Why were these people selected for the team?

2. What data need to be collected to evaluate this situation?

3. What are the potential outcomes for clients with uncontrolled diabetes?

4. Develop a flowchart of a typical hospital stay for a client with uncontrolled diabetes.

WEB SITES

jcaho.org/: Joint Commission on Accreditation of Healthcare Organizations
ahcpr.gov/: Agency for Healthcare Research and Quality
nursingworld.org: American Nurses Association
nursingworld.org/ancc/faqs.htm#bac: American Nurses Association Credentialing Center

REFERENCES

Allender, C., Egan, E., & Newman, M. (1995). An instrument for measuring differentiated nursing practice. *Nursing Management*, 26(4), 42–45.

American Organization of Nurse Executives (AONE). (1994). Differentiated competencies for nursing practice. *Nursing Management*, 25(9), 34.

Benson-Flynn, J. (2001). Incident reporting: Clarifying occurrences, incidents, and sentinel events. *Home Healthcare Nurse*, 19, 701–706.

Betta, P.A. (1992). Developing a successful ambulatory QA program. *Nursing Management*, 23(4), 31–33, 47–54.

Brook, R.H., Davis, A.R., & Kamberg, C. (1980). Selected reflections on quality of medical care evaluations in the 1980s. *Nursing Research*, 29(2), 127.

Capuano, T.A. (1995). Clinical pathways. *Nursing Management*, 26(1), 34–37.

Chang, C., Price, S., & Pfoutz, S. (2001). *Economics and Nursing*. Philadelphia: FA Davis.

Christensen, P., & Bender, L. (1994). Models of nursing care in a changing environment: Current challenges and future directions. *Orthopaedic Nursing*, 13(2), 64–70.

Clouten, K., & Weber, R. (1994). Patient–focused care...playing to win. *Nursing Management*, 25(2), 34–36.

Cole, L., & Houston, S. (1999). Structured care methodologies: Evolution and use in patient care delivery. *Outcomes Management for Nursing Practice*, 3(2), 53–60.

Crummer, M.B., & Carter, V (1993). Critical pathways: The pivotal tool. *Cardiovascular Nursing*, 7(4), 30–37.

Doenges, M.E., Moorhouse, M.F., & Geissler, A.C. (1997). *Nursing Care Plans: Guidelines for Individualizing Patient Care*, 4th ed. Philadelphia: FA Davis.

Donabedian, A. (1969). A guide to medical care administration. In *Medical Care Appraisal: Quality and Utilization*, vol. II. New York: American Public Health Association.

Donabedian, A. (1977). Evaluating the quality of medical care. *Milbank Memorial Fund Quarterly*, 44 (part 2), 166.

Donabedian, A. (1987). Some basic issues in evaluating the quality of health care. In Rinke, L.T. (ed.). *Outcome Measures in Home Care*. New York: National League of Nursing.

Duquette, A.M. (1991). Approaches to monitoring practice: Getting started. In Schroeder, P. (ed.). *Monitoring and Evaluation in Nursing*. Gaithersburg, MD: Aspen.

Flarey, D.L. (1995). *Redesigning Nursing Care Delivery*. Philadelphia: JB Lippincott.

Girard, N. (1994). The case management model of patient care delivery. *AORN Journal*, 60, 403–415.

Greenberg, L. (1994). Work redesign: An overview. *Journal of Emergency Nursing*, 20(3), 28A–32A.

Hansten, R., & Washburn, M. (2001). Outcomes-based care delivery. *American Journal of Nursing*, 101(2), 24A-D.

Harrison, J., Nolin, J., & Suero, E. (2004). The effect of case management on U.S. hospitals. *Nursing Economics*, 22(2), 64–70.

Heinrich, J. (2001). Nursing Workforce: Emerging Nurse Shortages due to Multiple Factors. Report to the Chairman, Subcommittee on Health, Committee on Ways and Means, House of Representatives, July 2001. ERIC Document ED 455 385.

Huber, D. (2000). *Leadership and Nursing Care Management*, 2nd ed. Philadelphia: WB Saunders.

Hunt, D.V. (1992). *Quality in America: How to Implement a Competitive Quality Program*. Homewood, IL: Business One Irwin.

Institute of Medicine. (2001). *Crossing the Quality Chasm: A New Health System for the 21st century*. National Academies Press. nap.edu/books/0309072808/html/

Irvine, D. (1998). Finding value in nursing care: A framework for quality improvement and clinical evaluation. *Nursing Economics*, 16(3), 110–118.

Johanssen, J.M. (1993). Update: Guidelines for treating hypertension. *American Nursing*, 93(3), 42–49.

Joint Commission on Accreditation of Healthcare Organizations (JCAHO). (1994). Framework for Improving Performance: A Guide for Nurses. Chicago: JCAHO.

Joint Commission on Accreditation of Healthcare Organizations (JCAHO). (2005). jcaho.com

Kido, V. (2001). The UAP dilemma. *Nursing Management*, 32(11), 27–29.

Koerner, J., Bunkers, L., Gibson, S., Jones, R., Nelson, B., & Santema, K. (1995). Differentiated practice: The evaluation of a professional practice model for integrated client care services. In Flarey, D.L. (ed.). *Redesigning Nursing Care Delivery*. Philadelphia: JB Lippincott.

Leebov, W. (1991). *The Quality Quest: A Briefing for Health Care Professionals*. Chicago: American Hospital Publishing.

Lichtig, L.K., Knauf, R.A., & Milholland, D.K. (1999). Some impacts of nursing on acute care hospital outcomes. *Journal of Nursing Administration*, 29(2), 25–33.

Long, L. (2003). Imbedding quality improvement into all aspects of nursing practice. *International Journal of Nursing Practice*, 9, 280–284.

Loveridge, C., & Cummings, S. (1996). *Nursing Management in the New Paradigm*. Gaithersburg, MD: Aspen.

Lynam, L. (1994). Case management and critical pathways: Friend or foe. *Neonatal Network*, 13(8), 48–51.

Lyon, J.C. (1993). Models of nursing care delivery and case management: Clarification of terms. *Nursing Economics*, 11(3), 163–169.

Manthey, M. (2001). A core incremental staffing plan. *Journal of Nursing Administration*, 31, 424–425.

Mark, B. A., Salyer, J., & Geddis, N. (1997). Outcomes research: Clues to quality and organizational effectiveness? *Nursing Clinics of North America*, 32, 589–601.

Mass, S., & Johnson, B. (November 1998). Case management and clinical guidelines. *Journal of Care Management*, 18–26.

McClure, M. (1991). Models of practice. In *Differentiating Nursing Practice*. Kansas City, MO: American Academy of Nursing.

McLaughlin, C., & Kaluzny, A. (2006). *Continuous Quality Improvement in Health Care*, 3rd ed. Massachusetts: Jones and Bartlett.

Nelson, M. (2002). Educating for professional nursing practice: Looking backward into the future. *Online Journal of Issues in Nursing*, May 31, 2002, nursingworld.org/ojin/topic18/tpc18_3.htm. Accessed on May 27, 2002.

Newell, M. (1996). *Using Nursing Case Management to Improve Health Outcomes*. Gaithersburg, MD: Aspen.

Nightingale, F., & Barnum, B.S. (1992). *Notes on Nursing: What It Is, and What It Is Not*, Commemorative Edition. Philadelphia: Lippincott-Raven.

Ray, G., & Hardin, S. (1995). Advanced practice nursing. *Nursing Management*, 26(2), 45–47.

Ritter-Teitel, J. (2002). The impact of restructuring on professional nursing practice. *Journal of Nursing Administration*, 32(1), 31–41.

Rogers, A.E., Hwang, W., Scott, L.D., Aiken, L.H., & Dinges, D.F. (2004). The working hours of hospital staff nurses and patient safety: Both errors and near errors are more likely to occur when hospital staff nurses work twelve or more hours at a stretch. *Health Affairs* 23(4), 202–212.

Scott, J., Sochalski, J., & Aiken, L. (1999). Review of magnet hospital research: Findings and implications for professional nursing practice. *Journal of Nursing Administration*, 29(1), 9–19.

Sharp, M. (1994). Every citizen deserves care and every patient deserves a nurse. *Nursing Management*, 25(9), 32–33.

Simpson, R. (2005). Patient and nurse safety. *Nursing Administration Quarterly*, 29(1), 97–101.

Strickland, O. (1997). Challenges in measuring patient outcomes. *Nursing Clinics of North America*, 32, 495–512.

Swansburg, R., & Swansburg, R. (2002). *Introduction to Management and Leadership for Nurse Managers*, 3rd ed. Boston: Jones and Bartlett.

Tappen, R.M. (2001). *Nursing Leadership and Management: Concepts and Practice*, 4th ed., Philadelphia: FA Davis.

Vena, C., & Oldaker, S. (1994). Differentiated practice: The new paradigm using a theoretical approach. *Nursing Administration Quarterly*, 19(1), 66–73.

Wakefield, M. (2003). Change drivers for nursing and health care. *Nursing Economics*, 21(3), 150–151.

Wayman, C. (1999). Hospital-based nursing case management: Role clarification. *Nursing Case Management*, 4, 236–241.

chapter 11

Time Management

OBJECTIVES

After reading this chapter, the student should be able to:

- Describe personal perceptions of time.

- Discuss the rationale for good time management skills.

- Set short- and long-term personal career goals.

- Analyze activities at work using a time log.

- Incorporate time management techniques into clinical practice.

- Organize work to make more effective use of available time.

- Set limits on the demands made on one's time.

- Create a personal calendar using a computerized calendar system.

OUTLINE

Coming onto the unit, Celia, the evening charge nurse, already knew that a hectic day was in progress. Scattered throughout the unit were clues from the past 12 hours. Two clients on emergency department stretchers had been placed outside observation rooms already occupied by clients who were admitted the previous day in critical condition. Stationed in the middle of the hall was the code cart, with its drawers opened and electrocardiograph paper cascading down the sides. Approaching the nurses' station, Celia found Guillermo buried deep in paperwork. He glanced at her with a face that had exhaustion written all over it. His first words were, "Three of your RNs called in sick. I called staffing for additional help, but only one is available. Good luck!"Celia surveyed the unit, looked at the number of staff members available, and reviewed the client acuity level of the unit. She decided not to let the situation upset her. She would take charge of her own time and reallocate the time of her staff. She began to reorganize her staff mentally according to their capabilities and alter the responsibilities of each member. Having taken steps to handle the problem, Celia felt ready to begin the shift.

Business executives, managers, students, and nurses know that time continues to be a valuable resource. Time cannot be saved and used later, so it must be used wisely now. As a new nurse, you may at times find yourself sinking in the "quicksand" of a time trap, knowing what needs to be done but just not having the necessary time to do it (Ferrett, 1996). In today's fast-paced health-care environment, time management skills are critical to a nurse's success. Learning to take charge of your time and to use it effectively and efficiently is the key to time management (Gonzalez, 1996). Many nurses believe they never have enough time to accomplish their tasks. Like the White Rabbit in *Alice in Wonderland*, they are constantly in a rush against time. Time management is simply organizing and monitoring time so that client care tasks can be scheduled and implemented in a timely and organized fashion (Bos & Vaughn, 1998).

▨ THE TYRANNY OF TIME

Newton stated that time was absolute and that it occurred whether the universe was there or not. Many years later, Einstein theorized that time has no independent existence apart from the order of events by which we measure it (Smith, 1994). It really does not matter which theory is correct because, as nurses, our pro-

fessional and personal lives are guided by time.

How often do you look at your watch during the day? Do you divide your day into blocks of time? Do you steal a quick glance at the clock when you come home after putting in a full day's work? Do you mentally calculate the amount of time left to complete the day's tasks of grocery shopping, driving in a car pool, making dinner, and leaving again to take a class or attend a meeting? In our society, calendars, clocks, watches, newspapers, television, and radio all remind us of our position in time. Our perception of time is important because it affects our use of time and our response to time (Box 11-1).

Computers complete operations in a fraction of a second, and speeds can be measured to the nanosecond. Time clocks that record the minute employees enter and leave work are commonplace, and few excuses for being late are really considered acceptable. Timesheets and schedules are part of most healthcaregivers' lives. Staff members are expected to

---

BOX 11-1

Time Perception

Webber (1980) collected a number of interesting tests of people's perception of time. You may want to try several of these:

◆ Do you think of time more as a galloping horseman or a vast motionless ocean?

◆ Which of these words best describes time to you: sharp, active, empty, soothing, tense, cold, deep, clear, young, or sad?

◆ Is your watch fast or slow? (You can check it with the radio.)

◆ Ask a friend to help you with this test. Go into a quiet room without any work, reading material, radio, food, or other distractions. Have your friend call you after 10 to 20 minutes have elapsed. Try to guess how long you were in that room.

◆ *Webber test results interpreted.* A person who has a circular concept of time would compare time with a vast ocean. A galloping horseman would be characteristic of a linear conception of time, emphasizing speed and motion forward. A fast-tempo, achievement-oriented person would describe time as clear, young, sharp, active, or tense rather than empty, soothing, sad, cold, or deep. These same fast-tempo people are likely to have fast watches and to overestimate the amount of time that they sat in a quiet room.

Adapted from Webber, R.A. (1980). *Time Is Money! Tested Tactics That Conserve Time for Top Executives.* New York: Free Press.

follow precisely set schedules and meet deadlines for virtually everything, from distributing medications to completing reports on time. Many agencies produce vast quantities of computer-generated data that can be analyzed to determine the amount of time spent on various activities.

Several fallacies exist regarding time management. One of the foremost is that time can be managed like other resources. Time is finite. There are only 24 hours in a day, so the amount of time available cannot be controlled, only how it is used (Brumm, 2004). Individual personality, culture, and environment all interact to influence human perceptions of time (Matejka & Dunsing, 1988). Everybody has an internal tempo (Chappel, 1970). Some internal tempos are quicker than others. Environment also affects the way people respond to time. A fast-paced environment influences most people to work at a faster pace, despite their internal tempo. For individuals with a slower tempo, this pace can cause discomfort. If you are a high-achievement–oriented person, you are likely to have already set some career goals for yourself and to have a mental schedule of deadlines for reaching these goals ("go on to complete my bachelor of science in nursing in 4 years; a master of science in nursing in 6 years").

Many health-care professionals are linear, fast-tempo, achievement-oriented people. Simply working at a fast pace, however, is not necessarily equivalent to achieving a great deal. Much energy can be wasted in rushing around and stirring things up but actually accomplishing very little. This chapter looks at ways in which you can use your time and energy wisely to accomplish your goals.

HOW DO NURSES SPEND THEIR TIME?

Nurses are the largest group of health-care professionals. Because of the number of nurses needed and the shift variations, attention concerning the efficiency and effectiveness of their time management is needed. Efficient nurses deliver care in an organized manner that makes best use of time, resources and effort. Effective care improves a situation.

Today's labor market for skilled health-care professionals remains tight. Institutions face new challenges of not "trimming the fat, but compensate[sic] for loss of muscle" (Baldwin, 2002, p. 1). Current shortages of nurses, radiology technicians, pharmacists, and other health-care specialists show all the signs of a long-term problem. Health-care institutions need to change their thinking on how to manage work. Most are looking toward technology to help cope with staffing shortages (Baldwin, 2002). For example:

A new graduate worked the 7 a.m. to 3 p.m. shift and rotated every third week to the 11 p.m. to 7 a.m. shift in a medical intensive care unit, working 7 days straight before getting 2 days off. It was not difficult to remain awake during the entire shift the first night on duty, but each night thereafter staying awake became increasingly difficult. After the 2 a.m. vital signs were taken and recorded, the new graduate inevitably fell asleep at the nurses' station. He was so tired that he had to check and recheck client medications and other procedures for fear of making a fatal error. He became so anxious over the possibility of injuring someone that sleep during the day became impossible. Because of his obsession with rechecking his work, he had difficulty completing tasks and was always behind at the end of the shift (of course, napping did not help his time management).

A number of studies have examined how nurses use their time, especially nurses in acute care. For example, a study by Arthur Andersen found that only 35% of nursing time is spent in direct client care (including care planning, assessment teaching, and technical activities). Lundgren and Segesten (2001) found that this increases to 50% when an all-RN staff is involved in client care delivery as the nurses spent less time supervising non-nursing personnel.

Documentation accounts for another 20% of nursing time. The remainder of time is spent on transporting clients, processing transactions, performing administrative responsibilities, and undertaking hotel services (Brider, 1992). Categories may change from study to study, but the amount of time spent on direct client care is usually less than half the workday. As hospitals continue to reevaluate the way they deliver health care, nurses are finding themselves more involved with tasks that are not directly client-related, such as determining quality improvement, developing critical pathways, and so forth. These are added to their already existing client care functions. The critical nursing shortage compounds this problem. The result is that, in some cases, nurses are able to meet only the highest priority client needs, particularly in certain clinical settings such as short-stay units or ambulatory care centers (Curry, 2002).

Any change in the distribution of time spent on various activities can have a considerable impact on client care and on the organization's bottom line. Prescott (1991) offered the following example: If more unit management responsibilities could be shifted from nurses to non-nursing personnel, about 48 minutes per nurse shift could be redirected to client care. In a large hospital with 600 full-time nurses, the result would be an additional 307 hours of direct client care *a day.* Calculating the results of this time-saving strategy in another way shows an even greater impact: the changes would contribute the equivalent of the work of 48 additional full-time nurses to direct client care.

Many health-care institutions are considering integrating units with similar patient populations and having them managed by a non-nurse manager, someone with business and management expertise and not necessarily nursing skills. However, as a group, nurses respect managers who have nursing expertise and who are able to perform as nurses. They believe that a nurse-manager has a greater understanding of both client and professional staff needs. To address these service concerns, many educational institutions have developed dual graduate degrees combining nursing and management.

ORGANIZING YOUR WORK

Setting Your Own Goals

It is difficult to decide how to spend your time because there are so many things that need time. A good first step is to take a look at the situation, and get an overview. Then ask yourself, "What are my goals?" Goals help clarify what you want and give you energy, direction, and focus. Once you know where you want to go, set priorities. This is not an easy task. Remem-

ber Alice's conversation with the Cheshire Cat in Lewis Carroll's *Alice in Wonderland:*

"Would you tell me please, which way I ought to go from here?" asked Alice.

"That depends a good deal on where you want to go to," said the Cat.

"I don't care where," said Alice.

"Then it doesn't matter which way you go," said the Cat. (Carroll, 1907).

How can you get somewhere if you do not know where you want to go? It is important to explore your personal and career goals. This can help you make decisions about the future.

This concept can be applied to day-to-day activities as well as help in career decisions. Ask yourself questions about what you want to accomplish over a particular period. Personal development skills include discipline, goal-setting, time management and organizational skills, self-monitoring, and a positive attitude toward the job (Bos & Vaughn, 1998). Many of the personal management and organizational skills related to the workplace focus on time management and scheduling. Most new nurses have the skills required to perform the job but lack the personal management skills necessary to get the job done, specifically when it comes to time management.

To help organize your time, set both short- and long-term goals. Short-term goals are those that you wish to accomplish within the near future. Setting up your day in an organized fashion is a short-term goal, as is scheduling a required Medical Errors or Domestic Violence course.

Long-term goals are those you wish to complete over a long time. Advanced education and career goals are examples. A good question to ask yourself is, "What do I see myself doing 5 years from now?" Every choice you make requires a different allocation of time (Moshovitz, 1993).

Alinore, a licensed practical nurse returning to school to obtain her associate's degree in nursing, faced a multitude of responsibilities. A wife, a mother of two toddlers, and a full-time staff member at a local hospital, Alinore suddenly found herself in a situation in which there just were not enough hours in a day. She became convinced that becoming a registered nurse was an unobtainable goal. When asked where she wanted to be in 5 years, she answered, "At this moment, I think, on an island in Tahiti!" Several instructors helped Alinore develop a time plan. First, she was asked to list what she did each day and how much time each task required. This list included basic child care, driving children to and from day care, shopping, cooking meals, cleaning, hours spent in the classroom, study hours, work hours, and time devoted to leisure. Once this was established, she was asked which tasks could be allocated to someone else (e.g., her husband), which tasks could be clustered (e.g., cooking for several days at a time), and which tasks could be shared. Alinore's husband was willing to assist with car pools, grocery shopping, and cleaning. Previously, Alinore never asked him for help. Cooking meals was clustered: Alinore made all the meals in 1 day and then froze and labeled them to be used later. This left time for other activities. Alinore graduated at the top of her class and subsequently completed her BSN. She became a clinical preceptor for other associate degree nursing students on a pediatric unit in a county hospital. She never did get to Tahiti, though.

Employers pay nurses for their time. Does that mean that nurses "sell" their time? If so, then nurses "own" their time. Looking at time from this perspective changes the point of view about time, as nurses then manage their own time to accomplish client care tasks.

Time management means handling time with a measure of proficiency. Therefore, time management means meeting client care needs skillfully during a nursing shift (Navuluri, 2001). Organizing work eliminates extra steps or serious delays in completing it. Organizing also reduces the amount of time spent in activities that are neither productive nor satisfying.

Working on the most difficult tasks when you have the most energy decreases frustration later in the day when you may be more tired and less efficient. To begin managing your time, develop a clear understanding of *how* you use your time. Creating a personal time inventory helps you estimate how much time you spend on typical activities. Keeping the inventory for a week gives a fairly accurate estimate of how you spend your time. The inventory also helps identify "time wasters" (Gahar, 2000).

MacKenzie (1990) identified 20 of the biggest time wasters. Some of these come directly from the work environment, whereas others are personal characteristics. To avoid time wasters, take control. It is important to prevent endless activities and other people controlling you. Every day, set priorities to help you meet your goals. Ten frequent activities that infringe on time can be found in Box 11-2.

BOX 11-2

Frequent Activities That Infringe on Time

Managing by crisis
Telephone calls
Poor planning
Taking on too much
Unexpected visitors
Improper delegation
Disorganization
Inability to say no
Procrastinating
Meetings

http://www.abanet.org/careercounsel/prelaw/5timeprelawtips.pdf

---

Lists

One of the most useful organizers is the "to do" list. You can make this list either at the end of every day or at the beginning of each day before you do anything else. Some people say they do it at the end of the day because something always interferes at the beginning of the next day. Do not include routine tasks because they will make the list too long and you will do them without the extra reminder.

If you are a team leader, place the unique tasks of the day on the list: team conference, telephone calls to families, discussion of a new project, or in-service demonstration on a new piece of equipment. You may also want to arrange these things to do in order of their priority, starting with those that must be done on that day. Ask yourself the following questions regarding the tasks on the list (Moshovitz, 1993):

◆ What is the relative importance of each of these tasks?

◆ How much time will each task require?

◆ When must each task be completed?

◆ How much time and energy have to be devoted to these tasks?

If you find yourself postponing an item for several days, decide whether to give it top priority the next day or drop it from the list as an unnecessary task.

The list should be in a user-friendly form: on your electronic organizer, in your pocket, or on

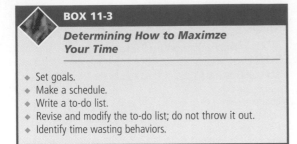

BOX 11-3

Determining How to Maximze Your Time

- Set goals.
- Make a schedule.
- Write a to-do list.
- Revise and modify the to-do list; do not throw it out.
- Identify time wasting behaviors.

a clipboard. Checking the list several times a day quickly becomes a good habit. Computerized calendar-creator programs help in setting priorities and guiding daily activities. Many of these are found on the Internet or intranet of an institution. These programs can be set to appear on the desktop when you turn on your computer to give an overview of the day, week, or month. This calendar acts as an automated to-do list. Your daily list may become your most important time manager (Box 11-3).

Long-Term Planning Systems

At the beginning of the semester, students are told the examination dates and when papers will be due. Many students find it helpful to enter the dates on a semester-long calendar so they can be seen at a glance. Then the students can see when clusters of assignments are due at the same time. This allows for advance planning or perhaps requests to change dates or get extensions.

Personal digital assistants (PDAs), or handheld organizers, have become quite popular. These devices allow both short-term and long-term scheduling. PDAs permit storing of personal notes and reminders, contact data, Internet access, and other program files. Handheld devices permit synchronization with personal computers and Internet-based calendars.

Schedules and Blocks of Time

Without some type of schedule, you are more likely to drift through a day or bounce from one activity to another in a disorganized fashion. Assignment sheets, worksheets, flow sheets, and critical pathways are all designed to help you plan client care and schedule your time effectively. The critical pathway is a guide to recommended treatments and optimal client outcomes (see Chapter 10). *Assignment sheets* indicate the clients for whom each staff member is responsible. *Worksheets* are then created to organize the daily care that must be given to the assigned clients (see Chapter 9 for examples of worksheets). *Flow sheets* are lists of items that must be recorded for each client.

Effective worksheets and flow sheets schedule and organize the day by providing reminders of various tasks and when they need to be done. The danger in using them, however, is that the more they divide the day into discrete segments, the more they fragment the work and discourage a holistic approach. If a worksheet becomes the focus of attention, the perspective of the whole and of the individuals who are your clients may be lost. Some activities must be done at a certain time. These activities structure the day or week to a great extent, and their timing may be out of your control. However, in every job there are tasks that can be done whenever you want to do them, as long as they are done.

In certain nursing jobs, reports and presentations are often required. For these activities, you may need to set aside blocks of time during which you can concentrate on the task. Trying to create and complete a report in 5- or 10-minute blocks of time is unrealistic. By the time you reorient yourself to the project, the time allotted is over, and nothing has been accomplished. Setting aside large blocks of time to do complex tasks is much more efficient.

Consider energy levels when beginning a big task. Start when levels are high and not at, say, 4:00 in the afternoon if that is when you find yourself winding down (Baldwin, 2002). For example, if you are a morning person, plan your demanding work in the morning. If you get energy spurts later in the morning or early afternoon, plan to work on larger or heavier tasks at that time. Nursing shifts may be designed in 8-, 10-, or 12-hour blocks. Many nurses working the night shifts (11 p.m. to 7 a.m. or 7 p.m. to 7 a.m.) find they have more energy a little later into their shift rather than at the beginning, whereas nurses working the day shifts (7 a.m. to 3 p.m. or 7 a.m. to 7 p.m.)

find they have the most energy at the beginning of their shift. Also, learn to delegate tasks that do not require professional nursing skills.

Some people go to work early to have a block of uninterrupted time. Others take work home with them for the same reason. This extends the workday and cuts into leisure time. The higher your stress level, the less effective you will be on the job—do not bring your work home with you. You need some time off to recharge your batteries (Turkington, 1996).

Filing Systems

Filing systems are helpful for keeping track of important papers. All professionals need to maintain copies of licenses, certifications, continuing education credits, and current information about their specialty area. Keeping these organized in an easily retrievable system saves time and energy when you need to refer to them. Using color-coded folders is often helpful. Each color holds documents that are related to one another. For example, all continuing education credits might be placed in a blue folder, anything pertaining to licensure in a yellow folder, and so on.

SETTING LIMITS

To set limits, it is necessary to identify your objectives and then arrange the actions needed to meet them in order of their priority (Haynes, 1991; Navuluri, 2001). The focus of time management exists on two levels: temporal and spatial. Nurses need to focus on client care needs during the shift (temporal) or within the boundaries of the working environment (spatial).

Saying No

Saying no to low-priority demands on your time is an important but difficult part of setting limits. Assertiveness and determination are necessary for effective time management. Learn to say no tactfully at least once a day (Hammerschmidt & Meador, 1993). Client care is a team effort. Effective time management requires you to look at other members of the team who may be able to take on the task.

The wisdom of time management is that we may have to let others help us manage our time, only to the extent that we never give up ownership of our time. In other words, although supervisors and managers tell you what to do, how you accomplish this remains up to you (Navuluri, 2001). Is it possible to say no to your supervisor or manager? It may not seem so at first, but many requests are negotiable. Requests sometimes are in conflict with career goals. Rather than sit on a committee in which you have no interest, respectfully decline, and volunteer for one that holds promise for you as well as meets the needs of your unit.

Can you refuse an assignment? Your manager may ask you to work overtime or to come in on your scheduled day off, but you can decline. You may not refuse to care for a group of clients or to take a report because you think the assignment is too difficult or unsafe. You may, however, discuss the situation with your supervisor and, together, work out alternatives. You can also confront the issue of understaffing by filing an unsafe staffing complaint. Failure to accept an assignment may result in accusations of abandonment.

Some people have difficulty saying no. Ambition keeps some people from declining any opportunity, no matter how overloaded they are. Many individuals are afraid of displeasing others and therefore feel obligated to continuously take on all forms of additional assignments. Still others have such a great need to be needed that they continually give of themselves, not only to clients but also to their coworkers and supervisors. They fail to stop and replenish themselves, and then they become exhausted. Remember, no one can be all things to all people at all times without creating serious guilt, anger, bitterness, and disillusionment. "Anyone who says it's possible has never tried it" (Turkington, 1996, p. 9).

Eliminating Unnecessary Work

Some work has become so deeply embedded in one's routines that it appears essential, although it is really unnecessary. Some nursing routines fall into this category. Taking vital signs, giving baths, changing linens, changing dressings, performing irrigations, and doing similar basic tasks are more often done according to schedule rather than according to client need, which may be much more or much less often than the routine specifies. Some of these tasks may appropriately be delegated to others:

◆ If clients are ambulatory, bed linens may not need to be changed daily. Incontinent and diaphoretic clients need to have fresh linens more frequently. Not all clients need a complete bed bath every day. Elderly clients have dry, fragile skin; giving them good mouth, facial, and perineal care may be all that is required on certain days. This should be included in the client's care plan.

◆ Much paperwork is duplicative, and some is altogether unnecessary. For example, is it necessary to chart nursing interventions in two or three places on the client record? Charting by exception, flow sheets, and computerized records are attempts to eliminate some of these problems.

◆ Socialization in the workplace is an important aspect in maintaining interpersonal relationships. When there is a social component to interactions in a group, the result is usually positive. However, too much socialization can reduce productivity; use judgment in deciding when socializing is interfering with work.

You may create additional work for yourself without realizing it. How often do you walk back down the hall to obtain equipment when it all could have been gathered at one time? How many times do you walk to a client's room instead of using the intercom, only to find that you need to go back to where you were to get what the client needs? Is the staff providing personal care to clients who are well enough to meet some of these needs themselves?

▧ STREAMLINING YOUR WORK

Many tasks cannot be eliminated or delegated, but they can be done more efficiently. There are many sayings in time management that reflect the principle of streamlining work.

"Work smarter, not harder" is a favorite one that should appeal to nurses facing increasing demands on time. "Never handle a piece of paper more than once" is a more specific one, reflecting the need to avoid procrastination in your work. "A stitch in time saves nine" reflects the degree to which preventive action saves time in the long run.

Avoiding Crisis Management

Crisis management occurs when people procrastinate or do not pay attention to their intuitions. The key to avoiding this is to anticipate possible problems and intervene before they become overwhelming. As a new nurse, it may be difficult to anticpate everything; however, there are some things that you can do by organizing your day. Several methods of working smarter and not harder are:

◆ Gather materials, such as bed linen, for all of your clients at one time. As you go to each room, leave the linen so that it will be there when you need it.

◆ While giving a bed bath or providing other personal care, perform some of the aspects of the physical assessment, such as taking vital signs, skin assessment, and parts of the neurological and musculoskeletal assessment. Prevention is always a good idea.

◆ If a client does not "look right," do not ignore your intuition. The client is probably having a problem.

◆ If you are not sure about a treatment or medication, ask before you proceed. It is usually less time-consuming to prevent a problem than it is to resolve one.

◆ When you set aside time to do a specific task that has a high priority, stick to your schedule and complete it.

◆ Do not allow interruptions while you are completing paperwork, such as transcribing orders.

What else can you do to streamline your work? A few general suggestions follow, but the first one, a time log, can assist you in developing others unique to your particular job. If you complete the log correctly, a few surprises about how you really spend your time are almost guaranteed.

Keeping a Time Log

Our perception of time is elastic. People do not accurately estimate the time they spend on any particular task; we cannot rely on our memories for accurate information about how we spend our time. The time log is an objective source of information. Most people spend a much smaller amount of their time on productive activities than they estimate. Once you see how large amounts of your time are spent, you will be able to eliminate or reduce the time spent on nonproductive or minimally productive activities (Drucker, 1967; Robichaud, 1986). For example, many nurses spend a great deal of time searching for or waiting for missing medications, equipment, or supplies. Before beginning client care, assemble all the equipment and supplies you will need, and check the client's medication drawer against the medication administration record so that you can order anything that is missing before you begin.

Figure 11-1 is an example of a time log in which you enter your activities every half hour. This means that you will have to pay careful attention to what you are doing so that you can record it accurately. Do not postpone recordkeeping; do it every 30 minutes. A 3-day sample may be enough for you to see a pattern emerging. It is suggested that you repeat the process again in 6 months, both because work situations change and to see if you have made any long-lasting changes in your use of time.

Reducing Interruptions

Everyone experiences interruptions. Some of these are welcome and necessary, but too many interfere with your work. A phone call from the laboratory with a critical value is a necessary interruption. Hobbs (1987) stated that necessary interruptions are not time wasters. Middle-level managers are interrupted every 8 minutes, and senior managers suffer interruptions every 5 minutes. Client care managers—nurses—seem to be interrupted every minute. Interruptions need to be kept to a minimum or eliminated, if possible. Closing the door to a client's room may reduce interruptions. You may have to ask visitors to wait a few minutes before you can answer their questions, although you must remain sensitive to their needs and return to them as soon as possible.

There is nothing wrong with asking a colleague who wants your assistance to wait a few minutes if you are engaged in another activity. Interruptions that occur when you are trying to pour medications or make calculations can cause errors. Physicians and other professionals often request nursing attention when nurses are involved with client care tasks. Find out if an unlicensed person may help. If not, ask the physician to wait, stating that you will be more than glad to help as soon as you complete what you are doing. Be courteous, but be firm; you are busy also.

Categorizing Activities

Clustering certain activities helps eliminate the feeling of bouncing from one unrelated task to another. It also makes your caregiving more holistic. You may, for example, find that documentation takes less time if you do it while you are still with the client or immediately after seeing a client. The information is still fresh in your mind, and you do not have to rely on notes or recall. Many health-care institutions have switched to computerized charting, with the computers placed at the bedside. This setup assists in documenting care and interventions while the nurse is still with the client. Also, try to follow a task through to completion before beginning another.

Finding the Fastest Way

Many time-consuming tasks can be done more efficiently by automation. Narcotic delivery systems that deliver the correct dose and electronically record the dose, the name of the client, and the name of the health-care personnel removing the medication are being used in

Activities	Comments
6:30	
7:00	
7:30	
8:00	
8:30	
9:00	
9:30	
10:00	
10:30	
11:00	
11:30	
12:00	
12:30	
1:00	
1:30	
2:00	
2:30	
3:00	
3:30	
4:00	
4:30	
5:00	
5:30	
6:00	
6:30	
7:00	

FIGURE 11-1 ◆ Time log. (Adapted from Robichaud, A.M. (1986).

many institutions. This system saves staff time in documentation and in performing a narcotic count at the end of each shift. Bar coding is another method used by health-care institutions. Bar coding allows for scanning certain types of client data, decreasing the number of paper chart entries (Baldwin, 2002; Meyer, 1992).

Efficient systems do not have to be complex. Using a preprinted color-coded sticker system helps identify clients who must be without food or fluids (NPO) for tests or surgery, those who require 24-hour urine collections, or those who require special cultures. The information need not be written or entered repeatedly if stickers are used.

Everyone talks about the amount of time wasted by physicians, nurses, and other clinicians in looking for such things as client charts, equipment, and even clients. Erica Drazen, vice president of First Consulting Group in Lexington, Massachusetts, suggested using more sophisticated wireless technology, similar to the car tracking systems used by law enforcement. Tiny transmitters can be activated from a central point to locate the items or individuals. Using electronic medical record systems decreases the amount of time spent looking for client records. By using the approved access codes, health-care personnel can obtain information from anywhere within the institution. This also minimizes time spent on paper charting.

Automating Repetitive Tasks

Developing techniques for repetitive tasks is similar to finding the fastest method, but it focuses on specific tasks that are repeated again and again, such as client teaching.

Many clients come to the hospital or ambulatory center for surgery or invasive diagnostic tests for same-day treatment. This does not give nurses much teaching time. Using videotapes and pamphlets as teaching aids can reduce the time needed to share the information, allowing the nurse to be available to answer individual questions and create individual adaptations. Many facilities are using these techniques

for cardiac rehabilitation, preoperative teaching, and infant care instruction. Computer-generated teaching and instruction guides permit clients to take the information home with them. This can decrease the number of phone calls requiring repetition of information.

The Rhythm Model for Time Management

Navuluri (2001) looked at time management in terms of a Rhythm Model—a PQRST pattern: Prioritize, Question, Recheck, Self-reliance, Treat. By prioritizing, you can accomplish the most important tasks first. Questioning permits you to look at events and tasks in terms of effectiveness, efficiency, and efficacy. Rechecking unfinished tasks quickly helps you to manage your time efficiently. Self-reliance allows you to know the difference between events that are within your control and those that are not, as well as realizing your limitations. No one knows better what you are capable of doing than you. Treats are part of life. It is okay to take a break or time out. It is important because doing so permits you to refresh. Table 11-1 summarizes the Rhythm Model for Time Management.

CONCLUSION

Time can be our best friend or our worst enemy, depending on our perspective and how we manage it. It is important to identify how you feel about time and to assess your own time management skills. Nursing requires that we perform numerous activities within what often seems to be a very brief time. Remember that there are only so many hours in the day. Knowing this can create stress. No one works well "under pressure." Learn to delegate. Learn to say, "I would really like to help you; can it wait until I finish this?" Learn to say no. Most of all, learn how to make the most of your day by working effectively and efficiently. Finally, remember that 8 hours should be designated as sleep time and several more as personal or leisure ("time off") time.

TABLE 11-1
The Rhythm Model for Time Management

PRIORITIZE	List tasks in order of importance. Remember that some tasks must occur at specific times, whereas others can occur at any time. Emergencies take precedence. Identify events controlled by you and events controlled by others. Use critical thinking skills to assign priorities.
QUESTION EFFECTIVENESS	Did the task produce the desired outcome?
EFFICIENCY	How can I accomplish the plan with the least expenditure of time? Is there a way to break this down into simpler tasks?
EFFICACY	Do I have the skill and ability to obtain the desired effect?
RECHECK	Mentally and physically recheck an unfinished or delegated task.
SELF-RELIANCE	Identify those tasks that are within your control and those that are not. Use critical thinking skills and adaptability to revise priorities. "Go with the flow."
TREAT	Treat yourself to a break when you can. Treat yourself to time off. Treat yourself to an educational experience: Commit yourself to excellence. Treat others courteously and with respect.

STUDY QUESTIONS

1 Develop a personal time inventory. Identify your time wasters. How do you think you can eliminate these activities?

2 Create your own client care worksheet. How does this worksheet help you organize your clinical day?

3 Keep a log of your clinical day. Which activities took the most time, and why? Which activities took the least time? What situations interfered with your work? What could you do to reduce the interference?

4 Identify a task that is done repeatedly in your clinical area. Think of a new, more efficient way to do that task. How could you implement this new routine? How could you evaluate its efficiency?

5 Consider how many interruptions you had during the day. How did you handle them? How did they interfere in your time management?

CRITICAL THINKING EXERCISE

Antonio was recently hired as a team leader for a busy cardiac step-down unit. Nursing responsibilities of the team leader, in addition to client care, include meeting daily with team members, reviewing all admissions and discharges for acuity and length of stay, and documenting all clients who exceed length of stay and the reasons. At the end of each month, the team leaders are required to meet with unit managers to review the client care load and team member performance. This is the last week of the month, and Antonio has a meeting with the unit manager at the end of the week. He is 2 weeks behind on staff evaluations and documentation of clients who exceeded length of stay. He is becoming very stressed over his team leader responsibilities.

1. Why do you think Antonio is feeling stressed?

2. Make a to-do list for Antonio.

3. Develop a time log for Antonio to use to analyze his activities.

4. How can Antonio organize and streamline his work?

SELF-ASSESSMENT

1 Create a weekly schedule using a computerized calendar found on the Internet.

2 If you have a PDA, show your classmates how you use this to keep dates, notes, and personal information.

3 Draw the Rhythm Model for Time Management (see Table 11-1). Using the information from your clinical experience, fill in the table.

4 Find a copy of MacKenzie's 20 Biggest Time Wasters. Do you have any of these characteristics? If so, how could you change to use your time more effectively?

REFERENCES

American Bar Association Career Resource Center (n.d.). Identifying & conquering time wasters. Retrieved December 20, 2005, from abanet.org/careercounsel

Baldwin, F.D. (2002). Making do with less. *Healthcare Informatics*, pp. 1–7. Online, March 2002.

Bos, C.S., & Vaughn, S. (1998). *Strategies for Teaching Students with Learning and Behavioral Problems*, 4th ed. Boston: Allyn & Bacon.

Brider, P. (1992). The move to patient-focused care. *American Journal of Nursing*, 92(9), 27–33.

Brumm, J. (2004). Time can be on your side. *Nursing Spectrum*. http://nursingspectrum.com/StudentsCorner/StudentFeatures/TimeSide.htm.

Chappel, E.D. (1970). *Culture and Biological Man: Exploration in Behavioral Anthropology*. New York: Holt, Rinehart, & Winston. (Reprinted as *The Biological Foundations of Individuality and Culture*. Huntingdon, NY: Robert Krieger, 1979.)

Carroll, L (1907) *Alice's Adventures in Wonderland*, Reprint 2002. New York: North-South Books.

Curry, P. (March 25, 2002). Pressure cooker: Hospital's emphasis on productivity increases stress for nurses and patients. *Nurseweek News*, http://www.nurseweek.com

Drucker, P.E. (1967). *The Effective Executive*. New York: Harper & Row.

Ferrett, S.K. (1996). *Connections: Study Skills for College and Career Success*. Chicago: Irwin Mirror Press.

Gahar, A. (2000). *Programming for College Students with Learning Disabilities*. (Grant No.: 84–078C) http://www.csbsju.edu

Gonzalez, S.I. (1996). Time management. *The Nursing Spectrum in Florida*, 6(17), 5.

Hammerschmidt, R., & Meador, C.K. (1993). *A Little Book of Nurses' Rules*. Philadelphia: Hanley & Belfus.

Haynes, M.E. (1991). *Practical Time Management*. Los Altos, CA: Crisp Publications.

Hobbs, S. (1987). Getting to grips with business plans, audit, and applications. *Nursing Standard*.

Lundgren, S. & Segesten, K. (2001). Nurses' use of time in a medical-surgical ward with all-RN staffing. *Journal of Nursing Management*, 9, 13–20.

MacKenzie, A. (1990). *The Time Trap*. New York: American Management Association.

Matejka, J.K., & Dunsing, R.J. (1988). Time management: Changing some traditions. *Management World*, 17(2), 6–7.

Meyer, C. (1992). Equipment nurses like. *American Journal of Nursing*, 92(8), 32–38.

Moshovitz, R. (1993). *How to Organize Your Work and Your Life*. New York: Doubleday.

Navuluri, R.B. (March 2001). Our time management in patient care. *Research for Nursing Practice*, pp. 1–8.

Prescott, P.A. (1991). Changing how nurses spend their time. *Image*, 23(1), 23–28.

Robichaud, A.M. (1986). Time documentation of clinical nurse specialist activities. *Journal of Nursing Administration*, 16(1), 31–36.

Smith, H.W. (1994). *The Ten Natural Laws of Successful Time and Life Management: Proven Strategies for Increased Productivity and Inner Peace*. New York: Warner Books.

Turkington, C.A. (1996). *Reflections for Working Women: Common Sense, Sage Advice, and Unconventional Wisdom*. New York: McGraw-Hill.

Webber, R.A. (1980). *Time Is Money! Tested Tactics That Conserve Time for Top Executives*. New York: Free Press.

Professional Issues

chapter 12

The Workplace

OBJECTIVES

After reading this chapter, the student should be able to:

- Recognize the compoments of nurse job satisfaction.

- Describe quality indicators related to safety and quality.

- Recognize threats to safety in the workplace.

- Identify agencies responsible for overseeing workplace safety.

- Describe methods of dealing with violence in the workplace.

- Identify the role of the nurse in dealing with terrorism and other disasters.

- Recognize situations that may reflect sexual harassment.

- Make suggestions for improving the physical and social environment.

- Understand the American Nurses Association Future Vision for Nursing.

OUTLINE

Almost half our waking hours are spent in the workplace. For this reason alone, the quality of the workplace environment is a major concern. Yet it is neglected to a surprising extent in many health-care organizations. It is neglected by administrators, who would never allow peeling paint or poorly maintained equipment but who leave their staff, their most costly and valuable resource, unmaintained and unrefreshed. The "do more with less" thinking that has predominated in many organizations places considerable pressure on staff and management alike (Chisholm, 1992). Improvement of the workplace environment is more difficult to accomplish under these circumstances, but it is more important than ever.

Much of the responsibility for enhancing the workplace rests with upper-level management, people who have the authority and resources to encourage organization-wide growth and change. Nurses, however, have begun to take more responsibility for identification of and problem solving for workplace issues. The American Nurses Association (ANA) core initiatives in 2005 focused on the health and safety of nurses and clients in the workplace. This chapter focuses on these issues, in addition to sexual harassment, impaired workers, enhancement of work life quality, diversity, and disabled workers.

WORKPLACE SAFETY

Safety is not a new concept in the workplace. Although guidelines for safe working conditions have existed since the time of the early Egyptians, the modern movement began during the Industrial Revolution. In 1913, the National Council for Industrial Safety (now the National Safety Council) was formed. The Occupational Safety and Health Act of 1970 created both the National Institute of Occupational Safety and Health (NIOSH) and the Occupational Safety and Health Administration (OSHA). The OSHA, part of the U.S. Department of Labor, is responsible for developing and enforcing workplace safety and health regulations. The NIOSH, part of the U.S. Department of Health and Human Services, provides research, information, education, and training in occupational safety and health. The National Safety Council partners with the OSHA to provide training in a variety of safety initiatives. The National Safety Council maintains that safety in the workplace is the responsibility of both the employer and the employee. The employer must ensure a safe, healthful work environment, and employees are accountable for knowing and following safety guidelines and standards (National Safety Council, 1992). All the ANA core initiatives in 2005 affected health and safety in the workplace (ANA, 2005).

Threats to Safety

Health care is the second-fastest-growing sector of the U.S. economy, employing more than 12 million workers. Women represent nearly 80% of the health-care workforce. Health-care workers face a wide range of hazards on the job, including needlestick injuries, back injuries, latex allergy, violence, and stress. Although it is possible to prevent or reduce health-care worker exposure to these hazards, health-care workers are actually experiencing increasing numbers of occupational injuries and illnesses; rates of occupational injury have risen over the past decade. By contrast, two of the most hazardous industries, agriculture and construction, are safer today than they were a decade ago. NIOSH-TIC-2 is a searchable bibliographical database of occupational safety and health publications, documents, grant reports, and journal articles supported in whole or in part by the NIOSH (cdc.gov/niosh/topics/health-care/).

In 1993, 300 of Brigham Young Hospital's 1000 staff nurses reported the following symptoms: hives; rashes; headache; dizziness; nausea; eye, nose, and throat irritation; menstrual irregularities; urticaria; cardiac and respiratory distress; hair loss; joint pain; and memory loss. The mysterious illness began with the operating room staff and soon spread to all areas of the hospital. The hospital, undergoing reconstruction, was soon given a diagnosis of "sick building syndrome." Several nurses became so sensitized to the chemicals floating in the hospital air that they have been on permanent leave since 1994 and may never be able to return to nursing (Himali, 1995).

In spring 2001, a Florida nurse with 20 years' psychiatric nursing experience died of head and face trauma. Her assailant, a former wrestler, had been admitted involuntarily in the early morning to the private mental health–care facility. An investigation found that the facility did not have a policy on workplace violence and no method of summoning help in an emergency (Arbury, 2002).

Six hundred thousand to one million needlestick injuries occur annually to U.S. health-care workers. Percutaneous exposure is the principal route for human immunodeficiency virus (HIV) and hepatitis B and C virus transmission. Additionally, infections such as tuberculosis, syphilis, malaria, and herpes can be transmitted through needlesticks.

Threats to safety in the workplace vary from one setting to another and from one individual to another. A pregnant staff member may be more vulnerable to risks from radiation; staff members working in the emergency room of a large urban public hospital are at more risk for HIV and tuberculosis than the staff members working in the newborn nursery. All staff members have the right to be made aware of potential risks. No worker should feel intimidated or uncomfortable in the workplace.

Reducing Risk

OSHA

The Occupational Safety and Health Act of 1970 and the Mine Safety and Health Act of 1977 were the first federal guidelines and standards related to safe and healthful working conditions. Through these acts, the NIOSH and OSHA were formed. OSHA regulations apply to most U.S. employers that have one or more employees and that engage in businesses affecting commerce. Under OSHA regulations, the employer must comply with standards for providing a safe, healthful work environment. Employers are also required to keep records of all occupational (job-related) illnesses and accidents. Examples of occupational accidents and injuries include burns, chemical exposures, lacerations, hearing loss, respiratory exposure, musculoskeletal injuries, and exposure to infectious diseases.

OSHA regulations provide for workplace inspections that may be conducted with or without prior notification to the employer. However, catastrophic or fatal accidents and employee complaints may also trigger an OSHA inspection. OSHA encourages employers and employees to work together to identify and remove any workplace hazards before contacting the nearest OSHA area office. If the employee has not been able to resolve the safety or health issue, the employee may file a formal complaint, and an inspection will be ordered by the area OSHA director (U.S. Department of Labor, 1995). Any violations found are posted where all employees can view them. The employer has the right to contest the OSHA decision. The law also states that the employer cannot punish or discriminate against employees for exercising their rights related to job safety and health hazards or participating in OSHA inspections (U.S. Department of Labor, 1995).

In the past, OSHA inspections focused especially on blood-borne pathogens, lifting and ergonomic (proper body alignment) guidelines, confined-space regulations, respiratory guidelines, and workplace violence. Since September 11, 2001, the OSHA has added protecting the worksite against terrorism (osha.gov). Table 12-1 lists the major categories of potential hazards found in hospitals as identified by the OSHA. The U.S. Department of Labor publishes fact sheets related to various OSHA guidelines and activities. They can be obtained from your employer, at the local public library, or via the Internet at osha.gov

Centers for Disease Control and Prevention

The Centers for Disease Control and Prevention (CDC) is the lead federal agency for protecting the health and safety of citizens both at home and abroad. The CDC partners with other agencies throughout the nation to investigate health problems, conduct research, implement prevention strategies, and promote safe and healthy environments. The CDC publishes continuous updates of recommendations for prevention of HIV transmission in the

TABLE 12-1
Potential Hospital Hazards

Hazard	Definition	Examples
BIOLOGICAL	Infectious/biological agents such as bacteria, viruses, fungi, parasites	Human immunodeficiency virus, vancomycin-resistant enterococcus, methicillin-resistant *Staphylococcus aureus*, hepatitis B virus, tuberculosis
CHEMICAL	Medications, solutions, and gases that are potentially toxic or irritating to the body system	Ethylene oxide, formaldehyde, glutaraldehyde, waste anesthetic gases, cytotoxic agents, pentamidine ribavirin
PSYCHOLOGICAL	Factors and situations encountered in or associated with the work environment that create or potentiate stress, emotional strain, and/or interpersonal problems	Stress, workplace violence, shiftwork, inadequate staffing, heavy workload, increased client acuity
PHYSICAL	Agents that cause tissue trauma	Radiation, lasers, noise, electricity, extreme temperatures, workplace violence
ENVIRONMENTAL, MECHANICAL, BIOMEDICAL	Factors within work environment that cause or potentiate accidents, injuries, strain, or discomfort	Tripping hazards, unsafe or unguarded equipment, air quality, slippery floors, confined spaces, obstructed work areas or passageways, awkward postures, localized contact stresses, temperature extremes, repetitive motions, lifting and moving clients

Adapted from osha.gov/SLTC/healthcarefacilities/hazards

workplace and universal precautions related to blood-borne pathogens as well as the most recent information on other infectious diseases in the workplace, such as tuberculosis and hepatitis. Currently, the CDC is targeting public health emergency preparedness and response related to biological and chemical agents and threats (cdc.gov/). Information can be obtained by consulting the *Mortality and Morbidity Weekly Report* (MMWR) in the library, via the Internet (cdc.gov/health/diseases), or through the toll-free phone number (800–311–3435). Interested health-care workers can also be placed on the CDC's mailing list to receive any free publications.

NIOSH

The NIOSH is part of the CDC and is the federal agency responsible for conducting research and making recommendations for the prevention of work-related disease and injury. Occupational hazards for health-care workers continue to be enormous health and economic problems. According to statistics from the NIOSH, more than 6.1 million illnesses and injuries occur in the workplace yearly, with more than 2.9 million lost workdays attributed

to occupational illnesses and inuries (cdc.gov/niosh/about).

Box 12-1 lists the most important federal laws enacted to protect individuals in the workplace.

ANA

When looking at agencies that are instrumental in dealing with workplace safety, the ANA must be included. The ANA is discussed more completely in Chapter 15. The ANA's history embodies advocacy for the nurse. As early as March 1994, the ANA Board of Directors launched the Nursing Safety & Quality Initiative. This initiative focuses on educating registered nurses about quality measurement as well as evaluating the safety and quality of client care. Coming out of this initiative was the publication of nursing-sensitive quality indicators. The initial 10 nursing-sensitive quality indicators for acute care settings are outlined in Table 12-2.

New indicators are added continually. Newer indications include staff mix, type of unit, number of staffed beds, urban versus rural, pediatric pain, restraint use, peripheral intravenous infiltrations, and client aggression. In 1998, the ANA funded the development of a

> **BOX 12-1**
>
> *Federal Laws Enacted to Protect the Worker in the Workplace*
>
> ◆ **Equal Pay Act of 1963:** Employers must provide equal pay for equal work regardless of sex.
> ◆ **Title VII of Civil Rights Act of 1964:** Employees may not be discriminated against in employment on the basis of race, color, religion, sex, or national origin.
> ◆ **Age Discrimination in Employment Act of 1967:** Private and public employers may not discriminate against persons 40 years of age or older except when a certain age group is a bona fide occupational qualification.
> ◆ **Pregnancy Discrimination Act of 1968:** Pregnant women cannot be discriminated against in employment benefits if they are able to discharge job responsibilities.
> ◆ **Fair Credit Reporting Act of 1970:** Job applicants and employees have the right to know of the existence and content of any credit files maintained on them.
> ◆ **Vocational Rehabilitation Act of 1973:** An employer receiving financial assistance from the federal government may not discriminate against individuals with disabilities and must develop affirmative action plans to hire and promote individuals with disabilities.
> ◆ **Family Education Rights and Privacy Act— Buckley Amendment of 1974:** Educational institutions may not supply information about students without their consent.
> ◆ **Immigration Reform and Control Act of 1986:** Employers must screen employees for the right to work in the United States without discriminating on the basis of national origin.
> ◆ **Americans With Disabilities Act of 1990:** Persons with physical or mental disabilities or who are chronically ill cannot be discriminated against in the workplace. Employers must make "reasonable accommodations" to meet the needs of the disabled employee. These include such provisions as installing foot or hand controls; readjusting light switches, telephones, desks, tables, and computer equipment; providing access ramps and elevators; offering flexible work hours; and providing readers for blind employees.
> ◆ **Family Medical Leave Act of 1993:** Employers with 50 or more employees must provide up to 13 weeks of unpaid leave for family medical emergencies, childbirth, or adoption.
> ◆ **Needlestick Safety and Prevention Act of 2001:** This act directed OSHA to revise the blood-borne pathogens standard to establish in greater detail requirements that employers identify and make use of effective and safer medical devices.
>
> Adapted from Strader, M., & Decker, P. (1995). *Role Transition to Patient Care Management.* Norwalk, CN: Appleton and Lange; osha.gov/needle-sticks/needlefact

national database related to these indicators (NDNQI). The database is located at the Midwest Research Insitute (MRI) and is managed jointly by the MRI and the University of Kansas School of Nursing. Currently, data are being collected from more than 60 hospitals across the United States. Each insitution can examine its own processes and benchmark against other facilities. The NDNQI Web site is nursingquality.org (nursingworld.org/readroom/fssafe99).

In 1999, the Commission on Workplace Advocacy was established as part of the ANA. The Commission consists of nine members, appointed by the ANA Board of Directors, and represent constituent member associations. Additionally, state member associations often offer their own workplace advocacy information. Issues such as collective bargaining, workplace violence, mandatory overtime, staffing ratios, conflict management, delegation, ethi-

cal issues, compensation, needlestick safety, latex allergies, pollution prevention, and ergonomics are addressed.

The ANA core initiatives focus on health and safety in the workplace (ANA, 2005). Each initiative will be discussed in this chapter.

◆ Nursing shortage
◆ Client safety/advocacy
◆ Workplace rights
◆ Appropriate staffing
◆ Workplace health and safety

For ANA information on these issues, a substantial resource is the ANA Web site (nursingworld.org).

Joint Commission on the Accreditation of Healthcare Organizations

The Joint Commission on the Accreditation of Healthcare Organizations (JCAHO) is an inde-

TABLE 12-2
ANA Quality Indicators in Acute Care Settings

Indicator	Definition
Mix of RNs, LPNs, UAP	Percentage of RN staff care hours as a total of all nursing care hours
Total nursing care hours provided per client day	Total number of productive hours worked by RN staff with direct client care responsibilities per day
Pressure ulcers	Total number of clients with stage I, II, III, or IV ulcers
Client falls	Rate per 1000 client days that patients experience an unplanned descent to the floor during the course of their day
Client satisfaction with pain management	Clients' opinion of how well nursing staff managed their pain
Client satisfaction with educational information	Client perception of hospital experience related to satisfaction with client education
Client satisfaction with overall care	Client perception of hospital experience related to satisfaction with overall care
Client satisfaction with nursing care	Client perception of hospital experience related to satisfaction with nursing care
Nosocomial infection rate	Number of laboratory-confirmed bacteremia cases associated with sites of central lines
Nurse staff satisfaction	Job satisfaction expressed by nurses working in hospital settings to all RNs in direct client care or middle management roles.

Adapted from nursingworld.org/readroom/fssfe99

pendent, nonprofit organization. Established more than 50 years ago, it is governed by a board that includes physicians, nurses, and consumers. The JCAHO evaluates the quality and safety of care for more than 15,000 health-care organizations. To maintain and earn accreditation, organizations must have an extensive on-site review by a team of Joint Commission health-care professionals at least once every 3 years. In March 2005, the JCAHO and Joint Commission Resources (JCR) announced the establishment of the Joint Commission International Center for Patient Safety. In order to evaluate the safety and the quality of care provided at U.S. accredited

health-care organizations, each year the Joint Commission establishes National Patient Safety Goals (NPSGs). These goals have specific requirements for protecting patients according to the type of facility such as ambulatory care and office-based surgery, assisted living, behavioral health care, critical access hospital, and home care. Examples of 2006 Critical Access Hospital and Hospital National Patient Safety Goals include (a) Improve the accuracy of patient identification and (b) Improve the safety of using medications. A total of nine goals are listed with specific requirements that must be met under each goal. Additional information related to JCAHO and patient safety was discussed in Chapter 10 (jcaho.org/general+public/patient+safety/patient+safety).

Institute of Medicine

The Institute of Medicine (IOM) is a private, nongovernmental organization that carries out studies at the request of many government agencies. The mission of the IOM is to improve the health of people everywhere; thus, the topics it studies are very broad (iom.edu). In 1996, the IOM began a quality initiative to assess the nation's health. Part of this initiative was the 2004 report: Keeping Patients Safe: Transforming the Work Environment of Nurses. The report identified concerns and issues related to organizational management, workforce deployment practices, work design, and organizational culture (Beyea, 2004). Each of these issues will be discussed in the section of this chapter on enhancing the quality of work life.

Programs

The primary objective of any workplace safety program is to protect staff members from harm and the organization from liability related to that harm.

The first step in development of a workplace safety program is to *recognize a potential hazard* and then take steps to control it. Based on OSHA regulations (U.S. Department of Labor, 1995), the employer must inform staff members of any potential health hazards and provide as much protection from these hazards as possible. In many cases, initial warnings come from the CDC, NIOSH, and other federal, state, and local agencies. For example, employers must provide tuberculosis testing and hepatitis B vaccine; protective equipment such as gloves, gowns, and masks; and immediate treatment after exposure for all staff members who may have contact with blood-borne pathogens. Employers are expected to remove hazards, educate employees, and establish institution-wide policies and procedures to protect their employees (Herring, 1994; Roche, 1993). Nurses who are not provided with latex gloves may refuse to participate in any activities involving blood or blood products. The employee cannot be subjected to discrimination in the workplace, and reasonable accommodations for safety against blood-borne pathogens must be provided. This may mean that the nurse with latex allergies is placed in an area where exposure to blood-borne pathogens is not an issue (Strader & Decker, 1995; U.S. Department of Labor, 1995). The OSHA also has information available on exposure to chemical or biological agents related to terrorism. Terrorism response exercises are conducted through the OSHA to train health-care workers on responding to terrorism threats (osha.gov/pls/oshaweb/owadisp.show_document?p_table=NEWS_RELEASES&p_id=11317).

The second step in a workplace safety program is a *thorough assessment of the amount of risk entailed*. Staff members, for example, may become very fearful in situations that do not warrant such fear. For example:

Nancy Wu is the nurse manager on a busy geriatric unit. Most clients require total care: bathing, feeding, and positioning. She has observed that several of the staff members working on the unit use poor body mechanics when lifting and moving the clients. In the last month, several of the staff members were referred to Employee Health for back pain. This week, she noticed that the clients seem to remain in the same position for long periods and are rarely out of bed or in a chair for the entire day. When she confronted the staff, the response was the same from all of them: "I have to work for a living. I can't afford to risk a back injury for someone who may not live past the end of the week." Nancy Wu was concerned about the care of the clients as well as the apparent lack of information her staff had about prevention of back injuries. She decided to seek assistance from the nurse practitioner in charge of Employee Health in order to develop a back injury prevention program.

Assessment of the workplace may require considerable data gathering to document the incidence of the problem and consultation with experts before a plan of action is drawn up. Health-care organizations often create formal committees, consisting of experts from within the institution and representatives from the affected departments, to assess these risks. It is important that staff members from various levels of the organization be allowed to offer input into an assessment of safety needs and risks.

The third step is to *create a plan* to provide optimal protection for staff members. It is not always a simple matter to protect staff members without interfering with the provision of client care. For example, some devices that can be worn to prevent transmission of tuberculosis interfere with communication with the client ("Federal agencies clash," 1993). Some attempts have been made to limit visits or withdraw home health-care nurses from high-crime areas, but this leaves homebound clients without care (Nadwairski, 1992). A threat assessment team that evaluates problems and suggests appropriate actions may reduce the incidence and severity of problems due to violent behavior, but it may also increase employees' fear of violence if not handled well. Developing a safety plan includes the following:

◆ Seeking evidence-based practices and recommendations related to the problem.

◆ Consulting federal, state, and local regulations.

◆ Distinguishing real from imagined risks.

◆ Seeking administrative support and enforcement for the plan.

◆ Calculating costs of a program.

The fourth and final stage in developing a workplace safety program is *implementing the program*. Educating the staff, providing the necessary safety supplies and equipment, and modifying the environment contribute to an effective program. Protecting client and staff confidentiality and monitoring adherence to control and safety procedures should not be overlooked in the implementation stage (CDC, 1992; "Federal agencies clash," 1993; Jankowski, 1992).

An example of a safety program is the one for health-care workers exposed to HIV instituted at the Department of Veterans Affairs Hospital, San Francisco (Armstrong, Gordon, & Santorella, 1995). An HIV exposure can be stressful for health-care workers and their loved ones. This employee assistance program includes up to 10 hour-long individual counseling sessions on the meaning and experience of this traumatic event. Additional counseling sessions for couples are also provided. Information about HIV and about dealing with acute stress reactions is provided. Counseling helps workers identify a plan to obtain assistance from their individual support systems, identify practice methods of dealing with blood-borne pathogens, and return to work. A systematic review related to needlestick injury provides evidence for the use of tissue adhesives.

In the past, the options for wound closure have been largely limited to sutures (needle and thread), staples, and adhesive tapes. Tissue adhesives (glues) offer the advantages that there are no sutures to remove later for the client and no risk of needlestick injury to the health-care worker. The adhesive is applied over the surgical wound and holds the edges together until healing has occurred. Adhesives have been compared with alternative methods of surgical wound closure in 8 RCTs involving 630 clients. There was no evidence of a difference in rates of wound dehiscence or infection after surgical incision closure with tissue adhesive or sutures or adhesive tape. The recommendation from the evidence was that health-care providers may consider the use of tissue adhesives for the closure of incisions in the operating room, and a protocol was published in 2004 (Coulthard, et al., 2004).

VIOLENCE

Violence in the workplace is a contemporary social issue. Newspapers and magazines have reported on numerous violent incidents; one of six violent crimes occurs in the workplace, and homicide is the second leading cause of workplace death (Edwards, 1999). According to the Census of Fatal Occupational Injuries, there were 551 workplace homicides and 5,703 workplace injuries in 2004. The rate of assaults

on hospital workers is much higher than the rate of assaults for all private-sector industries. The Bureau of Labor Statistics measures the number of assaults resulting in injury per 10,000 full-time workers. The overall private sector injury incidence rate is 2; the overall incidence rate for health service workers 9.3. Further broken down, the incidence rate for social service workers is 15, and the rate for nurses and personal care workers is 25 (bls. gov/news/release/cfoi.nr0).

The aggressor can be a disgruntled employee or employer, an unhappy significant other, or a person committing a random act of violence. Nurses have been identified as a group at risk for violence from clients, family members, and other staff members. Violence may also have negative organizational outcomes. Table 12-3 identifies some of the causes. Examples of violence include:

◆ **Threats.** Expressions of intent to cause harm, including verbal threats, threatening body language, and written threats

◆ **Physical assaults.** Slapping, beating, rape, homicide, and the use of weapons such as firearms, bombs, or knives

◆ **Muggings.** Assaults conducted by surprise with intent to rob (cdc.gov/niosh/pdfs/ 2002-101.pdf)

The circumstances surrounding health-care work contributes to workers' susceptibility to homicide and assault (Edwards, 1999; nursing-world.org/dlwa/osh/wp5;cdc.gov/niosh/pdfs /2002-101.pdf; osha.gov/pls/oshaweb/owas-rch.new_search_results?p_text=workplace%20 violence&p_title=&in_clause='FULL_SITE' &p_status=CURRENT&p_category=&p_log-ger=/pdf):

TABLE 12-3
Negative Organizational Outcomes Due to Workplace Violence
◆ Low worker morale
◆ Increased job stress
◆ Increased worker turnover
◆ Reduced trust of management
◆ Reduced trust of coworkers
◆ Hostile working environment

◆ Prevalence of handguns and other weapons among clients, families, friends.

◆ Increased use of hospitals for criminal holds and violent individuals.

◆ Increased number of acute and chronic mentally ill clients being released without follow-up care.

◆ Having routine contact with the public in unrestricted areas.

◆ Working alone or in small numbers.

◆ Working late or until the very early morning hours.

◆ Working in high-crime areas.

◆ Working in buildings with poor security.

◆ Treating weapon-carrying clients and families.

◆ Working with inexperienced staff.

◆ Working in units needing seclusion or restraint activities.

◆ Transporting clients.

◆ Clients waiting long times for service.

◆ Having overcrowded, uncomfortable waiting areas.

◆ Lacking staff training and policies for managing crises.

Nurses must know their workplace. For example (www/nursingworld.org/dlwa.osh/wp5?):

◆ How does violence from the surrounding community affect your workplace?

◆ Do services like trauma or acute psychiatric care increase the likelihood of violence?

◆ Does the facility's physical layout invite violence—for example, do doors open to the street? Are waiting rooms cramped?

◆ How frequently do assaultive incidents, threats, and verbal abuse occur? Where? Who is involved? Are incidents reported?

◆ Are current emergency response systems effective?

◆ Are postassaultive treatment and support available to staff?

◆ Are staffing patterns sufficient, and is the staff experienced?

In the beginning of the chapter, the nurse who was attacked and killed by a patient in April 2001 was mentioned. Although assaults that result in severe injury or death usually receive media coverage, most assaults on nurses by patients or coworkers are not reported by the nurse. Working in a health-care facility is considered to be the third most dangerous job in the United States (nursingworld.org/ajn/w001/jul/ISSUES):

Ms. Jones works on the evening shift in the emergency department (ED) at a large urban hospital. The ED frequently receives patients who have been victims of gunshot wounds, stabbings, and other gang-related incidents. Many of the patients entering the ED are high on alcohol or drugs. Ms. Jones has just interviewed a 21-year-old male client who is awaiting treatment as a result of a fight during an evening of heavy drinking. Because his injuries have been determined not to be life-threatening, he had to wait to see a doctor. "I'm tired of waiting. Let's get this show on the road," he screamed loudly as Ms. Jones walked by. "I'm sorry you have to wait, Mr. P., but the doctor is busy with another client and will get to you as soon as possible." She handed him a cup of juice she had been bringing to another client. He grabbed the cup, threw it in her face, and then grabbed her arm. Slamming her against the wall, he jumped off the stretcher and yelled obscenities at her. He continued to scream in her face until a security guard intervened.

Be aware of clues that may indicate a potential for violence (Box 12-2). These behaviors may occur in clients, family members, visitors, or even other staff members. Even clients with no history of violent behavior may react violently to medication or pain (Carroll & Sheverbush, 1996; Lanza & Carifio, 1991).

BOX 12-2

Behaviors Indicating a Potential for Violence

◆ History of violent behavior
◆ Delusional, paranoid, or suspicious speech
◆ Aggressive, threatening statements
◆ Rapid speech, angry tone of voice
◆ Pacing, tense posture, clenched fists, tightening jaw
◆ Alcohol or drug use
◆ Male gender, youth
◆ Policies that set unrealistic limits

Adapted from Kinkle, S. (1993). Violence in the ED: How to stop it before it starts. *American Journal of Nursing, 93*(7), 22–24; Carroll, C., & Sheverbush, J. (September 1996). Violence assessment in hospitals provides basis for action. *American Nurse,* 18.

TABLE 12-4
When an Assault Occurs: Placing Blame on Victims

Victim Gender
Women receive more blame than men.

Subject Gender
Female victims receive more blame from women than men.

Severity
The more severe the assault, the more often the victim is blamed.

Beliefs
The world is a just place, and therefore the person deserves the misfortune.

Age of Victim
The older the victim, the more he or she is held to blame.

Adapted from Lanza, M.L., & Carifio, J. (1991). Blaming the victim: Complex (nonlinear) patterns of causal attribution by nurses in response to vignettes of a patient assaulting a nurse. *Journal of Emergency Nursing*, 17, 299–309.

In the health-care industry, violence is underreported, and there are persistent misperceptions that assaults are part of the job and that the victim somehow caused the assault. Causes of underreporting may be a lack of institutional reporting policies and employee fear that the assault was a result of negligence or poor job performance (U.S. Department of Labor, 1995). Table 12-4 lists some of the faulty reasoning that leads to placing blame on the victim of the assault.

Actions to address violence in the workplace include (1) identifying the factors that contribute to violence and controlling as many as possible and (2) assessing staff attitudes and knowledge regarding violence in the workplace (Carroll & Sheverbush, 1996; Collins, 1994; Mahoney, 1991).

When you begin your new job, you may want to find out the policies and procedures related to violence in the workplace at your institution. Preventing an incident is better than having to intervene after violence has occurred. The following are suggestions to nurses about how to participate in workplace safety related to violence (nursingworld.org/osh/wp5/htm):

◆ *Participate in or initiate regular workplace assessments.* Identify unsafe areas and the factors within the organization that contribute

to assaultive behavior such as inadequate staffing, high activity times of day, invasion of personal space, seclusion or restraint activities, and lack of experienced staff. Work with management to make and monitor changes.

◆ *Be alert for suspicious behavior* such as verbal expressions of anger and frustration, threatening body language, signs of drug or alcohol use, or presence of a weapon. Assess clients or suspicious workers, clients, and visitors for potential violence. Evaluate each situation for potential violence. Keep an open path for exiting.

◆ *Maintain behavior that helps to defuse anger.* Present a calm, caring attitude. Do not match threats, give orders, or present with behaviors that may be interpreted as aggressive. Acknowledge the person's feelings.

◆ *If you cannot defuse the situation:* quickly remove yourself from it, call Security, and report the situation to management.

◆ *Know your clients.* Be aware of any history of violent behaviors, diagnoses of dementia, alcohol, or drug intoxication.

Box 12-3 lists some additional actions that can be taken to protect staff members and clients from violence in the workplace.

BOX 12-3
Steps Toward Increasing Protection From Workplace Violence

◆ Security personnel and escorts
◆ Panic buttons in medication rooms, stairwells, activity rooms, and nursing stations
◆ Bulletproof glass in reception, triage, and admitting areas
◆ Locked or key-coded access doors
◆ Closed-circuit television
◆ Metal detectors
◆ Use of beepers and/or cellular car phones
◆ Handheld alarms or noise devices
◆ Lighted parking lots
◆ Escort or buddy system
◆ Enforced wearing of photo identification badges

Adapted from Simonowitz, J. (1994). Violence in the workplace: You're entitled to protection. *RN*, 57(11), 61–63; nursingworld.org/dlwa/osh/wp6.

What if, in spite of all precautions, violence occurs? What should you do?:

◆ Report to your supervisor. Report threats as well as actual violence. Include a description of the situation; names of victims, witnesses, and perpetrators; and any other pertinent information.

◆ Call the police. Although the assault is in the workplace, nurses are entitled to the same rights as workers assaulted in another setting.

◆ Get medical attention. This includes medical care, counseling, and evaluation.

◆ Contact your collective bargaining unit or your state nurses association. Inform them if the problems persist.

◆ Be proactive. Get involved in policy making (nursingworld.org/ajn/2001/jul/issues).

SEXUAL HARASSMENT

A new supervisor was hired on the unit. After months of interviewing, the candidate selected was a young male nurse whom the staff members jokingly described as "a blond Tom Cruise." The new supervisor was an instant hit with the predominantly female executives and staff members. However, he soon found himself on the receiving end of sexual jokes and innuendoes. He had been trying to prove himself a competent supervisor, with hopes of eventually moving up to a higher management position. He viewed the behavior of the female staff members and supervisors as undermining his credibility, in addition to being embarrassing and annoying. He attempted to have the unwelcome conduct stopped by discussing it with his boss, a female nurse manager. She told him jokingly that it was nothing more than "good-natured fun" and besides, "men can't be harassed by women" (Outwater, 1994).

In spite of the requirement for workplace education related to sexual harassment, it still remains one of the most persistent problems. The reasons are complex, but sex role stereotypes and the unequal balance of power between men and women are major contributors. Unfortunately, underreporting of this problem is common even though the emotional costs of anger, humiliation, and fear are high (nursingworld.org/dlwa/wpr/wp3/htm).

The laws that prohibit discrimination in the workplace are based on the Fifth and Fourteenth Amendments to the Constitution, mandating due process and equal protection under the law. The Equal Employment Opportunity Commission (EEOC) oversees the administration and enforcement of issues related to workplace equality. Although there may be exemptions from any law, it is important that nurses recognize that there is significant legislation that prohibits employers from making workplace decisions based on race, color, sex, age, disability, religion, or national origin.

The employer may ask questions related to these issues but cannot make decisions about employment based on them. Behaviors that could be defined as sexual harassment are identified in Table 12-5. The EEOC issued a statement in 1980 that sexual harassment is a form of sex discrimination prohibited by Title VII of the Civil Rights Act of 1964. Two forms of sexual harassment are identified; both are based on the premise that the action is unwelcome sexual conduct:

1. **Quid pro quo.** Sexual favors are given in exchange for favorable job benefits or continuation of employment. The employee must demonstrate that he or she was required to endure unwelcome sexual advances to keep the job or job benefits and that rejection of these behaviors would have resulted in deprivation of a job or benefits. Example: The administrator approaches a nurse for a date in exchange for a salary increase 3 months before the scheduled review.
2. **Hostile environment.** This is the most common sexual harassment claim and

TABLE 12-5
Behaviors That Could Be Defined as Sexual Harassment

◆ Pressure to participate in sexual activities
◆ Asking about another person's sexual activities, fantasies, preferences
◆ Making sexual innuendoes, jokes, comments, or suggestive facial expressions
◆ Continuing to ask for a date after the other person has expressed disinterest
◆ Making sexual gestures with hands or body movements or showing sexual graffiti or visuals
◆ Making remarks about a person's gender or body

the most difficult to prove. The employee making the claim must prove that the harassment is based on gender and that it has affected conditions of employment or created an environment so offensive that the employee could not effectively discharge the responsibilities of the job (Outwater, 1994).

In 1993, the Supreme Court ruled that a plaintiff is not required to prove any psychological injury to establish a harassment claim. If the environment could be shown to be hostile or abusive, there was no further need to establish that it was also psychologically injurious. Although sexual harassment against women is more common, men can be victims as well.

Sexual harassment can cost an employer money, unfavorable publicity, expensive lawsuits, and large damage awards. Low morale caused by a hostile work environment can cause significant decreases in employee productivity, increased absenteeism, increases in sick leave and medical payments, and decreased job satisfaction.

In addition to Title VII, other legal protections include Title IX of the Education Amendments of 1972 and state fair employment statutes. Title IX of the Education Amendments of 1972 prohibits sex discrimination and sexual harassment in any educational program receiving financial assistance from the federal government. Students and employees are covered by this law. Most state fair employment statutes apply to public and private employers, employment agencies, and labor organizations. Often, state workers' compensation statutes provide remedies for employees who have been injured, either physically or psychologically, by sexual harassment in the workplace. Prohibition against sexual harassment in the workplace may also be included in collective bargaining agreements (nursingworld. org/readroom/position/workplac/wkharass).

Addressing the issue of sexual harassment in the workplace is important. As an employee, be familiar with the policies and procedures related to reporting sexual harassment incidents. If you supervise other employees, regularly review your agency's policies and procedures. Seek appropriate guidance from your Human Resources personnel. If an employee approaches you with a complaint, a confidential investigation of the charges should be initiated. Above all, do not dismiss any incidents or charges of sexual harassment involving yourself or others as "just having fun" or respond that "there is nothing anyone can do." Responses such as this can have serious consequences in the workplace (Outwater, 1994).

The ANA cites four tactics to fight sexual harassment (nursingworld.org/dlwa/wpr/ wp3/htm):

1. **Confront.** Indicate immediately and clearly to the harasser that the attention is unwanted. If you are in a union facility, ask the nursing representative to accompany you.
2. **Report.** Report the incident immediately to your supervisor. If the harasser is your supervisor, report the incident to a higher authority. File a formal complaint, and follow the chain of command.
3. **Document.** Document the incident immediately while it is fresh in your mind—what happened, when and where it occurred, and how you responded. Name any witnesses. Keep thorough records, and keep them in a safe place away from work.
4. **Support.** Seek support from friends, relatives, and organizations such as your state nurses association. If you are a student, seek support from a trusted faculty member or advisor. Additionally, your employer has a responsibility to maintain a harassment-free workplace. You should expect your employer to demonstrate commitment to creating a harassment-free workplace, provide strong written policies prohibiting sexual harassment and describing how employees will be protected, and educate all employees verbally and in writing.

LATEX ALLERGY

A nurse developed hives in 1987, nasal congestion in 1989, and asthma in 1992. She was diagnosed with latex allergy. Eventually she developed severe respiratory symptoms in the health-care environment even when she had no direct contact with latex. The nurse was forced to leave her occupation because of these health effects (Bauer, et al., 1993).

A midwife initially suffered hives, nasal congestion, and conjunctivitis. Within a year, she developed asthma, and 2 years later she went into shock after a routine gynecological examination during which latex gloves were used. The midwife also suffered respiratory distress in latex-containing environments when she had no direct contact with latex products. She was unable to continue working (Bauer, et al., 1993).

A physician with a history of seasonal allergies, runny nose, and eczema on his hands suffered severe runny nose, shortness of breath, and collapse minutes after putting on a pair of latex gloves. A cardiac arrest team successfully resuscitated him (Rosen, et al., 1993).

Latex products are manufactured from the milky fluid of the rubber tree. Latex allergy was first identified in the late 1970s. It has become such a major health problem in the workplace that both the OSHA and the ANA have devoted Web sites to the problem. It is estimated that currently 8% to 12% of health-care workers are sensitive to natural rubber latex products. Table 12-6 lists products commonly produced with latex.

Since the 1987 CDC recommendations for universal precautions, use of latex gloves has greatly increased exposure of health-care workers to natural rubber latex (NRL). The two major routes of exposure to NRL are skin and inhalation, particularly when glove powder acts as a carrier for NRL protein (OSHA latex alert at cdc.gov/niosh/latexalt). Reactions range from contact dermatitis, with scaling, drying, cracking, and blistering skin, to allergic contact dermatitis in the form of generalized hives. More serious generalized reactions can progress to generalized urticaria, rhinitis, wheezing, swelling, shortness of breath, and anaphylaxis. According to the NIOSH, the most common reaction to latex products is irritant contact dermatitis, the development of dry, itchy, irritated areas on the skin, usually the hands. This reaction is caused by irritation from wearing gloves and by exposure to the powders added to them.

Irritant contact dermatitis is not a true allergy. Allergic contact dermatitis (sometimes called *chemical sensitivity dermatitis*) results from the chemicals added to latex during harvesting, processing, or manufacturing. These chemicals can cause a skin rash similar to that of poison ivy. Neither irritant contact dermatitis nor chemical sensitivity dermatitis is a true allergy (cdc.gov/niosh/98-113).

Latex allergy should be suspected if an employee develops symptoms after latex exposures. A complete medical history can reveal latex sensitivity, and blood tests approved by the Food and Drug Administration are available to detect latex antibodies. Skin testing and glove-use tests are also available.

TABLE 12-6
Latex Equipment

Emergency Equipment	Personal Protective Equipment	Office Supplies	Hospital Supplies
Blood pressure cuffs	Gloves	Rubber bands	Anesthesia masks
Stethoscopes	Surgical masks	Erasers	Catheters
Disposable gloves	Goggles		Wound drains
Oral and nasal airways	Respirators		Injection ports
Endotracheal tubes	Rubber aprons		Rubber tops of multidose vials
Tourniquets			Dental dams
IV tubing			Hot water bottles
Syringes			Baby bottle nipples
Electrode pads			Pacifiers

Adapted from OSHA Latex allergy: osha-slc.gov/SLTC/latexallergy/index; and OSHA latex alert cdc.gov/niosh/latexalt?

Compete latex avoidance is the most effective approach. Medications may reduce allergic symptoms, and special precautions are needed to prevent exposure during medical and dental care. Encourage employees with a latex allergy to wear a medical alert bracelet.

Decreasing the potential for development of latex allergy consists of reducing unnecessary exposure to NRL proteins for all health-care workers. Many employees in a health-care setting, such as food handlers or gardeners, can use alternative gloves. If an employee must use NRL gloves, gloves with a lower protein content and those that are powder-free should be considered. Good housekeeping practices should be identified to remove latex-containing dust from the workplace. Employee education programs to ensure appropriate work practices and hand washing should be encouraged. Identification of employees with increased potential for latex allergies is not possible. However, clinical evidence indicates that certain workers may be at greater risk, including those with the following histories:

◆ History of allergies to pollens, grasses, and certain foods or plants (avocado, banana, kiwi, chestnut)

◆ History of multiple surgeries

Decrease the potential for latex allergy problems (cdc.gov/niosh/98-113):

◆ Evaluate any cases of hand dermatitis or other signs or symptoms of potential latex allergy.

◆ Use latex-free procedure trays and crash carts.

◆ Use nonlatex gloves for activities that do not involve contact with infectious materials.

◆ Avoid using oil-based creams or lotions, which can cause glove deterioration.

◆ Seek ongoing training and the latest information related to latex allergy.

◆ Wash, rinse, and dry hands thoroughly after removing gloves or between glove changes.

◆ Use powder-free gloves.

In spite of all precautions, what do you do if you develop a latex allergy? At this point, never wear latex gloves. Be aware of the following precautions (nursingworld.org/dlwa/osh/wp7):

◆ Avoid all types of latex exposure.

◆ Wear a medical alert bracelet.

◆ Carry an EPI-kit with auto-injectible epinephrine.

◆ Alert employers and colleagues to your latex sensitivity.

◆ Carry nonlatex gloves.

OSHA "Right to Know" laws require employers to inform health-care workers of potentially dangerous substances in the workplace. For continuing information on latex allergies, see the NIOSH home page at cdc.gov/niosh

Clients as well as workers are at risk and should be screened for allergies. Clients with a history of hay fever, food allergies (especially to bananas, avocados, potatoes, tomatoes), asthma, or eczema can be at risk. A thorough health history is vital. Treat any indication of potential latex sensitivity seriously (Society of Gastroenterology Nurses and Associates, 2001). In 2006, most health-care personnel are well aware of issues related to latex allergies. In recent years, the number of new cases of latex allergy has decreased due to improved diagnositic methods, improved education, and more accurate labeling of medical devices. Although current research does not demonstrate whether the amount of allergen released during shipping and storage into medications from vials with rubber closures is sufficient to induce a systemic allergic reaction, nurses should take special precautions when clients are identified as high risk for latex allergies. The nursing staff should work closely with the pharmacy staff to follow universal one-stick-rule precautions, which assume that every pharmaceutical vial may contain a natural rubber latex closure, and the nurse should remain with any client at the start of medication and keep frequent observations and vital signs for 2 hours (Hamilton, et al., 2005).

NEEDLESTICK INJURIES

In 1997, a 27-year-old nurse, Lisa Black, attended an in-service session on postexposure prophylaxis for needlesticks. A short time later, she was attempting to aspirate blood from a client's intravenous line. The client, in the advanced stages of acquired immunodeficiency syndrome, moved, and the needle went into Lisa's hand. Nine months later she tested positive for HIV and 3 months after that for hepatitis C. She continues to share her story with nurses everywhere in an effort to prevent this unfortunate accident from happening to one more nurse (Trossman, 1999a).

Although health-care workers are much more aware of needlestick injuries, the potential for these exposures to lead to diseases such as hepatitis B, hepatitis C, and HIV is still very high. Health-care workers still suffer between 600,000 and 1,000,000 injuries from needles and sharps on an annual basis, with more than 80% of these being preventable. Millions of dollars in savings can be seen after implementing safer needle devices. These devices add only $.28 to the cost of standard devices, but one case of a serious infection by a blood-borne pathogen can run in excess of one million dollars (nursingworld.org/readroom/fsneedle).

On April 18, 2001, the Needlestick Act, or revised Bloodborne Pathogens Standard, went into effect. The revised OSHA Bloodborne Pathogens Standard obligates employers to consider safer needle devices when they conduct their annual review of their exposure control plan. Frontline employees must be included in the annual review and updating of standards process. Stricter requirements are now in effect for annual review and updating to reflect changes in technology that eliminate or reduce exposure to blood-borne pathogens (osha.gov/needlesticks/needlefaq).

Your Employer's Responsibility

According to the current OSHA requirements, your employer must provide you with the following (ANA, 1993; nursingworld.org/dlwa/osh/wp2):

◆ Free hepatitis B vaccine.

◆ Protective equipment that fits you (gloves, gowns, goggles, masks).

◆ Immediate, confidential medical evaluation, treatment, and follow-up if you are exposed.

◆ Implementation of universal precautions institution-wide.

◆ Adequate sharps disposal.

◆ Proper removal of hazards from the workplace.

◆ Annual employee training.

Your Responsibility

What are your responsibilities related to this revised legislation? Each year your institution must review and update its blood-borne pathogen standards. You will need to take the time to learn new devices and make certain that the current safety requirements are enforced with employees. Be part of the solution—volunteer to participate in evaluation committees, or work on teams testing new devices. Follow these guidelines in your daily nursing practice (ANA, 1993; Brooke, 2001; nursingworld.org/dlwa/osh/wp2; Perry, 2001):

◆ Always use universal precautions.

◆ Properly use and dispose of sharps.

◆ Be immunized against hepatitis B.

◆ Immediately wash all exposed skin with soap and water.

◆ Flush affected eyes or mucous membranes with saline or water.

◆ Report all exposures according to your facility's protocol.

◆ If possible, know the HIV/hepatitis B virus status of your client.

◆ Comply with postexposure follow-up.

◆ Support others who are exposed.

◆ Become active in the safety committee—be a change agent.

◆ Educate others.

Although health-care providers are aware of the need to use gloves as a protection against blood-borne pathogens, only one evidence-based summary has been reported regarding blood-borne pathogens and glove safety. The summary explored double gloving versus single gloving in reducing the number of infections.

This includes postoperative wound infections or blood-borne infections in surgical clients and blood-borne infections in the surgical team and to determine if double gloving reduces the incidence of glove perforations compared with single gloving. A total of 18 randomized controlled trials met the inclusion criteria and were included in the review. There is clear evidence from this review that double gloving reduces the number of perforations to the innermost glove. There does not appear to be an increase in the number of perforations to the outermost glove when two pairs of gloves are worn. Korniewicz et al. (2004) participated in the first clinical trial to test the barrier integrity of nonlatex sterile surgical gloves after use in the operating room. During the 14-month study, more than 21,000 gloves were collected from more than 4000 surgical procedures. Based on their results, they concluded that nonlatex or intact latex gloves provide adequate barrier protection but that nonlatex gloves may tear more frequently than latex during use.

ERGONOMIC INJURIES

Occupational-related back injuries affect more than 75% of nurses over the lifetime of their career. Poor ergonomics are a safety factor for both nurses and clients, whose safe nursing care is already in jeopardy by the escalating nursing shortage (Durr, 2004).

Back Injuries

The most critical of ergonomic injuries are back injuries. Annually, 12% of nurses leave the profession as a result of back injuries, and more than 52% complain of chronic back pain. The problem with lifting a client is not just one of overcoming heavy weight. Size, shape, and deformities of the client as well as balance and coordination, combativeness, uncooperativeness, and contractures must be considered. Any unpredictable movement or resistance from the client can quickly throw the nurse off balance and result in a back injury. Environmental considerations such as space,

equipment interference, and unadjustable beds, chairs, and commodes also contribute to back injury risk (Edlich, Woodard, & Haines, 2001).

This issue of back injuries and other ergonomic-related injuries has become so severe that in July 2001 the OSHA began to develop a comprehensive approach to ergonomics. Public forums, meetings with stakeholder groups and individuals, and written comments were analyzed. Out of this work, a four-pronged comprehensive approach to ergonomics was developed to include (osha.gov/ergonomics/ergofact02):

1. Task- or industry-specific written guidelines
2. Enforcement
3. Outreach/assistance
4. Research

The OSHA issued an ergonomics guideline for the nursing home industry on March 13, 2003. The back injury guide for health-care workers (dir.ca.gov/dosh/dosh_publications/backinj.pdf) and the OSHA guidelines for nursing homes (osha.gov/ergonomics/guidelines/nursinghome/index) are comprehensive resources. Although guidelines are less than legislated standards, OSHA uses the General Duty Clause to cite employers for ergonomic hazards. Under this clause, employers must keep their workplaces free from recognized serious hazards, including ergonomic hazards. This requirement exists whether or not there are voluntary guidelines (osha.gov/ergonomics/FAQs-external).

Suggestions for decreasing back injuries for nurses (Slattery, 1998; Trossman, 1999b; Edlich, Woodard, & Haines, 2001) are:

◆ Participate on the safety committee as a nursing representative to develop written guidelines detailing transfer requirements.

◆ Work in teams if possible—do not be afraid to ask for help.

◆ Use transfer and lifting equipment.

◆ Consider environment such as size of room and proximity of beds and chair.

◆ Do back exercises.

Repetitive Stress Injuries

Repetitive stress injuries (RSIs) have been called the *workplace epidemic of the modern age.* RSIs usually affect people who spend long hours at computers, switchboards, and other worksites where repetitive motions are performed. The most common RSIs are carpal tunnel syndrome and mouse elbow. As technology increases in health-care facilities, the use of computers increases for all health-care personnel. Badly designed computer workstations present the highest risk of RSIs. Preventive measures (Krucoff, 2001) include the following:

◆ Keep the monitor screen straight ahead of you, about an arm's length away. Position the center of the screen where your gaze naturally falls.

◆ Align the keyboard so that the forearms, wrists, and hands are aligned parallel to the floor. Do not bend the hands back.

◆ Position the mouse directly next to you and on the same level as the keyboard.

◆ Keep thighs parallel to the floor as you sit on the chair. Feet should touch the floor and the chair back should be ergonomically sound.

◆ Vary tasks. Avoid long sessions of sitting. Do not use excessive force when typing or clicking the mouse.

◆ Keep fingernails short, and use fingertips when typing.

The ANA, supported by the Johnson & Johnson Foundation, has begun a campaign "Handle with Care." This initiative is aimed at preventing potentially career-ending back and other musculoskeletal injuries among nurses. The investment in a safe client-handling program may seem daunting due to the cost of equipment such as mechanical lifts, transfer aids, and ergonomic beds and chairs. However, the cost savings in time, reduction of injuries, and lost workdays, as well as improved quality of care for clients, make this a sound return on investment. Health-care facilities that have invested in these programs report cost savings in thousands of dollars both for direct costs of back injuries and lost workdays (nursingworld.org/handlewithcare/factsheet). In conjunction with the ANA, the Veterans Administration has developed a Patient Safety Center of Inquiry (patientsafetycenter.com/) to support clinicians in providing safe client care by designing and testing clinical innovations, technological solutions, and client safety improvement systems.

IMPAIRED WORKERS

Substance Abuse

Sue had been a nurse for 20 years. Current marital and family problems were affecting her at work. To ease the tension, she took a Xanax from a client's medication drawer. This seemed to ease her tension. She continued to take medications, working her way up to narcotic analgesics.

Bill had begun weekend binge-drinking in college. Ten years later, he still continues the habit several times during the month. He does not believe he is an alcoholic because he can "control" his drinking. After he begins showing up at work hungover and making medication errors, he is fired for the medication errors. At the exit interview, no mention is made of his drinking problem. The agency feared a lawsuit for defamation of character.

Mr. P., the unit manager, has noticed that Ms. J. has frequently been late for work. She arrives with a wrinkled uniform, dirty shoes, unkempt hair, and broken nails. Lately she has been overheard making terse remarks to clients such as, "Who do you think I am—your maid?" and spends longer and longer periods off the unit. The floor has a large number of surgical clients who receive intramuscular and oral medications for pain. Lately, Ms. J.'s clients continue to complain of pain even after medication administration has been charted. Ms. J. frequently forgets to waste her intramuscular narcotics in front of another nurse. Mr. P. is concerned that Ms. J. may be an impaired nurse.

As nursing education moved from the untrained nurse, embodied in the character of Sairey Gamp in the Dickens novel *Martin Chuzzlewit,* to the educated Florence Nightingale model, nurses were expected to be of good moral character. The problem of addiction among nurses was not discussed until the 1950s, with addicted nurses receiving little sympathy or treatment from their peers. Research on addicted medical professionals increased in the 1970s, with major help for nurses with addictive disease in 1980. At this time the National Nurses' Society on Addictions (NNSA) task force and the ANA task force on addictions and psychological functions jointly passed a resolution calling for acknowledgment of the problem and guidelines for impaired nurse programs (Heise, 2003).

Alcohol and drug abuse continue to be major health problems in this country. Health-care professionals are not immune to alcoholism or chemical dependency. In addition, various kinds of mental illnesses may also affect a nurse's ability to deliver safe, competent care. Impaired workers can adversely affect client care, staff retention, morale, and management time as team members try to pick up the slack for the impaired worker (Damrosch & Scholler-Jaquish, 1993). The most common signs of impairment are performed (Damrosch & Scholler-Jaquish, 1993; Blair, 2005):

◆ Witnessed consumption of alcohol or other substances on the job.

◆ Changes in dress, appearance, posture, gestures.

◆ Slurred speech, abusive/incoherent language.

◆ Reports of impairment or erratic behavior from clients and/or coworkers.

◆ Witnessed unprofessional conduct.

◆ Significant lack of attention to detail.

◆ Witnessed theft of controlled substances.

◆ Assigned clients routinely request pain medication within a short period of being medicated.

Most employers and state boards of nursing have strict guidelines related to impaired nurses. Impaired-nurse programs conducted by state boards of nursing work with the employer to assist the impaired nurse to remain licensed while receiving help for the addiction problem. It is important that you become aware of workplace issues surrounding the impaired worker, signs and symptoms of impairment, and the policies and reporting procedures concerning an impaired worker. Compassion from coworkers and supervisors is of utmost importance in assisting the impaired worker to seek help (Damrosch & Scholler-Jaquish, 1993; Sloan & Vernarec, 2001). The National Council of State Boards lists all state boards of nursing. Information on support

programs for impaired nurses can be obtained from each state board (ncsbn.org/regulation/nursingpractice_npa_pennrn.asp).

Upholding the standards of the nursing profession is everyone's responsibility. Often coworkers, noticing a change in another's behavior, become protective and take on more work to ease the burden of their coworker. Although it is difficult to report a colleague, covering up or ignoring the problem can cause serious risks for the client and the nurse. Many state boards make it mandatory for nurses to report suspected impaired coworkers Most states accept anonymous reports. In many states, state law requires hospitals and health-care providers to report impaired practitioners, but the law also grants immunity from civil liability if the report was made in good faith (Sloan & Vernarec, 2001; Blair, 2005).

Microbial Threats

Health-care workers are an at-risk group for several microbial threats. Severe acute respiratory syndromes (SARS) is a respiratory illness that has been reported in Asia, Europe, and North America. According to the World Health Organization, 8,098 people worldwide became sick with SARS during the 2003 outbreak. SARS begins with a high fever and mild respiratory symptoms. Other symptoms may include headache, an overall feeling of discomfort, and body aches. It is not uncommon for the person to have diarrhea and develop a dry cough. Most clients develop pneumonia. The virus that causes SARS is thought to be transmitted most readily by respiratory droplets. The virus also can spread when a person touches a surface or object contaminated with infectious droplets and then touches his or her mouth, nose, or eye(s). In addition, it is possible that the SARS virus might spread more broadly through the air (airborne spread) or by other ways that are not now known. The CDC provides current information on the handling of SARS in the workplace (cdc.gov).

Unlike the newer microbial threat SARS, tuberculosis (TB) was a leading cause of death among infectious diseases from the 19th into the mid-20th centuries. Although TB rates declined in the 1990s, they are currently on the rise as resources that were committed to fighting the disease were withdrawn. Unfortunately, a more serious form of TB, mutidrug-resistant tuberculosis (MDR-TB) is on the rise. Nurses often come in contact with persons with active TB. At times, clients do not know they are infected until coming to the hospital with another complaint. As with SARS, the CDC provides current information and guidelines for dealing with TB in the workplace (cdc.gov/nchstp/tb/pubs/TB_HIVcoinfection/default).

ENHANCING THE QUALITY OF WORK LIFE

In the prior edition of this book, the issues of rotating shifts, mandatory overtime, and staffing ratios were discussed. The continued nursing shortage enforces an awareness to "treat with kindess" the nurses who remain in the workforce.

Rotating Shifts

Safety in the workplace involves nurses working rotating shifts. Nurses who work permanently at night often readjust their sleep-wake cycle. However, even permanent nightworkers may be subjected to continuous sleep deprivation. Nurses who randomly rotate shifts throw off their circadian rhythm. Fatigue, the number one complaint of these nurses, is the result of the body never getting the chance to adapt to changing sleep-wake cycles. The literature links some of the world's worst disasters, such as the Chernobyl nulear reactor catastrophe and the Exxon Valdez oil spill, to rotating shift work and the changes in circadian rhythm. Other effects of shift work include a higher risk of miscarriage and premature labor, menstrual and digestive problems, and respiratory irritation. One of the most serious results of rotating night shifts is the increasing number of nurses affected by coronary heart disease (CHD). Studies indicate that nurses who rotate to nights for 6 years have a 70% greater risk of developing CHD than nurses who never rotated shifts due to the circadian effect of lowering of blood pressure and heart rate at night (Trossman, 1999b). Suggestions for nurses who rotate shifts:

◆ Try to schedule working the same shifts for an entire scheduling period instead of rotating different shifts in one schedule.

◆ Try to schedule to same days off within the schedule.

◆ If you become sleepy during the shift, take a walk or climb stairs.

◆ Limit caffeine intake, especially toward the end of the shift.

◆ If you work evenings or nights, do not eat a big meal at the end of the shift. This interferes with sleep.

◆ Try to sleep a continuous block of time instead of catching a few hours here and there.

◆ Make the room you are sleeping in as dark and noise-free as possible.

◆ Maintain good nutrition and an exercise program.

◆ Negotiate your schedule with your manager. If you and your colleagues feel strongly about eliminating rotating shifts, work together to make changes (Trossman, 1999b).

Mandatory Overtime

When nurses are routinely forced to work beyond their scheduled hours, they can suffer a range of emotional and physical effects. As client acuity and workloads increase, working overtime puts the client and the nurse at greater risk. Mandatory overtime is seen by nurses as a control issue. Working overtime should be a choice, not a requirement. In some facilities, nurses are being threatened with dismissal or charge of client abandonment if they refuse to participate in mandatory overtime (nursingworld.org/tan/98mayjun/ot).

The ANA presented the following message to the 107th Congress in 2001: "ANA opposes the use of mandatory overtime as a staffing tool. We urge you to support legislation that would ban the use of mandatory overtime through Medicare and Medicaid law. Nurses must be given the opportunity to refuse overtime if we believe that we are too fatigued to provide quality care." (nursingworld.org/gova/federal/legis/107/ovrtme). Dembe, Erickson, Delbros, and Banks (2005) analyzed the occurrence of occupational injury and illness between 1987 and 2000. After a review of 10,793 participants working at least 12 hours per day, working overtime was associated with a 23% increased work hazard and a 61% higher injury hazard rate compared with jobs without overtime. More recently, Rogers et al. (2004) found that nurses' error rates increase significantly during overtime, after 12 hours, and over more than 60 hours per week. Currently, there are no regulations governing nurses' work hours. About half of staff nurses are scheduled routinely to work 12-hour shifts and 85% of staff nurses routinely work longer than scheduled hours.

Staffing Ratios

Although some state nurses associations are calling for mandated staffing ratios, the issue is not clear-cut. What has become clear is that there is no "one size fits all" solution. In 2004, a review was conducted of peer-reviewed studies published between 1980 and 2003 of the effects of nurse staffing on client, nurse employee, and hospital outcomes. Again, the literature offered no support for specific nurse-client ratios. However, findings from 12 key studies stood out, citing specific effects of nurse staffing on client outcomes: incidences of failure to rescue, in-client mortality, pnuemonia, urinary tract infections, and pressure ulcers. Effects of nurse staffing levels on nurse employee outcomes included needlestick

injuries, nursing burnout, and nursing documentation, whereas hospital length of stay, financial outcomes, and direct nursing care were experienced by the hospital. Table 12-7 provides a matrix for staffing decision making.

Above all, the ANA recommends moving staffing away from an industrial model of measuring time and motion to a more professional model that would examine factors needed to provide quality care. Changes in staffing levels should be based on analysis of nursing-sensitive indicators (nursingworld. org/readroom/stffprnc).

Utilization of Unlicensed Assistive Personnel

Educational preparation and clinical experiences in practice for nurses differs for basic registered nurse (RN) education. The nursing shortage will continue to force health-care facilities to explore creative ways of providing safe and effective client care. This will most likely include RNs working with not only licensed practical nurses (LPNs) but also with unlicensed assistive personnel (UAP). The legal regulation of nursing practice is defined by each state nursing practice act; however, the ANA believes that "curricula for all RN programs should include content on supervision, delegation, assignment, and legal aspects regarding nursing's utilization of assistive personnel" (nursingworld.org/readroom/position/uap/uaprned).

Hospital workforce issues will continue to be influenced by economic changes, managed care and insurance issues, media forces, and the nursing shortage. Linda Aiken has been researching relationships between positive client, nurse, and agency outcomes and RN staffing, educational preparation, and organizational culture (Aiken, 2002, 2004). Nurses voice disillusionment with nursing practice and decreased loyalty to organizations. Nursing leaders in the 21st century must demonstrate a respect and value for their nursing staff, communicate effectively with all levels of the organization, maintain visibility, and establish participative decision making. As you move forward in your career, be part of the solution, not the problem (Ray, Turkel, & Marino, 2002).

TABLE 12-7
Matrix for Decision Making: Staffing

CLIENTS	Characteristics and number of clients requiring care
INTENSITY OF UNIT AND CARE	Intensity of individuals within the unit and across the unit; variability of care; admissions, discharges, transfers, volume
CONTEXT	Architecture of unit, technology available
EXPERTISE	Staff consistency, continuity, and cohesion; staff preparation and experience
OTHER	Quality improvement activities; nursing control of practice

Adapted from nursingworld.org/readroom/stffprnc

REPORTING QUESTIONABLE PRACTICES

Most employers have policies that encourage the reporting of behavior that may affect the workplace environment. Behaviors to report may include (ANA, 1994):

1. Endangering a client's health or safety.
2. Abusing authority.
3. Violating laws, rules, regulations, or standards of professional ethics.
4. Grossly wasting funds.

The Code for Nurses (ANA, 2001) is very specific about nurses' responsibility to report questionable behavior that may affect the welfare of a client:

When the nurse is aware of inappropriate or questionable practice in the provision of health care, concern should be expressed to the person carrying out the questionable practice and attention called to the possible detrimental effect on the client's welfare. When factors in the health-care delivery system threaten the welfare of the client, similar action should be directed to the responsible administrative person. If indicated, the practice should then be reported to the appropriate authority within the institution, agency, or larger system (ANA, 2001).

The sources of various federal and state guidelines governing the workplace are listed in Box 12-4.

Protection by the agency should be afforded to both the accused and the person doing the reporting. *Whistleblower* is the term used for an employee who reports employer violations to an outside agency. Do not assume that doing the right thing will protect you. Speaking up could get you fired unless you are protected by a union contract or other formal employment agreement. In May 1994, the U.S. Supreme Court ruled that nurses who direct the work of other employees may be considered supervisors and therefore may not be covered by the protections guaranteed under the National Labor Relations Act. This ruling may cause nurses to have no protection from retaliation if they report illegal practices in the workplace (ANA, 1995b). The 1995 brochure from the ANA (1995a), *Protect Your Patients—Protect Your*

BOX 12-4

Laws Governing Health-Care Practices

◆ State nurse practice acts
◆ Federal and state health regulations
◆ State and federal pharmacy laws for controlled substances
◆ OSHA
◆ State medical records and communicable disease laws
◆ Environmental laws regulating hazardous waste and air and water quality
◆ CDC guidelines
◆ Federal and state antidiscrimination laws
◆ State clinical laboratory regulations
◆ JCAHO regulations

Adapted from American Nurses Association. (1994). *Guidelines on Reporting Incompetent, Unethical, or Illegal Practices.* Washington, DC: ANA.

License, stated, "Be aware that reporting quality and safety issues may result in reprisals by an employer." Does this mean that you should never speak up? Case law, federal and state statutes, and the federal False Claims Act may afford a certain level of protection. Some states have whistleblower laws. They usually apply only to state employees or to certain types of workers. Although these laws may offer some protection, the most important point is to work through the employer's chain of command and internal procedures: (a) make sure that whistleblowing is addressed at your facility, either through a collective bargaining contract or workplace advocacy program; (b) contact your state nurses association to find out if your state offers whistleblower protection or has such legislation pending; (c) be politically active by contacting your state legislators and urge them to support a pending bill or by educating your elected state officials on the need for such protection for all health-care workers; and (d) contact your U.S. congressional representatives and urge them to support the Patient Safety Act (nursingworld.org/tan/98janfeb/nlrbmass).

It is the responsibility of professional nurses to become acquainted with the state and federal regulations, standards of practice and professional performance, and agency protocols and practice guidelines governing their practice. Lack of knowledge will not protect you from ethical and legal obligations. Your state nurses' association can help you seek information related to incompetent, unethical, or illegal practices. When you join your state association, you will gain access to an organization that has input into policies and procedures designed to protect the public.

Although not usually considered a "questionable practice," the ANA is concerned with the rights of disabled nurses. The Americans With Disabilities Act, enacted in 1990, makes it unlawful to discriminate against a qualified individual with a disability. The employer is required to provide reasonable accommodations for the disabled person. A reasonable accommodation is a modification or adjustment to the job, work environment, work schedule, or work procedures that enable a qualified person with a disability to perform the job. Both you and your employer may see information from the Equal Employment Opportunity Commission (EEOC) for information (nursingworld.org/dlwa/wpr/wp6).

TERRORISM AND OTHER DISASTERS

Since the attacks on the World Trade Center and the Pentagon, as well as the anthrax outbreaks and continued terrorist threats nationwide, concerns related to biological and chemical agents have surfaced. The CDC Web site (bt.cdc.gov/) supports ongoing information related to public health emergency preparedness and response. The ANA has published a position statement on work release during a disaster for employers. In addition, the ANA provides RNs with valuable information on how they can better care for their clients, protect themselves, and prepare their hospitals and communities to respond to acts of bioterrorism and natural disasters (nursingworld.org/news/disaster/). For example, many nurses worked with the ANA to provide support for the victims of Hurricane Katrina.

Your importance in emergency readiness and bioterrorism is important. Following are some suggestions for steps that can be implemented in the workplace (awhonn.org/HealthPolicyLegislative/BIOTERRORISM PREPAREDNESS/bioterrorism preparedness):

◆ Know the evacuation procedures and routes in your facility.

◆ Develop your knowledge of the most likely and dangerous biochemical agents.

◆ Monitor for unusual disease patterns, and notify appropriate authorities as needed.

◆ Know the backup systems available for communication and staffing in the event of emergencies.

◆ Know the disaster policies and procedures in your facility as well as state and federal laws that pertain to licensed personnel.

ENHANCING THE QUALITY OF WORK LIFE

Both the social and physical aspects of a workplace can affect the way in which people work and how they feel about their jobs. The social aspects include working relationships, a climate that allows growth and creativity, and cultural diversity.

Social Environment

Working Relationships

Many aspects of the social environment have received attention in earlier chapters. Team building, communicating effectively, and developing leadership skills are essential to the development of working relationships. The day-to-day interactions with one's peers and supervisors have a major impact on the quality of the workplace environment.

Support of One's Peers and Supervisors

Most employees keenly feel the difference between a supportive and a nonsupportive environment:

Ms. B. came to work already tired. Her baby was sick and had been awake most of the night. Her team expressed concern about the baby when she told them she had a difficult night. Each team member voluntarily took an extra client so that Ms. B. could have a lighter assignment that day. When Ms. B. expressed her appreciation, her team leader said, "We know you would do the same for us." Ms. B. worked in a supportive environment.

Ms. G. came to work after a sleepless night. Her young son had been diagnosed with leukemia, and she was very worried about him. When she mentioned her concerns, her team leader interrupted her, saying, "Please leave your personal problems at home. We have a lot of work to do, and we expect you to do your share." Ms. G. worked in a nonsupportive environment.

Support from peers and supervisors involves professional concerns as well as personal ones. In a supportive environment, people are willing to make difficult decisions, take risks, and "go the extra mile" for team members and the organization. In contrast, in a nonsupportive environment, they are afraid to take risks, avoid making decisions, and usually limit their commitment.

Involvement in Decision Making

The importance of having a voice in the decisions made about one's work and clients cannot be overstated. Empowerment is a related phenomenon. It is a sense of having both the ability and the opportunity to act effectively (Kramer & Schmalenberg, 1993). Empowerment is the opposite of apathy and powerlessness. Many actions can be taken to empower nurses: remove barriers to their autonomy and to their participation in decision making, publicly express confidence in their capability and value, reward initiative and assertiveness, and provide role models who demonstrate confidence and competence. The following illustrates the difference between empowerment and powerlessness:

Soon after completing orientation, Nurse A heard a new nurse aide scolding a client for soiling the bed. Nurse A did not know how incidents of potential verbal abuse were handled in this institution, so she reported it to the nurse manager. The nurse manager asked Nurse A several questions and thanked her for the information. The new aide was counseled immediately after their meeting. Nurse A noticed a positive change in the aide's manner with clients after this incident. Nurse A felt good about having contributed to a more effective client care team. Nurse A felt empowered and will take action again when another occasion arises.

A colleague of Nurse B was an instructor at a community college. This colleague asked nurse B if students would be welcome on her unit. "Of course," replied Nurse B. "I'll speak with my head nurse about it." When Nurse B did so, the response was that the unit was too busy to accommodate students. In addition, Nurse B received a verbal reprimand from the supervisor for overstepping her authority by discussing the placement of students. "All requests for student placement must be directed to the education department," she said. The supervisor directed Nurse B to write a letter of apology for having made an unauthorized commit-

ment to the community college. Nurse B was afraid to make any decisions or public statements after this incident. Nurse B felt alienated and powerless.

Professional Growth and Innovation

The difference between a climate that encourages staff growth and creativity and one that does not can be quite subtle. In fact, many people are only partly aware, if at all, whether they work in an environment that fosters professional growth and learning. Yet the effect on the quality of the work done is pervasive, and it is an important factor in distinguishing the merely good health-care organization from the excellent health-care organization.

Much of the responsibility for staff development and promotion of innovation lies with upper-level management, people who can sponsor seminars, conduct organization-wide workshops, establish educational policies, promote career mobility, develop clinical ladders, initiate innovative projects, and reward suggestions.

Some of the ways in which first-line managers can develop and support a climate of professional growth are to encourage critical thinking, provide opportunities to take advantage of educational programs, encourage new ideas and projects, and reward professional growth.

Encourage Critical Thinking

If you ever find yourself or staff members saying, "Don't ask why. Just do it!" you need to evaluate the type of climate in which you are functioning. An inquisitive frame of mind is relatively easy to suppress in a work environment. Clients and staff members quickly perceive a nurse's impatience or defensiveness when too many questions are raised. Their response will be to simply give up asking these questions.

On the other hand, if you support critical thinkers and act as a role model who adopts a questioning attitude, you can encourage others to do the same.

Seek Out Educational Opportunities

In most organizations, first-line managers do not have discretionary funds that can be allocated for educational purposes. However, they can usually support a staff member's request for educational leave or for financial support and often have a small budget that can be used for seminars or workshops.

Team leaders and nurse managers can make it either easier or more difficult for staff members to further their education. They can make things difficult for the staff member who is trying to balance work, home, and school responsibilities. Or they can pitch in and help lighten the load of the staff member who has to finish a paper or take an examination. Unsupportive supervisors have even attacked staff members who pursue further education, criticizing every minor error and blocking their advancement. Obviously, such behavior should be dealt with quickly by upper-level management because it is a serious inhibitor of staff development.

Encourage New Ideas

The increasingly rapid accumulation of knowledge in health care mandates continuous learning for safe practice. Intellectual curiosity is a hallmark of the professional.

Every move up the professional ladder should bring new challenges that enrich one's work (Roedel & Nystrom, 1987). As a professional, you can be a role model for an environment in which every staff member is both challenged and rewarded for meeting these challenges. Participating in brainstorming sessions, group conferences, and discussions encourages the generation of new ideas. Although new nurses may think that they have nothing to offer, it is important for them to participate in activities that encourage them to look at fresh, new ideas.

Reward Professional Growth

A primary source of discontent in the workplace is lack of recognition. Positive feedback and recognition of contributions are important rewards. Everyone enjoys praise and recognition. A smile, a card or note, or a verbal "thank you" goes a long way with coworkers in recognizing a job well done. Staff recognition programs have also been identified as a means to increase self-esteem, social gratification, morale, and job satisfaction (Hurst, Croker, & Bell, 1994).

Cultural Diversity

Ms. V. is beginning orientation for a new staff nurse position. She has been told that part of her orientation will be a morning class on cultural diversity. She says to the Human Resources person in charge of orientation, "I don't think I need to attend that class. I treat all people as equal. Besides, anyone living in the United States has an obligation to learn the language and ways of those of us who were born here, not the other way around."

Mr. M. is a staff nurse on a medical-surgical unit. A young man with HIV infection has been admitted. He is scheduled for surgery in the morning and has requested that his significant other be present for the preoperative teaching. Mr. M. reluctantly agrees but mumbles under his breath to a coworker, "It wouldn't be so bad if they didn't throw their homosexuality around and act like an old married couple. Why can't he act like a man and get his own preop instructions?"

Diversity in health-care organizations includes ethnicity, culture, gender, lifestyle, and career stages of employees. The composition of nurses in health care is changing to include more older workers, minorities, and men. Working with people who have different customs, traditions, communication styles, and beliefs can be exciting as well as challenging. Workforce diversity, in terms of age, gender, culture, ethnicity, race, primary language, physical capabilities, and lifestyle, presents a challenge to the workplace. An organization that fosters diversity in the workplace encourages respect and understanding of human characteristics and acceptance of the similarities and differences that make us human.

Often, when stressful situations arise, gender, age, and culture can contribute to misunderstandings. Davidhizer, Dowd, and Giger (1999) identified six important factors in their model for understanding cultural diversity:

1. **Communication.** Communication and culture are closely bound. Culture is transmitted through communication, and culture influences how verbal and nonverbal communication is expressed. Vocabulary, voice qualities, intonation, rhythm, speed, silence, touch, body postures, eye movements, and pronunciation differ among cultural groups and vary among persons from similar cultures. Using respect as a central core to a relationship, each one of us needs to

assess personal beliefs and communication variables of others in the workplace.

2. **Space.** Personal space is the area that surrounds a person's body. The amount of personal space individuals prefer varies from person to person and from situation to situation. Cultural beliefs also influence a person's personal space comfort zone. In the workplace, an understanding of coworkers' comfort related to personal space is important. Often, this comfort is relayed in nonverbal rather than verbal communication.

3. **Social organization.** In most cultures, the family is the most important social organization. For some people, the importance of family supersedes that of other personal, work, or national causes; for example, caring for a sick child overrides the importance of being on time or even coming to work, regardless of staffing needs or policies. Because the health-care industry employs a large number of women, the value of the family becomes an important issue in the workplace.

4. **Time.** Time orientation is often related to culture, environment, and family experiences. Some cultures are more past-oriented and focus on maintaining traditions, with little interest in goals. People from cultures with more of a present and future orientation may be more likely to engage in activities, such as returning to school or receiving certifications, that will enhance the future. Working with people who have different time orientations may cause difficulty in planning schedules and setting deadlines for the group.

5. **Environment control.** Environmental control consists of those activities that an individual plans to control nature. Environmental control is best understood through the psychological terms *internal* and *external locus of control*. Individuals with an external locus of control believe in fate or chance. People with an internal locus of control believe in developing plans and directing their environment. In the workplace, nurses are expected to operate from an internal locus of control. This approach may be different from

what a person has grown up with or how a client deals with illness.

6. **Biological variations.** More and more information is available to health-care workers about the variations among races in aspects such as body structure, skin color, genetic variations, susceptibility to disease, and psychological differences. JCAHO states that cultural factors must be assessed in developing materials for client education.

As you begin your career, be alert to the signs of cultural diversity or insensitivity where you work. Signs that increased sensitivity and responsiveness to the needs of a culturally diverse workforce are needed on your team or in your organization may include a greater proportion of minorities or women in lower-level jobs, lower career mobility and higher turnover rates in these groups, and acceptance or even approval of insensitivity and unfairness (Malone, 1993). Observe interaction patterns, such as where people sit in the cafeteria or how they cluster during coffee breaks. Are they mixing freely, or are there divisions by gender, race, language, or status in the organization (Moch & Diemert, 1987; Ward, 1992)? Other indications of an organization's diversity "fitness" include the following (Mitchell, 1995):

◆ The personnel mix reflects the current and potential population being served.

◆ Individual cultural preferences pertaining to issues of social distance, touching, voice volume and inflection, silence, and gestures are respected.

◆ There is awareness of special family and holiday celebrations important to people of different cultures.

◆ The organization communicates through action that people are individuals first and members of a particular culture second.

Effective management of cultural diversity requires considerable time and energy. Although organized cultural diversity programs are usually the responsibility of middle- and upper-level managers, you can play a part in raising awareness. You can be a culturally competent practitioner and a role model for others by becoming:

◆ Aware of and sensitive to your own culture-based preferences.

◆ Willing to explore your own biases and values.

◆ Knowledgeable about other cultures.

◆ Respectful of and sensitive to diversity among individuals.

◆ Skilled using and selecting culturally sensitive intervention strategies.

Physical Environment

Attention to the physical environment of the workplace is not as well developed as the social aspect, especially in nursing. The increasing focus on workplace ergonomics, such as modifications to various elements of the physical environment including floors, chairs, desks, beds, and workstations, to decrease the incidence of back and upper extremity injuries, has already been discussed The use of lighting, colors, and music to improve the workplace environment is increasing. Computer workstations designed to promote efficiency in the client care unit are becoming commonplace. Relocation of supplies and substations closer to client rooms to reduce the number of steps, improved visual and auditory scanning of clients from the nurses' station, better light and ventilation, a unified information system, and reduced need for client transport are all possible with changes in the physical environment.

Health-care pollution is a more recently identified problem. Dioxin emissions, mercury, and battery waste are often not disposed of properly in the hospital environment. Disinfectants, chemicals, waste anesthesia gases, and laser plumes that float in the air are other sources of pollution exposure for nurses. Nurses have a responsibility to be aware of these potential problems and identify areas in the hospital at risk. Rethinking product choices, such as avoiding the use of polyvinyl chloride or mercury products, providing convenient collection sites for battery and mercury waste, and making waste management education for employees mandatory, are starts toward a more pollution-free environment (Slattery, 1998). The purchase of recyled paper and products, waste treatment choices that

minimize toxic disinfectants, and waste disposal choices that reduce incineration to a maximum are needed. Nurses as professionals need to be aware of the consequences of the medical waste produced by the health sector, supporting continued education for both nurses and clients.

NURSING'S AGENDA FOR THE FUTURE

"Individuals choose nursing as a career, and remain in the profession, because of the opportunities for personal and professional growth, supportive work environments, and compensation commensurate with roles and responsibilities" (ANA. 2005). In order to reach the desired agenda for the future of nursing, 10 areas of concern that demand action were identified at the ANA Summit. Box 12-5 identifies the 10 areas of concern. By the time you finish this textbook, each of these domains will have been addressed. The question to you: Will you be part of the problem or part of the solution? I challenge you, as a member of this highly valued profession, to join us in being part of the solution.

CONCLUSION

Workplace safety is an area of increasing concern. Staff members have a right to be informed of any potential risks in the workplace. Employers have a responsibility to

---

BOX 12-5

Ten Domains of Nursing Agenda for the Future

◆ Leadership and planning
◆ Delivery systems
◆ Legislation/regulation/policy
◆ Professiona/nursing culture
◆ Recruitment/retention
◆ Economic value
◆ Work environment
◆ Public relations/communication
◆ Education
◆ Diversity

ANA. (2005). Nursing's Agenda for the Future nursingworld.org

provide adequate equipment and supplies to protect employees and to create programs and policies to inform employees about minimizing risks to the extent possible. Issues of workplace violence, sexual harassment, impaired workers, ergonomics and other workplace injuries, and terrorism should be addressed to protect both employees and clients. The IOM and JCAHO client safety initiatives will continue to affect the way nurses do business. Workplace issues related to nursing and positive client outcomes will continue to be discussed.

A social environment that promotes professional growth and creativity and a physical environment that offers comfort and maxi-mum work efficiency should be considered in improving the quality of work life. Cultural awareness, respect for the diversity of others, and increased contact between groups should be the goals of the workforce for the next century.

Many waking hours are spent in the workplace. It can offer a climate of companionship, professional growth, and excitement. Decades of research have consistently shown that high-quality nursing care reduces the rate of complications and lengths of stay in hospitals (ANA, 2005). Join the ANA and the other 2.7 million nurses to chart the course for nursing in 2010.

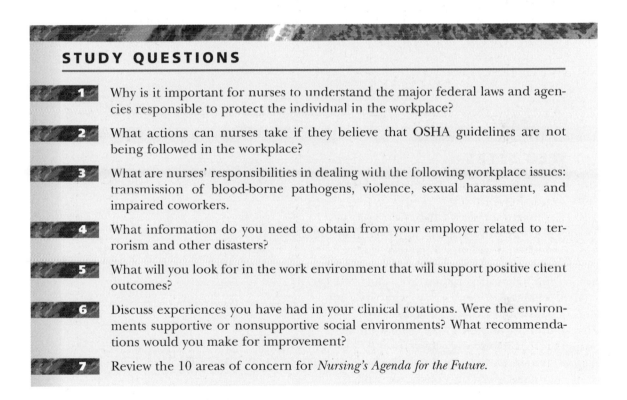

STUDY QUESTIONS

1 Why is it important for nurses to understand the major federal laws and agencies responsible to protect the individual in the workplace?

2 What actions can nurses take if they believe that OSHA guidelines are not being followed in the workplace?

3 What are nurses' responsibilities in dealing with the following workplace issues: transmission of blood-borne pathogens, violence, sexual harassment, and impaired coworkers.

4 What information do you need to obtain from your employer related to terrorism and other disasters?

5 What will you look for in the work environment that will support positive client outcomes?

6 Discuss experiences you have had in your clinical rotations. Were the environments supportive or nonsupportive social environments? What recommendations would you make for improvement?

7 Review the 10 areas of concern for *Nursing's Agenda for the Future.*

CRITICAL THINKING EXERCISE

You have been hired as a new RN on a busy pediatric unit in a large metropolitan hospital. The hospital provides services for a culturally diverse population including African-American, Asian, and Hispanic people. Family members often attempt alternative healing practices specific to their culture and bring special foods from home to entice a sick child to eat. One of the more

(Continued on following page)

experienced nurses said to you, "We need to discourage these people from fooling with all this hocus-pocus. We are trying to get their sick kid well in the time allowed under their managed care plans, and all this medicine-man stuff is only keeping the kid sick longer. Besides, all this stuff stinks up the rooms and brings in bugs." You have observed how important these healing rituals and foods are to the clients and families and believe that both the families and the children have benefited from this nontraditional approach to healing.

1. What are your feelings about nontraditional healing methods?

2. How should you respond to the experienced nurse?

3. How can you be a client advocate without alienating your coworkers?

4. What could you do to assist your coworkers in becoming more culturally sensitive to their clients and families?

5. How can health-care facilities incorporate both Western and nontraditional medicine? Should they do this? Why or why not?

WEB SITES

American Nurses Association (ANA):
nursingworld.org
nursingworld.org/dlwa/osh/wp5
nursingworld.org/ajn/w001/jul/ISSUES
nursingworld.org/dlwa/osh/wp2
nursingworld.org/readroom/position/workplac/wkharass
nursingworld.org/ajn/2001/jul/ISSUES
nursingworld.org/dlwa/wpr/wp3/htm
nursingworld.org/dlwa/osh/wp7
nursingworld.org/tan/98mayjun/ot
nursingworld.org/gova/federal/legis/107/ovrtme
nursingworld.org/about/summary/sum00/staffing
nursingworld.org/dlwa/osh/wp3
nursingworld.org/readroom/fssafe99
nursingworld.org/readroom/stff.prnc
nursingworld.org/tan/98/janfeb/nlrbmass
nursingworld.org/readroom/fsneedle
nursingworld.org/handlewithcare/factsheet

Association of Womens' Health, Obstetric and Neonatal Nurses (AWHONN):
awhonn.org/HealthPolicyLegislative/BIOTERRORISM PREPAREDNESS/bioterrorism preparedness
Bureau of Labor Statistics (BLS):
bls.gov/news/release/cfol.nro

Centers for Disease Control and Prevention (CDC):
cdc.gov/
cdc.gov/health/diseases
cdc.gov/niosh/about
cdc.gov/niosh/pdfs/2002-101.pdf
cdc.gov/niosh/98-113
bt.cdc.gov/
nursingworld.org/tan/01novdec/respond
cdc.gov/ncidod/sars/ic
cdc.gove/nchstp/tb/pubs/TBHIVconection/defact

Institute of Medicine (IOM):
iom.edu

Joint Commission on the Accreditation of Healthcare Organizations (JCAHO):
jcaho.org/generao+public+patient+safety/patient+safety

National Council State Boards of Nursing (NCSBN):
ncsbn.org/public/regulation/boards_of_nursing_board
ncsbn.org/regulation/nursingpractice_npa_pennra.asp

National Database of Nursing Quality Indicators (NDNQI):
nursingquality.org

National Institute for Occupational Safety and Health (NIOSH):
gov/niosh
gov/niosh/topics/healthcare
osha.gov
oshaslc.gov/SLTC/latexallergy/index
cdc.gov/niosh/latexalt/
osha.gov/media;oshnews/sept98/needles
osha.gov/SLTC/needlestick/index
osha.gov/needlesticks/needlefaq
osha.gov/needlesticks/needlefact
osha.gov/SLTC/workplaceviolence/index
osha.gov/ergonomics/ergofact02
osha.gov/ergonomics/FAQs-external
osha.gov/SLTC/healthcarefacilities/harzards
osha-slc.gov/SLTC/latexallergy/index
alertcdc.gov/niosh/latexalt
osha.gov/SLTC/needlestick/index
dr.ca.gov/dosh/cosh_publications/backing.pdf
osha.gov/ergonomics/guidelines/nursinghomes/index

Patient Safety Center of Inquiry:
patientsafetycenter.com

REFERENCES

Aiken L.H., Clarke S.P., Sloane D.M., et al. (2002) Hospital nurse staffing and patient mortality, nurse burnout, and job dissatisfaction. *JAMA*, 288(16), 1987–1991.

Aiken, L.H. (2004). Nurse Burnout and Patient Satisfaction, *JAMA*, 42(2), 57–66.

American Nurses Association. (1993). *HIV, Hepatitis-B, Hepatitis-C: Blood-Borne Diseases*. Washington, DC: ANA.

American Nurses Association. (1994). *Guidelines on Reporting Incompetent, Unethical, or Illegal Practices*. Washington, DC: ANA.

American Nurses Association. (1995a). *Protect Your Patients—Protect Your License*. Washington, DC: ANA.

American Nurses Association. (1995b). *The Supreme Court Has Issued the Ultimate Gag Order for Nurses.* Washington, DC: ANA.

American Nurses Association. (2001). *Code for Nurses.* Washington, DC: ANA.

American Nurses Association. (2005). *Nursings' Agenda for the Future.* Washington, DC: ANA.

Arbury, S. (2002). Healthcare workers at risk. *Job Safety and Health Care Quarterly,* 13(2), 30–31.

Armstrong, K., Gordon, R., & Santorella, G. (1995). Occupational exposure of healthcare workers to HIV. *Social Work in Health Care,* 21(3), 61–80.

Bauer, X., Ammon, J., Chen, Z., Beckman, W., & Czuppon, A.B. (1993). Health risk in hospitals through airborne allergens for patients pre-sensitized to latex. *Lancet,* 342, 1148–1149.

Beyea, S. (2004). A critical partnership-safety for nurses and patients. *AORN,* 79(6), 1299–1302.

Blair, D. (2005). Spot the signs of drug impairment. *Nursing Management,* 36(2), 20–21, 52.

Brooke, P. (2001). The legal realities of HIV exposure. *RN,* 64(12), 71–73.

Carroll, C., & Sheverbush, J. (September 1996). Violence assessment in hospitals provides basis for action. *American Nurse,* 18.

Centers for Disease Control and Prevention (CDC). (1992). Surveillance for occupationally acquired HIV infection—United States, 1981–1992. *MMWR,* 41(43), 823–825.

Chisholm, R.F. (1992). Quality of working life: A crucial management perspective for the year 2000. *Journal of Health and Human Resources Administration,* 15(1), 6–34.

Collins, J. (1994). Nurses' attitudes toward aggressive behavior following attendance at "The Prevention and Management of Aggressive Behavior Programme." *Journal of Advanced Nursing,* 20, 117–131.

Coulthard, P, Worthington, H., Esposito, M., van der Est, M., & van Wahl (2004). Tissue adhesives for closures of surgical incisions. *Cochrane Database of Systemic Reviews,* Issue 2.

Damrosch, S., & Scholler-Jaquish, A. (1993). Nurses' experiences with impaired nurse coworkers. *Applied Nursing Research,* 6(4), 154–160.

Davidhizar, R., Dowd, S., Giger, J. (1999). Managing diversity in the healthcare workplace. *Health Care Supervisor,* 17(3), 51–62.

Dembe, A.E., Erickson, J.B., Delbros, R.G., & Banks, S.M. (2005). The impact of overtime and long work hours on occupational injuries and illness: New evidence from the US Occupational and Environmental Medicine, 62(9), 588–597.

Durr, L. (2004). Commission on Workforce Issues: What nurses should expect in the workplace: The ANA Bill for Rights for Registered Nurses. *Virginia Nurses Today,* 12(2), 17.

Edlich, R., Woodard, C., & Haines, M. (2001). Disabling back injuries in nursing personnel. *Journal of Emergency Nursing,* 27(2), 150–155.

Edwards, R. (1999). Prevention of workplace violence. *Aspen's Advisor for Nurse Executives,* 14(8), 8–12.

Hamilton, R., Brown, R., Veltri, M, Feroli, R., Primeau, M,

Schauble, J, & Adkinson, N. (2005). Administering pharaceuticals to latex allergy patients from vials containing natural rubber latex closures. *Americal Journal Health Systems Pharmacy,* 62, 1822–1827.

Heise, B. (2003). The historical context of addictions within the nursing profession. *Journal of Addictions Nursing,* 14, 117–124.

Herring, L.H. (1994). *Infection Control.* New York: National League for Nursing.

Himali, U. (1995). Caring for the caregivers. *American Nurse,* 27(6), 8.

Hurst, K.L., Croker, P.A., & Bell, S.K. (1994). How about a lollipop? A peer recognition program. *Nursing Management,* 25(9), 68–73.

Jankowski, C.B. (1992). Radiation protection for nurses: Regulations and guidelines. *Journal of Nursing Administration,* 22(22), 30–34.

Kinkle, S. (1993). Violence in the ED: How to stop it before it starts. *American Journal of Nursing,* 93(7), 22–24.

Korniewicz, M., Garzon, L., Seltzer, J., & Feinleib, M. (2004). Failure rates in nonlatex surgical gloves. *American Journal of Infection Control,* 32(5), 268–273.

Kramer, M., & Schmalenberg, C. (1993). Learning from success: Autonomy and empowerment. *Nursing Management,* 24(5), 58–64.

Krucoff, M. (2001). How to prevent repetitive stress injury in the workplace. *American Fitness,* 19(1), 31.

Lanza, M.L., & Carifio, J. (1991). Blaming the victim: Complex (nonlinear) patterns of casual attribution by nurses in response to vignettes of a patient assaulting a nurse. *Journal of Emergency Nursing,* 17(5), 299–309.

Mahoney, B. (1991). The extent, nature, and response to victimization of emergency nurses in Pennsylvania. *Journal of Emergency Nursing,* 17, 282–292.

Malone, B.L. (1993). Caring for culturally diverse racial groups: An administrative matter. *Nursing Administration Quarterly,* 17(2), 21–29.

Mitchell, A. (1995). Cultural diversity: The future, the market, and the rewards. *Caring,* 14(12), 44–48.

Moch, S.D., & Diemert, C.A. (1987). Health promotion within the nursing work environment. *Nursing Administration Quarterly,* 11(3), 9–12.

Nadwairski, J.A. (1992). Inner-city safety for home care providers. *Journal of Nursing Administration,* 22(9), 42–47.

National Safety Council. (1992). *Accident Prevention Manual for Business and Industry.* Chicago: National Safety Council.

OSHA. (1989, January 26). OSHA's Safety and Health Program Management Guidelines. *Federal Register* 54(16), 3904–3916.

Outwater, L.C. (1994). Sexual harassment issues. *Caring,* 13(5), 54–56, 58, 60.

Pennsylvania Bar Institute. (1996). Legal Definition of Sexual Harassment: *de.psu.edu/harass/legal/define*

Perry, J. (2001). Attention all nurses! New legislation puts safer sharps in your hands. *American Journal of Nursing,* 101(9), 24AA–24CC.

Ray, M., Turkel, M., & Marino, F. (2002). The transformative process for nursing in workforce redevelopment. *Nursing Administration Quarterly,* 26(2), 1–14.

Roche, E. (23 February 1993). Nurses' risks and their rights. *Vital Signs,* 3.

Roedel, R.S., & Nystrom, P.C. (1987). Clinical ladders and job enrichment. *Hospital Topics,* 65(2), 22–24.

Rogers, A.E., Hwang, W., Scott, L.D., Aiken, L.H., & Dinges, D.F. (2004). The working hours of hospital staff nurses and patient safety: Both errors and near errors are more likely to occur when hospital staff nurses work twelve or more hours at a stretch. *Health Affairs* 23(4), 202–212.

Rosen, A., Isaacson, D., Brady, M., & Corey J.P. (1993). Hypersensitivity to latex in health care workers: Report of five cases. *Otolaryngology—Head and Neck Surgery,* 109, 731–734.

Simonowitz, J. (1994). Violence in the workplace: You're entitled to protection. *RN,* 57(11), 61–63

Slattery, M. (September/October 1998). Caring for ourselves to care for our patients. *American Nurse,* 12–13.

Sloan, A. (2002). Legally speaking: Whistleblowing: Proceed with caution. *RN,* 65(1), 67–68, 70, 80–81.

Sloan, A., & Vernarec, E. (2001). Impaired nurses: Reclaiming careers. *Medical Economics,* 64(2), 58–64.

Society of Gastroenterology Nurses and Associates. (2001). Guidelines for preventing sensitivity and allergic reactions to natural rubber latex in the workplace. *Gastroenterology Nursing,* 24(2), 88–94.

Strader, M.K., & Decker, P.J. (1995). *Role Transition to Patient Care Management.* Norwalk, CN: Appleton & Lange.

Trossman, S. (May/June 1999a). When workplace threats become a reality. *American Nurse,* 1, 12.

Trossman, S. (September/October 1999b). Working 'round the clock. *American Nurse,* 1–2.

U.S. Department of Labor (OSHA). (1995). *Employee Workplace Rights and Responsibilities.* OSHA 95–35.

Ward, L.B. (27 December 1992). In culturally diverse work place, language may alienate. *Miami Herald.*

chapter 13

Work-Related Stress and Burnout

OBJECTIVES

After reading this chapter, the student should be able to:

- Identify signs and symptoms of stress, reality shock, and burnout.

- Describe the impact of stress, reality shock, and burnout on the individual and the health-care team.

- Evaluate his or her own and colleagues' stress levels.

- Develop strategies to manage personal and professional stresses.

OUTLINE

CONSIDER THE STATISTICS

Fifty years ago, the term *personal anxiety* was never used to describe stress. In the decades since, stress has become the most common psychological complaint and a widespread health problem. In the last decade alone, approximately 28,000 studies have been published on the subject of stress and over 1000 studies on the subject of burnout (Pines, 2004, p. 66).

In the workplace, stress is usually defined from a "demand-perception-response" perspective—that stress is related to both the perception of the demands being made on the individual and that individual's perception of the ability to meet those demands. When there is a mismatch between the two the stress response is triggered. The stress threshold, or hardiness, depends on the individual's characteristics, experiences, coping mechanisms, and the circumstances of the event (McVicar, 2003).

The phrase "this is so stressful" is frequently used to describe negative work and personal situations. However, in reality, some stress responses are positive (eustress). The stress response is not a single event but a continuum, ranging from feeling of eustress to mild/moderate distress to severe distress. It is the severe and prolonged distress that causes people to emotionally "burn out" and experience serious physiological and psychological disturbances. Table 13-1 describes the continuum of the stress response. ·

STRESS

Effects of Stress

Hans Selye first explored the concept of stress in the 1930s. Selye (1956) defined *stress* as the nonspecific response of the body to any demands made on it. His description of the general adaptation syndrome (GAS) has had an enormous influence on our present day notions about stress and its effect on human beings. The GAS consists of three stages:

1. **Alarm.** The body awakens to the stressor, and there is a slight change below the normal level of resistance.

2. **Resistance.** The body adjusts to the stressor and tries to restore balance.
3. **Exhaustion.** As the stressor continues, the body energy falls below the normal level of resistance, and illness may occur.

Most people think of stress as work pressure, rush-hour traffic, or sick children. These are triggers to the stress response, the actual body reaction to the daily factors mentioned. As identified by Selye, *stress* is the fight-or-flight response in the body, caused by adrenaline and other stress hormones, causing physiological changes such as increased heart rate and blood pressure, faster breathing, dilated pupils, increased blood sugar, and dry mouth.

Currently, stress is assessed on four levels: environmental, social, physiological, and psychological. *Environmental stressors* include weather, pollens, noise, traffic, and pollution. *Social stressors* include deadlines, finances, work responsibilities and interactions, and multiple demands on time and attention. *Physiological stressors* include illness, aging, injuries, lack of exercise, poor nutrition, and inadequate sleep. *Psychological stressors* are human thoughts: how the brain interprets changes in the environment and the body and determines when the body turns on the fight-or-flight response (Davis, Eshelman, & McCay, 2000).

Epidemiological research has shown that long-term stress contributes to cardiovascular disease, hypertension, ulcers, substance abuse, immune system disorders, emotional disturbances, and job-related injuries (Crawford, 1993; Lusk, 1993).

Responses to Stress

"Whether the stress you experience is the result of major life changes or the cumulative effect of minor everyday hassles, it is how you respond to these experiences that determines the impact stress will have on your life" (Davis, Eshelman, & McCay, 2000).

Some people manage potentially stressful events more effectively than others (Crawford, 1993; Teague, 1992). Perceptions of events and the subsequent stress responses vary considerably from one person to another. A client crisis that one nurse considers stressful, for example,

	Eustress	Distress	Severe Distress
TABLE 13-1 **Stress Continuum**			
Psychological	Fear/excitement Increased level of arousal/mental acuity	Feelings of uneasiness, apprehension, sadness, depression, pessimism, listlessness Lack of self esteem Negative attitude Increased use of alcohol/smoking/drugs Decreased interest in sexual activity Procrastination/unable to complete tasks	Burnout Emotional exhaustion/depersonalization and disengagement Isolation
Physiological	Autonomic nervous system response: increased blood pressure/heart rate; increased metabolic rate; release of cortisol; quicker reaction times	Prolonged elevated blood pressure/pulse Indigestion Bowel disturbances Weight gain or loss Reduced immunity Fatigue/low energy Poor sleep habits Headache Trembling hands, fingers, body Dry mouth and throat	Clinical hypertension Coronary artery disease Gastric disorders Menstrual problems
Individual Response	**Adaptive** Increased alertness Focus totally on the situation Able to respond quickly to changes Energized for fight or flight preparation	Varies among individuals but usually *maladaptive* Absenteeism Apathy Callousness Cynicism Defensiveness	Varies among individuals but usually *severely maladaptive,* possible life-threatening

Adapted from Martin, K. (May 1993). To cope with stress. *Nursing 93*, 39–41, with permission; Gollszek, A. (1992). *Sixty-Six Second Stress Management: The Quickest Way to Relax and Ease Anxiety.* Far Hills, NJ: New Horizon; and McVicar, A. (2003). Workplace stress in nursing: A literature review. *Journal of Advanced Nursing*, 44(6), 633–642.

may not seem stressful at all to a coworker. The following is an example:

A new graduate was employed on a busy telemetry floor. Often, when clients were admitted, they were in acute distress, with shortness of breath, diaphoresis, and chest pain. Family members were distraught and anxious. Each time the new graduate had to admit a client, she experienced a "sick-to-her-stomach" feeling, tightness in the chest and throat, and difficulty concentrating. She was afraid that she would miss something important and that the client would die during the admission. The more experienced nurses seemed to handle each admission with ease, even when the client's physical condition was severely compromised.

Selye also differentiated between "good" stress and "bad" stress. In 1974, Selye stated: "Stress is the spice of life. Since stress is associated with all types of activity, we could not avoid most of it only by never doing anything" (Lenson, 2001, p. 5). Good stress can push people to perform better and accomplish more. What makes an event "good stress" or "bad stress"? Lenson (2001) identified seven factors:

1. People can exert a high level of control over the outcomes of good stresses. With bad stresses, there is little or no control.
2. Positive feelings are experienced in processing good stress. With bad stress, negative or ambivalent feelings occur.
3. Good stress helps achieve positive goals. No desirable outcomes occur with bad stress.
4. There is a feeling of eagerness when

anticipating the work that needs to be done to process the good stressors.

5. Bad stress leaves feelings of exhaustion and avoidance.

6. Good stress helps growth; bad stress is limiting. Good stress improves interpersonal relationships; bad stress makes these relationships worse.

7. Processing all stress requires human action.

▚ THE REAL WORLD

Today's health-care system has adopted the corporate mindset. Both the new graduate and the seasoned professional continue to experience redesigning, changing staffing models, complex documentation requirements, continued nursing shortages, and the expectation that work does not end when the employee goes home (Trossman, 1999). Most agencies expect new graduates to come to the work setting able to organize their work, set priorities, and provide leadership to ancillary personnel. New graduates often say, "I had no idea that nursing would be this demanding." Even though nursing programs of study are designed to help students prepare for the demands of the work setting, new nurses still need to continue to learn on the job. In fact, experienced nurses will tell you that what you learn in school is only the beginning; it provides you with the fundamental knowledge and skills needed to continue to grow and develop as you practice nursing in various capacities and work settings. Graduation signals not the end of learning but the beginning of a journey toward becoming an expert nurse (Benner, 1984).

Right now you are probably thinking, "Nothing can be more stressful than going to school. I can't wait to go to work and not have to study for tests, go to the clinical agency for my assignment, do client care plans," and so forth. In most associate degree programs, students are assigned to care for one to three clients a day, working up to six or seven clients under a preceptor's supervision by the end of their program. Compare this with your "next clinical rotation," your first real job as a nurse.

You may work 7 to 10 days in a row on 8- to 12-hour shifts, caring for 10 or more clients. You may also have to supervise several technicians or licensed practical nurses. These drastic changes from school to employment cause many to experience what is called *reality shock* (Kraeger & Walker, 1993; Kramer, 1981).

Initial Concerns

The first few weeks on a new job are the "honeymoon" phase. The new employee is excited and enthusiastic about the new position. Coworkers usually go out of their way to make the new person feel welcome and overlook any problems that arise. Everything seems rosy. Unfortunately, honeymoons do not last forever. The new graduate is soon expected to behave just like everyone else and discovers that expectations for a professional employed in an organization are quite different from expectations for a student in school. Those behaviors that brought rewards in school are not necessarily valued by the organization. In fact, some of them are criticized. The new graduate who is not prepared for this change feels confused, shocked, angry, and disillusioned. The tension of the situation can become almost unbearable if it is not resolved. Table 13-2 provides a list of ongoing and newer workplace stresses

Graduate nurses in the first 3 months of employment identified concerns related to skills, personal and professional roles, client care management, the shocks of bad experiences, the affirmations of good experiences, constructive evaluation, knowledge of the unit routine, and school versus work priorities (Godinez, Schweiger, Gruver, & Ryan, 1999; Heslop, 2001).

Well-supervised orientation programs are very helpful for newly licensed nurses. In this era of the nursing shortage, the orientation program may be cut short and the new nurse required to function on his or her own very quickly. One way to minimize initial work stress is to ask questions about the orientation program: How long will it be? Whom will I be working with? When will I be on my own? What happens if at the end of the orientation I still need more assistance?

TABLE 13-2
Stress in the Workplace

Ongoing Sources	Newer Sources
Conflict with physicians	Terrorism
Work overload/work is devalued	Changes in technology
Role conflict	Downsizing
Ineffective, hostile, incompetent supervisors and/or peers	Constant changes in nursing care delivery
	Work-home conflicts
Lack of personal job fit, inadequate preparation, recognition, or clear job description	Elder and child care issues
	Workplace violence
Poor work control/fear and uncertainty related to career progress	Lawsuits related to job stress
Age, gender, racial, religious discrimination	Demands of accreditation/compliance issues
Dealing with death and dying clients/families	Pressure for immediate results
Salary	Colleagues' inexperience

Adapted from DeFrank, R., & Ivancevich, J. (1998). Stress on the job: An executive update. *Academy of Management Executives*, 12(3), 55; McVicar, A. (2003). Workplace stress in nursing: A literature review. *Journal of Advanced Nursing*, 44(6), 633–642; and Hall, D. (2004). Work-related stress of registered nurses in a hospital setting. *Journal for Nurses in Staff Development*, 20(1), 6–14

Differences in Expectations

The enthusiasm and eagerness of the first new job quickly disappear as reality sets in. Regardless of the career one chooses, there is no perfect job. The problem begins when reality and expectations collide. After 2 to 3 months, the new nurse begins to experience a formal separation from being a student and embraces the professional reality of the nursing role. To cope with reality, several facts of work life need to be recognized (Goliszek, 1992, pp. 36, 46):

1. Expectations are usually distortions of reality. Unless you accept this and react positively, you will go through life experiencing disappointment. As a student, you had only two or three patients to care for, and you are very surprised to hear on your first full day of orientation that you have five clients. Although you did hear the nurses talking about their caseload while you were a student, you expected to continue to have 2 or 3 clients for at least the next 4 months.

2. To some extent, you need to fit yourself into your work, not fit the work to suit your needs or demands. Having a positive attitude helps to maintain flexibility and a sense of humor. Your first position is at a physician's office. He is ready to retire, and his client load is dwindling. You wanted to apply for a position in acute care, but you have a very active social life and did not want to work weekends. The current position is not very challenging, and you are concerned that you might be unemployed soon. You are starting to miss the acute care environment. Go back to your SWOT analysis. Evaluate your current strengths, weaknesses, opportunities, and threats. Where do you see yourself in 1 year? 5 years? How will you fit yourself into your work to meet your goals?

3. Regardless of the job, the way you perceive events on the job will influence how you feel about your work. Your attitude will affect whether work is a pleasant or unpleasant experience. Health care is not easy. Sick people can be cranky and demanding. Health-care agencies continue to want to do more with less. How you perceive your contribution to the health-care system will definitely influence your reality.

4. Feelings of helplessness and powerlessness at work cause frustration and unrelieved job stress. If you go to work every day feeling that you do not make a difference, it is time to reevaluate your position and your goals.

What are these differences in expectations? Kramer (1981), who studied reality shock for many years, found a number of them, which are listed in Table 13-3.

Ideally, health care should be comprehensive. It should not only meet all of a client's needs but also be delivered in a way that

TABLE 13-3
Professional Ideals and Work Realities

Professional Ideals	Work Realities
Comprehensive, holistic care	Mechanistic, fragmented care
Emphasis on quality of care	Emphasis on efficiency
Explicit expectations	Implicit (unstated) expectations
Balanced, frequent feedback	Intermittent, often negative feedback
Assignments that "make sense"	

Adapted from Kramer, M. (January 27–28, 1981). Coping with reality shock. Workshop presented at Jackson Memorial Hospital, Miami, FL.

considers the client as a whole person, a member of a particular family that has certain unique characteristics and needs, and a member of a particular community. Most health-care professionals, however, are not employed to provide comprehensive, holistic care. Instead, they are asked to give medications, provide counseling, make home visits, or prepare someone for surgery, but rarely to do all these things. These tasks are divided among different people, each a specialist, for the sake of efficiency rather than continuity or effectiveness.

When efficiency is the goal, the speed and amount of work done are rewarded rather than the quality of the work. This also creates a conflict for the new graduate, who was allowed to take as much time as needed to provide good care while in school.

Expectations are also communicated in different ways. In school, an effort is made to provide explicit directions so that students know what they are expected to accomplish. In many work settings, however, instructions on the job are brief, and many expectations are left unspoken. New graduates who are not aware of these expectations may find that they have unknowingly left tasks undone or are considered inept by coworkers. The following is an example:

Brenda, a new graduate, was assigned to give medications to all her team's clients. Because this was a fairly light assign-ment, she spent some time looking up the medications and explaining their actions to the clients receiving them. Brenda also straightened up the medicine room and filled out the order forms, which she thought would please the task-oriented team leader. At the end of the day, Brenda reported these activities with some satisfaction to the team leader. She expected the team leader to be pleased with the way she used the time. Instead, the team leader looked annoyed and told her that whoever passes out medications always does the blood pressures too and that the other nurse on the team, who had a heavier assignment, had to do them. Also, because supplies were always ordered on Fridays for the weekend, it would have to be done again tomorrow, so Brenda had in fact wasted her time.

Additional Pressures on the New Graduate

The first job a person takes after finishing school is often considered a proving ground where newly gained knowledge and skills are tested. Many people set up mental tests for themselves that they feel must be passed before they can be confident of their ability to function. Passing these self-tests also confirms achievement of identity as a practitioner rather than a student.

At the same time, new graduates are undergoing testing by their coworkers, who are also interested in finding out whether the new graduate can handle the job. The new graduate is entering a new group, and the group will decide whether to accept this new member. The group is usually reasonable, but sometimes new graduates are given tasks they are not ready to handle. If this happens, Kramer (1981) recommended that new graduates refuse to take the test rather than fail it. Another opportunity for proving themselves will soon come along.

Additional problems, such as dealing with resistant staff members, cultural differences, and age differences, may also occur. Above all, the experience of loss is frequently described by new graduates. Losses are described as the following (Boychuk, 2001):

◆ The ideal world of caring and curing they had come to know through their education.

◆ Their innocence.

◆ The familiarity of academia.

◆ The protection of clinical supervision by nursing instructors.

◆ Externally set boundaries of care and safety.

◆ A sense of collegiality and trusted relationships with peers.

◆ Grounded feedback.

Resolving the Problem

Before considering ways to resolve these problems, some less successful ways of coping with these problems are listed.

◆ **Abandon professional goals.** When faced with reality shock, some new graduates abandon their professional goals and adopt the organization's operative goals as their own. This eliminates their conflict but leaves them less effective caregivers. It also puts the needs of the organization before their needs or the needs of the client and reinforces operative goals that might better be challenged and changed.

◆ **Give up professional ideals.** Others give up their professional ideals but do not adopt the organization's goals or any others to replace them. This has a deadening effect; they become automatons, believing in nothing related to their work except doing what is necessary to earn a day's pay.

◆ **Leave the profession.** Those who do not give up their professional ideals try to find an organization that will support them. Unfortunately, a significant proportion of those who do not want to give up their professional ideals escapes these conflicts by leaving their jobs and abandoning their profession. Kramer and Schmalenberg (1993) stated that there would be fewer shortages of nurses if more health-care organizations met these ideals.

Instead of focusing on the bad stress, new nurses can meet the transition to professional nursing by adapting to good stress:

◆ **Develop a professional identity.** Opportunities to challenge one's competence and develop an identity as a professional can begin in school. Success in meeting these challenges can immunize the new graduate against the loss of confidence that accompanies reality shock.

◆ **Learn about the organization.** The new graduate who understands how organizations operate will not be as shocked as the naive individual. When you begin a new job, it is important to learn as much as you can about the organization and how it really operates. This not only saves you some surprises but also gives you some ideas about how to work within the system and how to make the system work for you.

◆ **Use your energy wisely.** Keep in mind that much energy goes into learning a new job. You may see many things that you think need to be changed, but you need to recognize that to implement change requires your time and energy. It is a good idea to make a list of these things so that you do not forget them later when you have become socialized into the system and have some time and energy to invest in change.

◆ **Communicate effectively.** Deal with the problems that can arise with coworkers. The same interpersonal skills you use in communicating with clients can be effective in dealing with your coworkers.

◆ **Seek feedback often and persistently.** Seeking feedback not only provides you with needed information but also pushes the people you work with to be more specific about their expectations of you.

◆ **Develop a support network.** Identify colleagues who have held onto their professional ideals with whom you can share your problems and the work of improving the organization. Their recognition of your work can keep you going when rewards from the organization are meager. A support network is a source of strength when resisting pressure to give up professional ideals and a source of power when attempting to bring about change. Developing your skills can help to prevent the problems of reality shock.

◆ **Find a mentor.** A mentor is someone more experienced within or outside the organization who provides career development support, such as coaching, sponsoring advancement, providing challenging assignments, protecting protégés from adversity, and promoting positive visibility. Mentors provide guidance to new graduates as they change from student to professional nurse. Mentors can also assume psychosocial functions, such as personal support, friendship, acceptance, role modeling, and counseling. Many organizations have preceptors for the new employee. In many instances, the preceptor will become your mentor. However, the mentor role is much more encompassing than the preceptor role. The mentor relationship is a voluntary one and is built on mutual respect and development of the mentee. Table 13-4 identifies responsibilities of the mentor and mentee in this relationship (Scheetz, 2000; Simonetti & Ariss, 1999).

You have made it through the first 6 months of employment, and you are finally starting to feel like a "real" nurse. You are beginning to realize that a stress-free work environment is probably impossible to achieve. Shift work, overtime, distraught families, staff shortages, and pressure to do more with less continue to contribute to the stresses placed on nurses. An inability to deal with this continued stress will eventually lead to burnout.

TABLE 13-4
Mentor and Mentee Responsibilities

Mentor Responsibilities	Mentee Responsibilities
Has excellent communication and listening skills	Demonstrates eagerness to learn
Shows sensitivity to needs of nurses, clients, and workplace	Participates actively in the relationship by keeping all appointments and commitments
Able to encourage excellence in others	Seeks feedback and uses it to modify behaviors
Able to share and provide counsel	Demonstrates flexibility and an ability to change
Exhibits good decision-making skills	Is open in the relationship with mentor
Shows an understanding of power and politics	Demonstrates an ability to move toward independence
Demonstrates trustworthiness	Able to evaluate choices and outcomes

BURNOUT

Definition

The ultimate result of unmediated job stress is burnout. The term *burnout* became a favorite buzzword of the 1980s and continues to be part of today's vocabulary. Herbert Freudenberger formally identified it as a leadership concern in 1974. The literature on job stress and burnout continues to grow as new books, articles, workshops, and videotapes appear regularly. A useful definition of *burnout* is the "progressive deterioration in work and other performance resulting from increasing difficulties in coping with high and continuing levels of job-related stress and professional frustration" (Paine, 1984, p. 1).

More than 20 years of research on nursing work environments point to personal, job, and organizational factors that contribute to dissatisfaction and ultimately burnout (McLennan, 2005). Ultimately, nurse burnout affects clients' satisfaction with their nursing care. Eight hundred and twenty nurses and 621 clients were surveyed from 20 hospitals across the United States (Vahey, et al., 2004). The results of this study showed that units characterized by nurses as having adequate staff, good administrative support for nursing care, and good relations between doctors and nurses were twice as likely as other units to report high satisfaction with nursing care. The level of nurse burnout on these units also affected client satisfaction.

Much of the burnout experienced by nurses has been attributed to the frustration that arises because care cannot be delivered in the ideal manner they learned in school. For those whose greatest satisfaction comes from caring for clients, anything that interferes with providing the highest quality care causes work stress and feelings of failure.

People who expect to derive a sense of significance from their work enter their professions with high hopes and motivation and relate to their work as a calling. When they feel that they have failed, that their work is meaningless, that they make no difference in the world—they start feeling helpless and hopeless and eventually burn out (Pines, 2004, p. 67).

The often unrealistic and sometimes sexist image of nurses in the media adds to this frustration. Neither the school ideal nor the media image is realistic, but either may make nurses feel dissatisfied with themselves and their jobs, keeping stress levels high (Corley, et al., 1994; Fielding & Weaver, 1994; Grant, 1993; Kovner, Hendrickson, Knickman, & Finkler, 1994; Malkin, 1993; Nakata & Saylor, 1994; Skubak, Earls, & Botos, 1994; Pines, 2004).

Sharon had wanted to be a nurse for as long as she could remember. She married early, had three children, and put her dreams of being a nurse on hold. Now her children are grown, and she finally realized her dream by graduating last year from the local community college with a nursing degree. However, she has been feeling overwhelmed at work, critical of coworkers and clients, and argumentative with supervisors. She is having difficulty adapting to the restructuring changes at her hospital and goes home angry and frustrated every day. She cannot stop working for financial reasons but is seriously thinking of quitting nursing and taking some computer classes. "I'm tired of dealing with people. Maybe machines will be more friendly and predictable." Sharon is experiencing burnout.

Aspects

Goliszek (1992) identified four stages of the burnout syndrome:

1. **High expectations and idealism.** At the first stage, the individual is enthusiastic, dedicated, and committed to the job and exhibits a high energy level and a positive attitude.
2. **Pessimism and early job dissatisfaction.** In the second stage, frustration, disillusionment, or boredom with the job develops, and the individual begins to exhibit the physical and psychological symptoms of stress.
3. **Withdrawal and isolation.** As the individual moves into the third stage, anger, hostility, and negativism are exhibited. The physical and psychological stress symptoms worsen. Through stage three, simple changes in job goals, attitudes, and behaviors may reverse the burnout process.
4. **Irreversible detachment and loss of interest.** As the physical and emotional stress symptoms become severe, the individual exhibits low self-esteem, chronic absen-

teeism, cynicism, and total negativism. Once the individual has moved into this stage and remains there for any length of time, burnout is inevitable. Regardless of the cause, experiencing burnout leaves an individual emotionally and physically exhausted.

Stressors Leading to Burnout

Personal Factors

Some of the personal factors influencing job stress and burnout are age, gender, number of children, education, experience, and favored coping style. For example, the fact that many nurses are single parents raising families alone adds to the demands of already difficult days at work. Married nurses may have the additional stress of dual-career homes, causing even more stress in coordinating work and vacation schedules as well as day-care problems. Baby boomers are finding they need to care for elderly parents along with their children (DeFrank & Ivancevich, 1998). Competitive, impatient, and hostile personality traits have also been associated with emotional exhaustion and subsequent burnout (Borman, 1993). Most experienced nurses will tell you that they separate their home from work when dealing with work-related stressors and that they try but usually fail to leave their work-related stressors in the workplace (Hall, 2004).

Job-Related Conditions

Job-related stress is broadly defined by the National Institute for Occupational Safety and Health as the "harmful physical and emotional responses that occur when the requirements of the job do not match the capabilities, resources, or needs of the worker" (http://www.cdc.gov/niosh/homepage.html). Since the prior edition of this text, the threat of terrorism has been added to the list of job-related conditions that contribute to job-related stress. Box 13-1 lists some of these conditions, which were discussed in Chapter 12.

Human Service Occupations

People who work in human service organizations consistently report lower levels of job sat-

---

BOX 13-1

Five Sources of Job Stress That Can Lead to Burnout

1. **Intrinsic factors.** Characteristics of the job itself, such as the multiple aspects of complex client care that many nurses provide, lack of autonomy.
2. **Organizational variables.** Characteristics of the organization, such as limited financial resources, staffing, workload, and models of care delivery.
3. **Reward system.** The way in which employees are rewarded or punished, particularly if these are obviously unfair.
4. **Human resources system.** In particular, the number and availability of opportunities for staff development, salary and benefits, organizational policies.
5. **Leadership.** The way in which managers relate to their staff, particularly if they are unrealistic, uncaring, or unfair; communication patterns with supervisors and coworkers.

Adapted from Carr, K., & Kazanowski, M. (1994). Factors affecting job satisfaction of nurses who work in long-term care. *Journal of Advanced Nursing,* 19, 878–883; Crawford, S. (1993). Job stress and occupational health nursing. *American Association of Occupational Health Nurses Journal,* 41, 522–529; Duquette, A., Sandhu, B., & Beaudet, L. (1994). Factors related to nursing burnout: A review of empirical knowledge. *Issues in Mental Health Nursing,* 15, 337–358; and Best, M. & Thurston, N. (2004). Measuring nurse job satisfaction, *Journal of Nursing Administration,* 34(6), 283–290.

---

isfaction than do people working in other types of organizations. Much of the stress experienced by nurses is related to the nature of their work: continued intensive, intimate contact with people who often have serious and sometimes fatal physical, mental, emotional, and/or social problems. Efforts to save clients or help them achieve a peaceful ending to their lives are not always successful. Despite nurses' best efforts, many clients get worse, not better. Some return to their destructive behaviors; others do not recover but die. The continued loss of clients alone can lead to burnout. Even exposure to medicinal and antiseptic substances, unpleasant sights, and high noise levels can cause stress for some people. Health-care providers experiencing burnout may become cynical and even hostile toward their coworkers and colleagues (Carr & Kazanowski, 1994; Dionne-Proulx & Pepin, 1993; Goodell & Van Ess Coeling, 1994; Stechmiller & Yarandi, 1993; Tumulty, Jernigan, & Kohut, 1994).

In some instances, human service professionals also experience lower pay, longer hours, and more extensive regulation than do professionals in other fields. Inadequate advancement opportunities for women and minorities in lower-status, lower-paid positions are apparent in many health-care areas.

Conflicting Demands

Meeting work-related responsibilities and maintaining a family and personal life can increase stress when there is insufficient time or energy for all of these. As mentioned in the section on personal factors, both the single and the married parent are at risk because of the conflicting demands of their personal and work lives. The perception of balance in one's life is a personal one.

There appear to be some differences in the way that men and women find a comfortable balance. Men often define themselves in terms of their separateness and their career progress; women are more likely to define themselves through attachment and connections with other people. Women who try to focus on occupational achievement and pursue personal attachments at the same time are likely to experience conflict in both their work and personal lives. In addition, society evaluates the behaviors of working adult men and women differently. "When a man disrupts work for his family, he is considered a good family man, while a woman disrupting work for family risks having her professional commitment questioned" (Borman, 1993, p. 1).

Closely tied to conflicting demands is the decision to come to work when ill. Nurses who come to work when ill describe tension associated with making this decision: tension between the nurse and the supervisor, tension between the nurse and the team members, and tension in the nurse due to responsibilities between self and others. As you move forward in your career, be proactive in working with team members and your supervisors in helping yourself and others find balance in the workplace (Crout, Change, & Cioffi, 2005).

Technology

Decisions related to changes in technology are often made without input from employees.

These same employees are then required to adapt and cope with the changes. How many of the following changes have you had to adapt to: e-mail, voice mail, fax machines, computerized charting, desktop computers, cellular phones? Often, employees feel that their role has become secondary to technology (DeFrank & Ivancevich, 1998).

Lack of Balance in Life

When personal interests and satisfactions are limited to work, a person is more susceptible to burnout; trouble at work becomes trouble with that individual's whole life. A job can become the center of someone's world, and that world can become very small. Two ways out of this are to set limits on the commitment to work and to expand the number of satisfying activities and relationships outside of work.

Many people in the helping professions have difficulty setting limits on their commitment. This is fine if they enjoy working extra hours and taking calls at night and on weekends, but if it exhausts them, then they need to stop doing it or risk serious burnout. For example, when you are asked to work another double shift or the third weekend in a row, you can say no. At the same time as you are setting limits at work, you can expand your outside activities so that you live in a large world in which a blow to one part can be cushioned by support from other parts. If you are the team leader or nurse manager, you also need to recognize and accept staff members' need to do this as well. Ask yourself the following questions:

◆ Do I exercise at least three times weekly?

◆ Do I have several close friends that I see regularly?

◆ Do I have a plan for my life and career that I have told someone about?

◆ Do I have strong spiritual values that I carry out in practice regularly?

◆ Do I have some strong personal interests that I regularly enjoy?

Studies have shown that the two best indicators of customer satisfaction were related to employee satisfaction and employee work-life balance. Well-rounded employees have a different perspective on life and are perceived by employers as more trustworthy and more grounded in reality. Ultimately, you do not have to give up your personal life to excel in your professional life (Farren, 1999).

Consequences

Certain combinations of personal and organizational factors can increase the likelihood of burnout. Finding the right fit between your preferences and the characteristics of the organization for which you work can be keys to preventing burnout. Health care demands adaptable, innovative, competent employees who care about their clients, desire to continue learning, and try to remain productive despite constant challenges. Unfortunately, these are the same individuals who are prone to burnout if preventive action is not taken (Lickman, Simms, & Greene, 1993; McGee-Cooper, 1993).

Burnout has financial, physical, emotional, and social implications for the professional, the clients, and the organization. Burnout can happen to anyone, not just to people with a history of emotional problems. In fact, it is not considered an emotional disturbance in the sense that depression is but, instead, a reaction to sustained organizational stressors (Duquette, Sandhu, & Beaudet, 1994).

The shortage of professional nurses is predicted to continue for at least another 10 years. Two of the main causes of the shortage are individuals not entering the profession and nurses leaving. As discussed, one reason for leaving is burnout. A recent study of 106 nurses demonstrated that the three dimensions of burnout (emotional exhaustion, depersonalization, and personal accomplishment) were correlated with work excitement. Work excitement is defined as "personal enthusiasm and commitment for work evidenced by creativity, receptivity to learning, and ability to see opportunity in everyday situations" (Sadovich, 2005, p. 91). Work excitement factors include: work arrangements, variable work experiences, the work environment, and growth and development opportunities. As you pursue your nursing career, consider looking for positions that support a favorable work environment.

A Buffer Against Burnout

The idea that personal hardiness provides a buffer against burnout has been explored in recent years. *Hardiness* includes the following:

◆ A sense of personal control rather than powerlessness.

◆ Commitment to work and life's activities rather than alienation.

◆ Seeing life's demands and changes as challenges rather than as threats.

The hardiness that comes from having this perspective leads to the use of adaptive coping responses, such as optimism, effective use of support systems, and healthy lifestyle habits (Duquette, Sandhu, & Beaudet, 1994; Nowak & Pentkowski, 1994). In addition, letting go of guilt, fear of change, and the self-blaming, wallowing-in-the-problem syndrome will help you buffer yourself against burnout (Lenson, 2001).

You might be asking yourself, "What can I possibly do as a new graduate? I don't even have a job yet, let alone understand the politics of health-care organizations." It is never too early to understand yourself—what triggers stressful situations for you, how you respond to stress, and how you manage it.

STRESS MANAGEMENT

Although you cannot always control the demands placed on you, you can learn to manage your reactions to them and to make healthy lifestyle choices that better prepare you to meet those demands.

ABCs of Stress Management

Frances Johnston (1994) suggested using the ABCs of stress management (awareness, belief, and commitment) in order to have as constructive a response to stress as possible. See Box 13-2.

Awareness

How do you know that you are under stress and may be beginning to burn out? The key is being honest with yourself. Asking yourself the questions in Box 13-3 and answering them

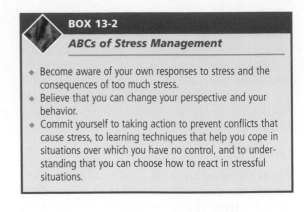

BOX 13-2

ABCs of Stress Management

◆ Become aware of your own responses to stress and the consequences of too much stress.

◆ Believe that you can change your perspective and your behavior.

◆ Commit yourself to taking action to prevent conflicts that cause stress, to learning techniques that help you cope in situations over which you have no control, and to understanding that you can choose how to react in stressful situations.

honestly is one way to assess your personal risk. To further analyze your responses to stress, you may also want to answer the questions in Box 13-4. The answers to these questions require some thought. You do not have to share your answers with others unless you want to, but you do need to be completely honest with yourself when you answer them or the exercise will not be worth the time spent on it. Try to determine the sources of your stress (Goliszek, 1992):

◆ Is it the *time of day* you do the activity?

◆ Is it the *reason* you do the activity?

◆ Is it the *way* you do the activity?

◆ Is it the *amount of time* you need to do the activity?

Belief

Now that you have done the "A" part of stress management, you are ready to move on to "B," which is belief in yourself. Your relationship with your inner self may be the most important relationship of all. Building your self-image and self-esteem will enable you to block out negativism (Davidhizar, 1994). You must also believe that your destiny is not inevitable but that change is possible. Be honest with yourself. Truly value your life. Ask yourself, "If I could live 1 more month, what would I do?"—and start doing it (Johnston, 1994).

Commitment

As you move forward to step "C," you will need to make a commitment to continuing to work on stress recognition and reduction. Once you have recognized the warning signs of stress and

---

BOX 13-3

Assessing Your Risk for Burnout

- Do you feel more fatigued than energetic?
- Do you work harder but accomplish less?
- Do you feel cynical or disenchanted most of the time?
- Do you often feel sad or cry for no apparent reason?
- Do you feel hostile, negative, or angry at work?
- Are you short-tempered? Do you withdraw from friends or coworkers?
- Do you forget appointments or deadlines? Do you frequently misplace personal items?
- Are you becoming insensitive, irritable, and short-tempered?
- Do you experience physical symptoms, such as headaches or stomachaches?
- Do you feel like avoiding people?
- Do you laugh less? Feel joy less often?
- Are you interested in sex?

- Do you crave junk food more often?
- Do you skip meals?
- Have your sleep patterns changed?
- Do you take more medication than usual? Do you use alcohol or other substances to alter your mood?
- Do you feel guilty when your work is not perfect?
- Are you questioning whether the job is right for you?
- Do you feel as though no one cares what kind of work you do?
- Do you constantly push yourself to do better, yet feel frustrated that there is no time to do what you want to do?
- Do you feel as if you are on a treadmill all day?
- Do you use holidays, weekends, or vacation time to catch up?
- Do you feel as if you are "burning the candle at both ends"?

Adapted from Golin, M., Buchlin, M., & Diamond, D. (1991). *Secrets of Executive Success*. Emmaus, PA: Rodale Press; and Goliszek, A. (1992). *Sixty-Six Second Stress Management: The Quickest Way to Relax and Ease Anxiety*. Far Hills, NJ: New Horizon.

---

impending burnout and have gained some insight into your personal needs and reactions to stress, it is time to find the stress management techniques that are right for you.

The stress management techniques in the next section are divided into physical and mental health management for ease in reading and remembering them. However, bear in mind that this is really an artificial division and that mind and body interact continuously. Stress affects both mind and body, and you need to care for both if you are going to be successful in managing stress and preventing burnout.

Physical Health Management

Nurses spend much of their time teaching their clients the basics of keeping themselves healthy. However, many fail to apply these principles in their own lives. Some of the most important aspects of health promotion and stress reduction are reviewed in this section: deep breathing, good posture, rest, relaxation, proper nutrition, and exercise (Davidhizar, 1994; Posen, 2000; Wolinski, 1993).

Deep Breathing

Most of the time people use only 45% of their lung capacity when they breathe. Remember all the times you instructed your clients to "take a few deep breaths"? Practice taking a few slow, deep, "belly" breaths. When faced with a stressful situation, people often hold their breath for a few seconds. This reduces the amount of oxygen delivered to the brain and causes them to feel more anxious. Anxiety can lead to faulty reasoning and a feeling of losing control.

BOX 13-4

Questions for Self-Assessment

- What does the term *health* mean to me?
- What prevents me from living this definition of health?
- Is health important to me?
- Where do I find support?
- Which coping methods work best for me?
- What tasks cause me to feel pressured?
- Can I reorganize, reduce, or eliminate these tasks?
- Can I delegate or rearrange any of my family responsibilities?
- Can I say no to less important demands?
- What are my hopes for the future in terms of:
  Career?
  Finances?
  Spiritual life and physical needs?
  Family relationships?
  Social relationships?
- What do I think others expect of me?
- How do I feel about these expectations?
- What is really important to me?
- Can I prioritize in order to have balance in my life?

Often you can calm yourself by taking a few deep breaths. Try it right now. Don't you feel better already?

Good Posture

A common response to pressure is to slump down into your chair, tensing your upper torso and abdominal muscles. Again, this restricts blood flow and the amount of oxygen reaching your brain. Instead of slumping, imagine a hook on top of your head pulling up your spine; relax your abdomen, and look up. Now, shrug your shoulders a few times to loosen the muscles, and picture a sunny day at the beach or a walk in the woods. Do you feel more relaxed?

Rest

Sleep needs vary with the individual. Find out how much sleep you need, and work on arranging your activities so that you get enough sleep. Fatigue in the human body is no different than fatigue in anything else. Starting out small, a fatigue fracture may remain unnoticed until a catastrophic failure occurs. Several studies indicate the consequences of fatigue:

◆ Subjects who had gone 17 to 19 hours without sleep ranked on testing as equal or or worse than someone with a blood alcohol level of 0.05%.

◆ 24% of 2259 adults surveyed cited fatigue as the primary reason for a recent visit to the doctor.

◆ 16% to 60% of all traffic accidents are related to fatigue.

Fatigue is a mulitdimensional symptom. Origins of fatigue may be biological, psychological, and/or behavioral in nature. What can you do to ward off workplace fatigue?

1. Spot the pattern. Be aware of a weekend state or decrease in strength, an interruption in the ability to perform activities of daily living, or an overabundance in conditions or behaviors that contribute to fatigue such as physical or mental stress, sleep loss, or drug use.
2. Identify precursors. Are you pushing yourself continuously beyond the healthy limits of your phsical and/or mental capabilities? If you do this continually, you are bound to encounter fatigue.
3. Recognize the signs. Emotional outbursts, clumsiness, loss of sensory motor control, weariness, and exhausion all may indicate fatigue.
4. Discern the results. Physical and mental disorders, physical injuires, collapse, and even death may be the catastrophic consequences of fatigue. Be aware of the symptoms of fatigue in yourself and others. Plan how to care for yourself. Be supportive to your coworkers to safeguard against fatigue in others (Smith, 2004).

Relaxation and Time Out

Many people have found that relaxation with guided imagery or other forms of meditation decreases both the physiological and psychological impact of chronic stress. Guided imagery has been used in competitions for many years, in golf, ice skating, baseball, and other sports. Research studies have shown that creation of a mental image of the desired results enhances one's ability to reach the goal. Positive behavior or goal attainment is enhanced even more if you imagine the details of the process of achieving your desired outcome (Vines, 1994). Box 13-5 lists useful relaxation techniques.

Imagine taking the National Council License Examination. You sit down at the computer, take a few deep breaths, and begin. Visualize yourself reading the questions, smiling as you identify the correct answer, and hitting the Enter key after recording your answer. You complete the examination, feeling confident that you were successful. A week later, you go to your

> **BOX 13-5**
> *Useful Relaxation Techniques*
>
> ◆ Guided imagery
> ◆ Yoga
> ◆ Transcendental meditation
> ◆ Relaxation tapes or music
> ◆ Favorite sports or hobbies
> ◆ Quiet corners or favorite places

mailbox and find a letter waiting for you: "Congratulations, you have passed the test and are now a licensed registered nurse." You imagine telling your family and friends. What an exciting moment!

Taking breaks and time out during the day for a short walk or a refreshment (not caffeine) break or just to daydream can help de-stress you during the day. Just as we have circadian rhythms during the night, we have circadian rhythms during the day. These cycles are peaks of energy with troughs of low energy. Watching for these low energy cycles and taking breaks at that time will help to keeping stress from building up.

Proper Nutrition

New research results endorsing the benefits of healthful eating habits seem to appear almost daily. Although the various authorities may prescribe somewhat different regimens, ultimately it appears that too little or too much of any nutrient can be harmful. Many people do not realize that simply decreasing or discontinuing caffeine can help decrease a stress reaction in the body. Some general guidelines for good nutrition are in Box 13-6.

Exercise

Regular aerobic exercise for 20 minutes three times a week is recommended for most people. The exercise may be walking, swimming, jogging, bicycling, stair-stepping, or low-impact aerobics. Whichever you choose, work at a pace that is comfortable for you and increase it gradually as you become conditioned. Do not overdo it. The experience should leave you feeling invigorated, not exhausted.

The physiological benefits of exercise are well known. Exercise may not eliminate the stressors in life, but it is an important element in a healthy lifestyle. Exercise has been shown to improve people's mood and to induce a state of relaxation through the reduction of physiological tension. Regular exercise decreases the energy from the fight-or-flight response discussed in the beginning of this chapter.

Exercise can also be a useful distraction, allowing time to regroup before entering a stressful situation again (Long & Flood, 1993). It is important to choose an exercise that you enjoy doing and that fits into your lifestyle. Perhaps you could walk to work every day or pedal an exercise bicycle during your favorite television program. It is not necessary to join an expensive club or to buy elaborate equipment or clothing to begin an exercise program. It is necessary to get up and get moving, however.

Some people recommend an organized exercise program to obtain the most benefit. For some, however, the cost or time required may actually contribute to their stress. For others, the organized program is an excellent motivator. Find out what works for you.

Keep your exercise plan reasonable. Plan for the long haul, not just until you get past your next performance evaluation or lose that extra 5 pounds.

Mental Health Management

Mental health management begins with *taking responsibility for your own thoughts and attitudes.* Do not allow self-defeating thoughts to dominate your thinking. You may have to remind yourself to stop thinking that you have to be perfect all the time. You may also have to adjust your expectations and become more realistic. Do you always have to be in control? Does everything have to be perfect? Do you have a difficult time delegating? Are you constantly frustrated because of the way you perceive situations? If you answer yes to many of these ques-

BOX 13-6

Guidelines for Good Nutrition

- Eat smaller, more frequent meals for energy. Six small meals are more beneficial than three large ones.
- Eat foods that are high in complex carbohydrates, contain adequate protein, and are low in fat content. Beware of fad diets!
- Eat at least five servings of fruits and vegetables daily.
- Avoid highly processed foods.
- Avoid caffeine.
- Use salt and sugar sparingly.
- Drink plenty of water.
- Make sure you take enough vitamins, including C, B, E, beta carotene, and calcium; and minerals, including copper, manganese, zinc, magnesium, and potassium.

Adapted from Bowers, R. (1993). Stress and your health. *National Women's Health Report*, 15(3), 6.

tions, you may be setting yourself up for failure, resentment, low self-esteem, and burnout. Give yourself positive strokes, even if no one else does (Davidhizar, 1994; Posen, 2000; Wolinski, 1993).

Realistic Expectations

One of the most common stressors in life is having unrealistic expectations. Expecting family members, coworkers, and your employer to be perfect and meet your every demand on your time schedule is setting yourself up for undue stress.

Reframing

Reframing is looking at a situation in many different ways. When you can reframe stressful situations, they often become less stressful or at least more understandable. If you have an extremely heavy workday and believe it is due to the fact that your nurse manager created it for personal reasons, the day becomes much more stressful than if you realize that, unfortunately, all institutions are short-staffed.

Humor

Laughter relieves tension. Humor is a wonderful way to reduce stress both for yourself and your clients. Remember, however, that humor is very individual, and what may be funny to you may be hurtful to your client or coworker.

Social Support

Much research has been done to show that the presence of social support and the quality of relationships can significantly influence how quickly people become ill and how quickly they recover. A sense of belonging and community, an environment where people believe they can share their feelings without fear of condemnation or ridicule, helps to maintain a sense of well-being. Having friends with whom to share hopes, dreams, fears, and concerns and with whom to laugh and cry is paramount to mental health and stress management. In the work environment, coworkers who are trusted and respected become part of social support systems (Wolinski, 1993). Box 13-7 lists some additional tips for coping with work stress.

Nurses are professional caregivers. Many years ago, Carl Rogers (1977) said that you can-

---

BOX 13-7

Coping With Daily Work Stress

- Spend time on outside interests, and take time for yourself.
- Increase professional knowledge.
- Identify problem-solving resources.
- Identify realistic expectations for your position. Make sure you understand what is expected of you; ask questions if anything is unclear.
- Assess the rewards your work can realistically deliver.
- Develop good communication skills, and treat coworkers with respect.
- Join rap sessions with coworkers. Be part of the solution, not part of the problem.
- Do not exceed your limits—you do not always have to say yes!
- Deal with other people's anger by asking yourself, "Whose problem is this?"
- Recognize that you can teach other people how to treat you.

---

not care for others until you have taken care of yourself. The word *selfish* may bring to mind someone who is greedy, self-centered, and egotistical, but to take care of yourself, you have to be *creatively selfish*. Learn to nurture yourself so that you will be better able to nurture others.

Stress reduction, relaxation techniques, exercise, and good nutrition are all helpful in keeping energy levels high. However, although they can prepare people to cope with the stresses of a job, they are not solutions to the conflicts that lead to reality shock and burnout. It is more effective to resolve the problem than to treat the symptoms (Lee & Ashforth, 1993). Box 13-8 lists the keys already discussed to physical and mental health management.

BOX 13-8

Keys to Physical and Mental Health Management

- Deep breathing
- Posture
- Rest
- Relaxation
- Nutrition
- Exercise
- Realistic expectations
- Reframing
- Humor
- Social support

BOX 13-9

Ten Daily De-Stress Reminders

◆ Express yourself! Communicate your feelings and emotions to friends and colleagues to avoid isolation and share perspectives. Sometimes, another opinion helps you see the situation in a different light.

◆ Take time off. Taking breaks, or doing something unrelated to work, will help you feel refreshed as you begin work again.

◆ Understand your individual energy patterns. Are you a morning or an afternoon person? Schedule stressful duties during times when you are most energetic.

◆ Do one stressful activity at a time. Although this may take advanced planning, avoiding more than one stressful situation at a time will make you feel more in control and satisfied with your accomplishments.

◆ Exercise! Physical exercise builds physical and emotional

resilience. Do not put physical activities "on the back burner" as you become busy.

◆ Tackle big projects one piece at a time. Having control of one part of a project at a time will help you to avoid feeling overwhelmed and out of control.

◆ Delegate if possible. If you can delegate and share in problem solving, do so. Not only will your load be lighter, but others will be able to participate in decision making.

◆ It's okay to say no. Do not take on every extra assignment or special project.

◆ Be work-smart. Improve your work skills with new technologies and ideas. Take advantage of additional job training.

◆ Relax. Find time each day to consciously relax and reflect on the positive energies you need to cope with stressful situations more readily.

Adapted from Bowers, R. (1993). Stress and your health. *National Women's Health Report*, 15(3), 6.

CONCLUSION

You already know that the work of nursing is not easy and may sometimes be very stressful. Yet nursing is also a profession filled with a great deal of personal and professional satisfaction. Periodically ask yourself the questions designed to help you assess your stress level and risk for burnout, and review the stress management techniques described in this chapter.

There is no one right way to manage stress and avoid burnout. Rather, by managing small segments of each day, you will learn to identify and manage your stress. This chapter contains many reminders to help you de-stress during the day (Box 13-9). You can also help your colleagues do the same. If you find yourself in danger of job burnout during your career, you will have learned how to bring yourself back to a healthy, balanced position.

Ultimately, you are in control. Every day you are faced with choices. By gaining power over your choices and the stress they cause, you empower yourself. Instead of being preoccupied with the past or the future, acknowledge the present moment and say to yourself (Davidson, 1999):

◆ I choose to relish my days.

◆ I choose to enjoy this moment.

◆ I choose to be fully present to others.

◆ I choose to fully engage in the activity at hand.

◆ I choose to proceed at a measured, effective pace.

◆ I choose to acknowledge all I have achieved so far.

◆ I choose to focus on where I am and what I am doing.

◆ I choose to acknowledge that this is the only moment in which I can take action.

People cannot live in a problem-free world, but they can learn how to handle stress. Using the suggestions in this chapter, you will be able to adopt a healthier personal and professional lifestyle. The self-assessment worksheet, Coping with Stress, can help you manage stress and help you understand your responses better. The worksheet, Values Clarification, will help you identify how to begin to change taking into account what is most important to you.

Coping with Stress

Before you begin to change how you deal with stress, consider how you currently manage stress. Below are some of the more common ways of coping with stressful events. Identify those that you use.

	Never/Seldom	Sometimes	Frequently
1. I ignore my own needs and just work harder.			
2. I seek out family/friends for support.			
3. I eat more than usual.			
4. I do some sort of exercise.			
5. I get irritable and take it out on others.			
6. I take time to relax, breathe, and unwind.			
7. I smoke cigarettes or drink caffeinated beverages.			
8. I confront my stress and work to change it.			
9. I withdraw emotionally and just go through the motions of the day.			
10. I change my outlook on the problem and try and put it in a better perspective.			

	Never/Seldom	Sometimes	Frequently
11. I sleep too much.			
12. I take time off.			
13. I go shopping.			
14. I use humor to take the edge off.			
15. I increase my alcohol intake.			
16. I get involved in a hobby.			
17. I take prescription drugs to help me relax or sleep.			
18. I maintain a healthy diet.			
19. I ignore the problem.			
20. I pray, meditate, or enhance my spiritual life.			
21. I worry and become anxious.			
22. I try to focus on the things I can control and accept the things I can't.			

The even numbered items tend to be more constructive tactics than the odd numbered items.
Source: Adapted from Davis, M., Eshelman, E., & McCay, M. (2000). *The Relaxation & Stress Reduction Workbook,* 5th ed. San Jose, Calif.: New Harbinger Publications.

CHAPTER 13 SELF-ASSESSMENT
Values Clarification

The first step in managing your time is to decide what is most worthwhile or desirable for you. Some of the values that are important to people are career, health, home, family, spirituality, finances, leisure, learning, creativity, happiness, peace of mind, communication. You may identify others. In this exercise, list the values that are most important to you. List all of them, not in any particular order.

_____   _____

_____   _____

_____   _____

_____   _____

_____   _____

Next, think carefully about how important each value is to you and rank order them. You will find that this list comes in handy when you have difficulty choosing between two or more alternatives. If family and leisure rank very high, you many not want to consider a position where you have unscheduled hours or many on-call responsibilities.

1.	6.
2.	7.
3.	8.
4.	9.
5.	10.

Source: Adapted from Davis, M., Eshelman, E., & McCay, M. (2000). *The Relaxation & Stress Reduction Workbook,* 5th ed. San Jose, Calif.: New Harbinger Publications.

Evidence-Based Practice

This systematic review and meta-analysis, completed in 2003, consisted of 500 studies of job satisfaction with 267,995 employees in a large variety of organizations and demonstrated a strong correlation between job satisfaction and mental and physical health. Aspects of mental health, i.e., burnout, lowered self-esteem, anxiety, and depression, were identified. Cardiovascular disease was the main physical illness showing a correlation between job satisfaction and physical health. These relationships demonstrated that job satisfaction level is an important factor influencing health of workers.

Additional examples can be found in:
    Bernsier, D. (1998). A study of coping: Successful recovery from severe burnout and other reactions to severe work-related stress. *Work & Stress*, 12(1), 50–65.
    Boey, K.W. (1999). Distressed and stress-resistant nurses. *Issues in Mental Health Nursing*, 20(1), 33–54.
    Ekstedt, M. (2005). Lived experiences of the time preceding burnout. *Journal of Advanced Nursing*, 49(1), 59–67.
    Ruggeriero, J. (2005). Health, work variables, and job satisfaction among nurses. *Journal of Nursing Administration*, 35(5), 254–263.

Faragher, E., Cass, M, & Cooper, C. (2003). The relationship between job satisfaction and health: A meta-analysis. *Journal of Occupational and Environmental Medicine*, 62: 105–112.

STUDY QUESTIONS

1 Discuss the characteristics of health-care organizations that may lead to burnout among nurses. Which of these have you observed in your clinical rotations? How could they be changed or eliminated?

2 How can a new graduate adequately prepare for reality shock? Based on your responses to the questions in Boxes 13-3 and 13-4, what plans will you make to prepare yourself for your new role?

3 What qualities would you look for in a mentor? What qualities would you demonstrate as a mentee? Can you identify someone you know who might become a mentor to you?

4 What are the signs of stress, reality shock, and burnout? How are they related?

5 How can you help colleagues deal with their stress?

6 Identify the physical and psychological signs and symptoms you exhibit during stress. What sources of stress are most likely to affect you? How do you deal with these signs and symptoms?

7 Develop a plan to manage stress on a long-term basis.

CRITICAL THINKING EXERCISE

Shawna, the "new kid on the block," has been working from 7 a.m. to 3 p.m. on an infectious disease floor since obtaining her RN license 4 months ago. Most of the staff she works with have been there since the unit opened 5 years ago. On a typical day, the staffing consists of a nurse manager, two RNs, an LPN, and

(Continued on following page)

one technician for approximately 40 clients. The majority of the clients are HIV-positive with multisystem failure. Many are severely debilitated and need help with their activities of daily living. Although the staff members encourage family members and loved ones to help, most of them are unavailable because they work during the day. Several days a week, the nursing students from Shawna's community college program are assigned to the floor.

Tina, the nurse manager, does not participate in any direct client care, saying that she is "too busy at the desk." Laverne, the other RN, says the unit depresses her and that she has requested a transfer to pediatrics. Lynn, the LPN, wants to "give meds" because she is "sick of the clients' constant whining," and Sheila, the technician, is "just plain exhausted." Lately, Shawna has noticed that the other staff members seem to avoid the nursing students and reply to their questions with annoyed, short answers. Shawna is feeling alone and overwhelmed and goes home at night worrying about the clients, who need more care and attention. She is afraid to ask Tina for more help because she does not want to be considered incompetent or a complainer. When she confided in Lynn about her concerns, Lynn replied, "Get real—no one here cares about the clients or us. All they care about is the bottom line! Why did a smart girl like you choose nursing in the first place?"

1. What is happening on this unit in leadership terms?

2. Identify the major problems and the factors that contributed to these problems.

3. What factors might have contributed to the behaviors exhibited by Tina, Lynn, and Sheila?

4. How would you feel if you were Shawna?

5. Is there anything Shawna can do for herself, for the clients, and for the staff members?

6. What do you think Tina, the nurse manager, should do?

7. How is the nurse manager reacting to the changes in her staff members?

8. What is the responsibility of administration?

9. How are the clients affected by the behaviors exhibited by all staff members?

REFERENCES

Benner, P. (1984). *From Novice to Expert*. Menlo Park, CA: Addison-Wesley.

Best, M., & Thurston, N. (2004). Measuring nurse job satisfaction, *Journal of Nursing Administration*, 34(6), 283–290.

Borman, J. (1993). Chief nurse executives balance their work and personal lives. *Nursing Administration Quarterly*, 18(1), 30–39.

Bowers, R. (1993). Stress and your health. *National Women's Health Report*, 15(3), 6.

Boychuk, J. (2001). Out in the real world: Newly graduated nurses in acute-care speak out. *Journal of Nursing Administration*, 31, 426–439.

Carr, K., & Kazanowski, M. (1994). Factors affecting job satisfaction of nurses who work in long-term care. *Journal of Advanced Nursing*, 19, 878–883.

Corley, M., Farley, B., Geddes, N., Goodloe, L., & Green, P. (1994). The clinical ladder: Impact on nurse satisfaction and turnover. *Journal of Nursing Administration,* 24(2), 42–48.

Crawford, S. (1993). Job stress and occupational health nursing. *American Association of Occupational Health Nurses Journal,* 41, 522–529.

Crout, L., Change, E., & Cioffi, J.(2005). Why do registered nurses work when ill? *Journal of Nursing Administration,* 35(1), 23–28.

Davidhizar, R. (1994). Stress can make you or break you. *Advance Practice Nurse,* 10(1), 17.

Davidson, J. (1999). *Managing Stress,* 2nd ed. New York: Pearson Education Macmillan Company.

Davis, M., Eshelman, E., & McCay, M. (2000). *The Relaxation and Stress Reduction Workbook,* 5th ed. California: New Harbinger Publications.

DeFrank, R., & Ivancevich, J. (1998). Stress on the job: An executive update. *Academy of Management Executives,* 12(3), 55.

Dionne-Proulx, J., & Pepin, R. (1993). Stress management in the nursing profession. *Journal of Nursing Management,* 1, 75–81.

Duquette, A., Sandhu, B., & Beaudet, L. (1994). Factors related to nursing burnout: A review of empirical knowledge. *Issues in Mental Health Nursing,* 15, 337–358.

Faragher, E., Cass, M., & Cooper, C. (2003). The relationship between job satisfaction and health: A meta-analysis. *Journal of Occupational and Environmental Medicine,* 62, 105–112.

Farren, C. (1999). Stress and productivity: What tips the scale? *Strategy and Leadership,* 27(1), 36.

Fielding, J., & Weaver, S. (1994). A comparison of hospital and community-based mental health nurses: Perceptions of their work environment and psychological health. *Journal of Advanced Nursing,* 19, 1196–1204.

Freudenberger, H.J. (1974). Staff burn-out. *Journal of Social Issues,* 30(1), 159.

Godinez, G., Schweiger, J., Gruver, J., & Ryan, P. (1999). Role transition from graduate to staff nurse: A qualitative analysis. *Journal for Nurses in Staff Development,* 15(3), 97–110.

Golin, M., Buchlin, M., & Diamond, D. (1991). *Secrets of Executive Success.* Emmaus, PA: Rodale Press.

Goliszek, A. (1992). *Sixty-Six Second Stress Management. The Quickest Way to Relax and Ease Anxiety.* Far Hills, NJ: New Horizon.

Goodell, T., & Van Ess Coeling, H. (1994). Outcomes of nurses' job satisfaction. *Journal of Nursing Administration,* 24(11), 36–41.

Grant, P. (1993). Manage nurse stress and increase potential at the bedside. *Nursing Administration Quarterly,* 18(1), 16–22.

Hall, D. (2004). Work-related stress of registered nurses in a hospital setting. *Journal for Nurses in Staff Development,* 20(1), 6–14.

Heslop, L. (2001). Undergraduate student nurses: Expectations and their self-reported preparedness for the graduate year role. *Journal of Advanced Nursing,* 36, 626–634.

Johnston, F. (May-June 1994). Stress can kill. *Today's OR Nurse,* 5–6.

Kovner, C., Hendrickson, G., Knickman, J., & Finkler, S. (1994). Nurse care delivery models and nurse satisfaction. *Nursing Administration Quarterly,* 19(1), 74–85.

Kraeger, M., & Walker, K. (1993). Attrition, burnout, job dissatisfaction and occupational therapy manager. *Occupational Therapy in Health Care,* 8(4), 47–61.

Kramer, M. (January 27–28, 1981). Coping with reality shock. Workshop presented at Jackson Memorial Hospital, Miami, FL.

Kramer, M., & Schmalenberg, C. (1993). Learning from success: Autonomy and empowerment. *Nursing Management,* 24(5), 58–64.

Lee, R.T., & Ashforth, B.E. (1993). A further examination of managerial burnout: Toward an integrated model. *Journal of Organizational Behavior,* 14(1), 3–20.

Lenson, B. (2001). *Good Stress—Bad Stress.* New York: Marlowe and Company.

Lickman, P., Simms, L., & Greene, C. (1993). Learning environment: The catalyst for work excitement. *Journal of Continuing Education in Nursing,* 24, 211–216.

Long, B., & Flood, K. (1993). Coping with work stress: Psychological benefits of exercise. *Work and Stress,* 7(2), 109–119.

Lusk, S. (1993). Job stress. *American Association of Occupational Health Nurses Journal,* 41, 601–606.

Malkin, K.F. (1993). Primary nursing: Job satisfaction and staff retention. *Journal of Nursing Management,* 1, 119–124.

Martin, K. (May 1993). To cope with stress. *Nursing 93,* 39–41.

McGee-Cooper, A. (September-October 1993). Shifting from high stress to high energy. *Imprint,* 93(5), 61–69.

McLennan, M. (2005). Nurses' views on work enabling factors. *Journal of Nursing Administration,* 35(6), 311–318.

McVicar, A. (2003). Workplace stress in nursing: A literature review. *Journal of Advanced Nursing,* 44(6), 633–642.

Nakata, J., & Saylor, C. (1994). Management style and staff nurse satisfaction in a changing environment. *Nursing Administration Quarterly,* 18(3), 51–57.

National Institute for Occupational Safety and Health (NIOSH) http://www.cdc.gov/niosh/homepage.html, accessed on July 27, 2002.

Nowak, K., & Pentkowski, A. (1994). Lifestyle habits, substance use, and predictors of job burnout in professional women. *Work and Stress,* 8(1), 19–35.

Paine, W.S. (1984). Professional burnout: Some major costs. *Family and Community Health,* 6(4), 1–11.

Pines, A. (2004). Adult attachment styles and their relationship to burnout: A preliminary, cross-cultural investigation. *Work & Stress,* 18(1), 66–80.

Posen, D. (2000). Stress management for patient and physician. http://www.mentalhealth.com/mag1/p51-str.html.

Rogers, C. (1977). *Carl Rogers on Personal Power.* New York: Dell.

Sadovich, J. (2005). Work excitement in nursing: An examination between work excitement and burnout. *Nursing Economics,* 23(2), 91–96.

Scheetz, L.J. (2000). *Nursing Faculty Secrets*. Philadelphia: Hanley & Belfus.

Selye, H. (1956). *The Stress of Life*. New York: McGraw-Hill.

Simonetti, J., & Ariss, S. (1999). The role of a mentor. *Business Horizons*, 42(6), 56–73.

Skubak, K., Earls, N., & Botos, M. (1994). Shared governance: Getting it started. *Nursing Management*, 25(5), 80I-J, 80N, 80P.

Smith, B. (October 2004). Test your stamina for workplace fatique. *Nursing Management*, 38–40.

Stechmiller, J., & Yarandi, H. (1993). Predictors of burnout in critical care nurses. *Heart Lung*, 22, 534–540.

Teague, J.B. (1992). The relationship between various coping styles and burnout among nurses. *Dissertation Abstracts International*, 1994.

Trossman, S. (July/August 1999). Stress! It's everywhere! And it can be managed! *American Nurse*, 1.

Tumulty, G., Jernigan, E., & Kohut, G. (1994). The impact of perceived work environment on job satisfaction of hospital staff nurses. *Applied Nursing Research*, 7(2), 84–90.

Vahey, D., Aiken, L., Sloane, D., Clarke, S. & Vargas, D. (2004). Nurse burnout and patient satisfaction. *Medical Care*, 42(2), II-57-II-66.

Vines, S. (1994). Relaxation with guided imagery. *American Association of Occupational Health Nurses Journal*, 42, 206–213.

Wolinski, K. (1993). Self-awareness, self-renewal, self management. *AORN Journal*, 58, 721–730.

chapter 14

Your Nursing Career

OBJECTIVES

After reading this chapter, the student should be able to:

◆ Evaluate personal strengths, weaknesses, opportunities, and threats using a SWOT analysis.

◆ Develop a résumé including objectives, qualifications, skills experience, work history, education, and training.

◆ Compose job search letters including cover letter, thank-you letter, and acceptance and rejection letters.

◆ Discuss components of the interview process.

◆ Discuss the factors involved in selecting the right position.

◆ Explain why the first year is critical to the planning of a career.

OUTLINE

Health care is one of the largest and fastest growing industries in the United States. By the year 2008 health services employment is projected to increase to 13,600,00, with more than 2,800,000 new jobs (Zedlitz, 2003, p. vii).

By now, you have invested considerable time, expense, and emotion into preparing for your new career. Your educational preparation, technical and clinical expertise, interpersonal and management skills, personal interests and needs, and commitment to the nursing profession will contribute to meeting your career goals. Changes in technology and the anticipated lengthy nursing shortage will continue to affect the way in which nursing care is delivered. However, as these changes eventually work out, nurses will continue to play a major role in the delivery of health care. Successful nurses view nursing as a lifetime pursuit, not as an occupational stepping stone. As a professional nurse, "the sky is the limit" in terms of the opportunities and challenges.

What steps are important in strategizing your career path? This chapter deals with a most important endeavor: finding and keeping your first nursing position. The chapter begins with planning your initial search; developing a strengths, weaknesses, opportunities, and threats (SWOT) analysis; searching for available positions; and researching organizations. Also included is a section on writing a résumé and employment-related information about the interview process and selecting the first position.

GETTING STARTED

By now at least one person has said to you, "Nurses will never be out of a job." This statement is only one of several career myths. These myths include the following (Miller, 2003):

1. "Good workers do not get fired." They may not get fired, but many good workers have lost their positions during restructuring and downsizing.
2. "Well-paying jobs are available without a college degree." Yes, you many know one or two people who have well-paying and exciting positions without having a college degree. However, even if entrance into a career path does not require a college education, the potential for career advancement is minimal without that degree. In many health-care agencies, a baccalaureate degree in nursing is required for an initial management position.
3. "Go to work for a good company, and move up the career ladder." This statement assumes that people move up the career ladder due to longevity in the organization. In reality, the responsibility for career advancement rests on the employee, not the employer.
4. "Find the 'hot' industry and you will always be in demand." Nursing is projected to continue to be one of the "hottest industries" well into the next decade. A nurse who performs poorly will never be successful, no matter what the demand.

Many students attending college today are adults with family, work, and personal responsibilities. On graduating with an associate degree in nursing, you may still have student loans and continued responsibilities for supporting a family. If this is so, you may be so focused on job security and a steady source of income that the idea of career planning has not even entered your mind. You might even assume that your goal is just to "get the first job." The correct goal is to find a job that fits *you,* one that is a good first step on the path to a lifelong career in nursing. It is also not too early to begin formal planning of your career. You will most likely work well in excess of 70,000 hours in a lifetime outside the home. Do you want to spend all this time devoted to a carreer that is not fulfilling?

SWOT Analysis

Many students assume that their first position will be as a staff nurse on a medical-surgical floor. They see themselves as "putting in their year" and then moving on to what they really want to do. However, as the health-care system continues to evolve and reallocate resources, this may no longer be the automatic first step for new graduates. Instead, new graduates should focus on long-term career goals and the different avenues by which they can be reached.

Many times, your past experiences will be an asset in presenting your abilities for a particular position. A SWOT analysis plan, borrowed from the corporate world, can guide you through your own internal strengths and weaknesses, and an analysis of external opportunities and threats that may help or hinder your job search and career planning. The SWOT analysis is really an in-depth look at what will make you truly happy in your work. Although you have already made the decision to pursue nursing, knowing your strengths and weaknesses can help you select the work setting that will be personally satisfying (Ellis, 1999). Your SWOT analysis may include the following factors (Pratt, 1994):

Strengths

- ◆ Relevant work experience.
- ◆ Advanced education.
- ◆ Product knowledge.
- ◆ Good communication and people skills.
- ◆ Computer skills.
- ◆ Self-managed learning skills.
- ◆ Flexibility.

Weaknesses

- ◆ Poor communication and people skills.
- ◆ Inflexibility.
- ◆ Lack of interest in further training.
- ◆ Difficulty adapting to change.
- ◆ Inability to see health care as a business.

Opportunities

- ◆ Expanding markets in health care.
- ◆ New applications of technology.
- ◆ New products and diversification.
- ◆ Increasing at-risk populations.

Threats

- ◆ Increased competition among health-care facilities.
- ◆ Changes in government regulation.

Take some time to personalize the preceding SWOT analysis. What are *your* strengths? What are the things *you* are not so good at? What weaknesses do *you* need to minimize or what strengths do *you* need to develop as you begin your job search? What opportunities and threats exist in the health-care community *you* are considering? Doing a SWOT analysis will help you make an initial assessment of the job market. It can be used again after you narrow down your search for that first nursing position.

In addition to completing a SWOT analysis, there are several other tools that can help you learn more about yourself. Two of the most common instruments are the Strong Interest Inventory (SII) and the Myers-Briggs Type Indicator (MBTI). The SII compares the individual's interests with the interests of those who are successful in a large number of occupational fields in the areas of (1) work styles, (2) learning environment, (3) leadership style, and (4) risk-taking/adventure. Completing this inventory can assist you to discover what work environment might be best suited to your interests.

The MBTI is a widely used indicator of personality patterns. This self-report inventory provides information about individual psychological-type preferences on four dimensions:

1. Extroversion (E) or Introversion (1)
2. Sensing (S) or Intuition (N)
3. Thinking (T) or Feeling (F)
4. Judging (J) or Perceiving (P)

Although there are many factors that influence behaviors and attitudes, the MBTI summarizes underlying patterns and behaviors common to most people. Both instruments should be administered and interpreted by a qualified practitioner. Most university and career counseling centers are able to administer these instruments. If you are unsure of just where you fit in the workplace, you might explore these instruments with your college or university.

Beginning the Search

It is no longer true for many nursing graduates that once they have a degree, they can get a job anywhere. However, even with a nationwide nursing shortage predicted to last for at least 10 years, hospital mergers, emphasis on increased staff productivity, budget crises, staffing shifts, and changes in job market availability affect the numbers and types of nurses employed in various facilities and agencies. Instead of focusing on long-term job security, the career-secure employee focuses on becoming a career survivalist. A career survivalist focuses on the person, not the position. Consider the following career survivalist strategies (Waymon & Baber, 1999):

◆ **Be psychologically self-employed.** Your career belongs to you, not to the person who signs your paycheck. Security and advancement on the job are up to you. Security may be elusive, but opportunities for nurses are growing every day.

◆ **Learn for employability.** Take personal responsibility for your career success. Learn not only for your current position but also for your next position. Employability in health care today means learning technology tools, job-specific technical skills, and people skills such as the ability to negotiate, coach, work in teams, and make presentations.

◆ **Plan for your financial future.** Ask yourself, "How can I spend less, earn more, and manage better?" Often, people make job decisions based on financial decisions, which makes them feel trapped instead of secure.

◆ **Develop multiple options.** The career survivalist looks at multiple options constantly. Moving up is only one option. Being aware of emerging trends in nursing, adjacent fields, lateral moves, and special projects presents other options.

◆ **Build a safety net.** Networking is extremely important to the career survivalist. Joining professional organizations, taking time to build long-term nursing relationships, and getting to know other career survivalists will make your career path more enjoyable and successful.

What do employers think you need to be ready to work for them? Besides passing the National Council Licensure Examination (NCLEX), employers cite the following skills as desirable in job candidates (Shingleton, 1994).

Oral and Written Communication Skills

◆ Ability to assume responsibility.
◆ Interpersonal skills.
◆ Proficiency in field of study/technical competence.
◆ Teamwork ability.
◆ Willingness to work hard.
◆ Leadership abilities.
◆ Motivation, initiative, and flexibility.
◆ Critical thinking and analytical skills.
◆ Computer knowledge.
◆ Problem-solving and decision-making abilities.
◆ Self-discipline.
◆ Organizational skills.

Active job searches may include looking in a variety of places (Beatty, 1991; Hunsaker, 2001):

◆ Public employment agencies.
◆ Private employment agencies.
◆ Human resource departments.
◆ Information from friends or relatives.
◆ Newspapers; professional journals.
◆ College and university career centers.
◆ Career and job fairs.
◆ Internet Web sites.
◆ Other professionals (networking).

In recent years, three trends have emerged related to recruiting. First, employers are using more creativity by using alternative sources to increase diversity of employees. They are commonly running advertisements in minority newspapers and magazines and recruiting nurses at minority organizations. Second, employers are using more temporary help as a way to "look at" potential employees. Nursing staffing agencies are common in most areas of the county. Third, the Internet is being used more frequently for advertising and recruitment (Hunsaker, 2001).

Regardless of where you begin your search, explore the market vigorously and thoroughly.

Looking only in the classified ads on Sunday morning is a limited search. Instead, speak to everyone you know about your job search. Encourage classmates and colleagues to share contacts with you, and do the same with them. Also, when possible, try to speak directly with the person who is looking for a nurse when you hear of a possible opening. The people in human resources (personnel) offices may reject a candidate on a technicality that a nurse manager would realize does not affect that person's ability to handle the job if he or she is otherwise a good match for the position. For example, experience in day surgery prepares a person to work in other surgery-related settings, but a human resources interviewer may not know this.

Try to obtain as much information as you can about the available position. Is there a match between your skills and interests and the position? Ask yourself whether you are applying for this position because you really want it or just to gain interview experience. Be careful about going through the interview process and receiving job offers only to turn them down. Employers may share information with one another, and you could end up being denied the position you really want. Regardless of where you explore potential opportunities, Miller (2003, p. 100) identifies the following "pearls of widom" from career nurses:

◆ Know yourself.
◆ Seek out mentors and wise people.
◆ Be a risk taker.
◆ Never, ever stop learning.
◆ Understand the business of health care.
◆ Involve yourself in community and professional organizations.
◆ Network.
◆ Understand diversity.
◆ Be an effective communicator.
◆ Set short- and long-term goals and continually strive to achieve them.

Researching Your Potential Employer

You have spent time taking a look at yourself and the climate of the health-care job market.

You have narrowed your choices to the organizations that really interest you. Now is the time to find out as much as possible about these organizations.

Ownership of the company may be public or private and foreign-owned or American-owned. The company may be local or regional, a small corporation or a division of a much larger corporation. Depending on the size and ownership of the company, information may be obtained from the public library, chamber of commerce, government offices, or company Web site. A telephone call or letter to the corporate office or local human resources department may also generate valuable information on organizations of interest (Crowther, 1994). Has the organization recently gone through a merger, a reorganization, or downsizing? Information from current and past employees is valuable and may provide you with more details about whether the organization might be suitable for you. Be wary of gossip and half-truths that may emerge, however, because they may discourage you from applying to an excellent health-care facility. In other words, if you hear something negative about an organization, check it out for yourself.

Often, individuals jump at work opportunities before doing a complete assessment of the culture and politics of the institution.

The first step in assessing the culture is to review a copy of the company's mission statement. The mission statement reflects what the institution considers important to its public image. What are the core values of the institution?

A look at the department of nursing philosophy and objectives indicates how the nursing department defines nursing and outlines the objectives for the department; in other words, it identifies what the important goals are for nursing. The nursing philosophy and goals should reflect the mission of the organization. Where is nursing administration on the organizational chart of the institution? To whom does the chief nursing administrator report? Although much of this information may not be obtained until an interview, a preview of how the institution views itself and the value it places on nursing will help you to decide if your philosophy of health care and nursing is compatible with that of a particular organization. To find out more about a specific health-care facility, you can (Zedlitz, 2003):

- ◆ Talk to nurses currently employed at the facility.
- ◆ Access the Internet Web site for information on the mission, philosophy, and services.
- ◆ Check the library for newspaper and magazine articles related to the facility.

WRITING A RÉSUMÉ

Your résumé is your personal data sheet and self-advertisement. It is the first impression the recruiter or your potential employer will have of you. Through the résumé you are selling yourself: your skills, talents, and abilities. You may decide to prepare your own résumé or have it prepared by a professional service. Regardless of who prepares it, the purpose of a résumé is clear: to get a job interview. Many people dislike the idea of writing a résumé. After all, how can you sum up your entire career in a single page? You want to scream at the printed page, "Hey, I'm bigger than that! Look at all I have to offer!" However, this one-page summary has to work well enough to get you the position you want. Chestnut (1999) summarized résumé writing by stating, "Lighten up. Although a very important piece to the puzzle in your job search, a résumé is not the only ammunition. What's between your ears is what will ultimately lead you to your next career" (p. 28). Box 14-1 summarizes reasons for preparing a well-considered, up-to-date résumé.

Although you labor intensively over preparing your résumé, most job applications live or die within 10 to 30 seconds as the receptionist or applications examiner decides whether your résumé should be forwarded to the next step or rejected. The initial screening is usually done by non-nursing personnel. Some beginning helpful tips include: (Marino, 2000):

- ◆ Keep the résumé to one or two pages. Do not use smaller fonts to cram more information on the page. Proofread, proofread, proofread. Typing errors, misspelled words,

---

BOX 14-1

Reasons for Preparing a Résumé

- ◆ Assists in completing an employment application quickly and accurately
- ◆ Demonstrates your potential
- ◆ Focuses on your strongest points
- ◆ Gives you credit for all your achievements
- ◆ Identifies you as organized, prepared, and serious about the job search
- ◆ Serves as a reminder and adds to your self-confidence during the interview
- ◆ Provides initial introduction to potential employers in seeking the interview
- ◆ Serves as a guide for the interviewer
- ◆ Functions as a tool to distribute to others who are willing to assist you in a job search

Adapted from Marino, K. (2000). *Resumes for the Health Care Professional.* New York: John Wiley & Sons; and Zedlitz, R. (2003). *How to Get a Job in Health Care.* New York: Delmar Learning.

---

and poor grammar can damage your chances of obtaining an interview.

- ◆ Your educational background goes at the end of the résumé, unless you are a recent graduate and your degree is stronger than your experience or you are applying for a job at an educational institution.
- ◆ State your objective. Although you know very well what position you are seeking, the receptionist doing the initial screening does not want to take the time to determine this. Tailor your resume to the insitution and position to which you are applying.
- ◆ Employers care about what you can do for them and your potential future success with their company. Your résumé must answer that question.

Essentials of a Résumé

Résumés most frequently follow one of four formats: standard, chronological, functional, or a combination. Regardless of the type of résumé, basic elements of personal information, education, work experience, qualifications for the position, and references should be included (Marino, 2000; Zedlitz, 2003):

- ◆ **Standard.** The standard résumé is organized by categories. By clearly stating your personal information, job objective, work experience, education and work skills, memberships, honors, and special skills, the employer can easily have a "snapshot" of the person requesting entrance into the workforce. This is a useful résumé for first-time employees or recent graduates.

◆ **Chronological.** The chronological résumé lists work experiences in order of time, with the most recent experience listed first. This style is useful in showing stable employment without gaps or many job changes. The objective and qualifications are listed at the top.

◆ **Functional**. The functional résumé also lists work experience but in order of importance to your job objective. List the most important work-related experience first. This is a useful format when you have gaps in employment or lack direct experience related to your objective. Figure 14-1 demonstrates a functional résumé that could be used for seeking initial employment as a registered nurse (RN).

Delores Wheatley
5734 Foster Road
Middleton, Indiana 46204
(907) 123-4567

Objective: Position as staff registered nurse on medical-surgical unit

HIGHLIGHTS OF QUALIFICATIONS
High School Diploma, 2001
Coral Ridge High School
Dolphin Beach, Florida

Associate of Science Degree in Nursing, 2006
Howard Community College (HCC)
Middleton, Indiana
Currently enrolled in the following courses at HCC:
30-hour IV certification course
8-hour phlebotomy course
16-hour 12-lead EKG course

EXPERIENCE
Volunteer, Association for the Blind, 1998-2001
Nursing Assistant, Howard Community Hospital, 2001-2006
  (summer employment)
Special Olympics Committee, 2003-2006

QUALIFICATIONS
Experience with blind and disabled children
Pediatric inpatient experience
Ability to work as part of an interdisciplinary team
Experience with families in crisis

FIGURE 14-1 ◆ Sample functional résumé.

◆ **Combination**. The combination résumé is a popular format, listing work experience directly related to the position but in a chronological order.

Most professional recruiters and placement services agree on the following tips in preparing a résumé (Anderson, 1992; Rodriguez & Robertson, 1992):

◆ *Make sure your résumé is readable.* Is the type large enough for easy reading? Are paragraphs indented or bullets used to set off information, or does the entire page look like a gray blur? Using bold headings and appropriate spacing can offer relief from lines of gray type, but be careful not to get so carried away with graphics that your résumé becomes a new art form. The latest trends with résumé writing are using fonts such as Ariel or Century New Gothic over the standard Times New Roman (James, 2003). The paper should be an appropriate color such as cream, white, or off-white. Use easily readable fonts and a laser printer. If a good computer and printer are not available, most printing services prepare résumés at a reasonable cost.

◆ *Make sure the important facts are easy to spot.* Education, current employment, responsibilities, and facts to support the experience you have gained from previous positions are important. Put the strongest statements at the beginning. Avoid excessive use of the word "I." If you are a new nursing graduate and have little or no job experience, list your educational background first. Remember that positions you held before you entered nursing can frequently support experience that will be relevant in your nursing career. Ensure you let your prospective employer know how you can be contacted.

◆ *Do a spelling and grammar check.* Use simple terms, action verbs, and descriptive words. Check your finished résumé for spelling, style, and grammar errors. If you are not sure how something sounds, get another opinion.

◆ *Follow the don'ts.* Do not include pictures, fancy binders, salary information, or hobbies (unless they have contributed to your work experience). Do not include personal information such as weight, marital status, and number of children. Do not repeat information just to make the résumé longer. A good résumé is concise and focuses on your strengths and accomplishments.

No matter which format you use, it is essential to include the following (Parker, 1989):

◆ A clearly stated job objective.
◆ Highlighted qualifications.
◆ Directly relevant skills experience.
◆ Chronological work history.
◆ Relevant education and training.

How to Begin

Start by writing down every applicable point you can think of in the preceding five categories. Work history is usually the easiest place to begin. Arrange your work history in reverse chronological order, listing your current job first. Account for all your employable years. Short lapses in employment are acceptable, but give a brief explanation for longer periods (e.g., "maternity leave"). Include employer, dates worked (years only, e.g., 2001–2002), city, and state for each employer you list. Briefly describe the duties and responsibilities of each position. Emphasize your accomplishments, any special techniques you learned, or changes you implemented. Use action verbs, such as those listed in Table 14-1, to describe your accomplishments. Also cite any special awards or committee chairs. If a previous position was not in the health field, try to relate your duties and accomplishments to the position you are seeking.

Education

Next, focus on your education. Include the name and location of every educational institution you attended; the dates you attended; and the degree, diploma, or certification attained. Start with your most recent degree. It is not necessary to include your license number

TABLE 14-1			
Action Verbs			
Management Skills	*Communication Skills*	*Accomplishments*	*Helping Skills*
Attained	Collaborated	Achieved	Assessed
Developed	Convinced	Adapted	Assisted
Improved	Developed	Coordinated	Clarified
Increased	Enlisted	Developed	Demonstrated
Organized	Formulated	Expanded	Diagnosed
Planned	Negotiated	Facilitated	Expedited
Recommended	Promoted	Implemented	Facilitated
Strengthened	Reconciled	Improved	Motivated
Supervised	Recruited	Instructed	Represented
		Reduced (losses)	
		Resolved (problems)	
		Restored	

Adapted from Parker, Y. (1989). *The Damn Good Résumé Guide.* Berkeley, CA: Ten Speed Press.

because you will give a copy of the license when you begin employment. If you are still waiting to sit the NCLEX, you need to indicate when you are scheduled to sit the examination. If you are seeking additional training, such as for intravenous certification, include only what is relevant to your job objective.

Your Objective

It is now time to write your job objective. Write a clear, brief job objective. To accomplish this, ask yourself: What do I want to do? For whom, or with whom? When? At what level of responsibility? For example (Parker, 1989):

- **What:** RN.
- **For whom:** Pediatric patients.
- **Where:** Large metropolitan hospital.
- **At what level:** Staff.

A new graduate's objective might read: "Position as staff nurse on a pediatric unit" or "Graduate nurse position on a pediatric unit." Do not include phrases such as "advancing to neonatal intensive care unit." Employers are trying to fill current openings and do not want be considered a stepping stone in your career.

Skills and Experience

Relevant skills and experience are included in your résumé not to describe your past but to present a "word picture of you in your proposed new job, created out of the best of your past experience" (Parker, 1989, p. 13; Impollonia, 2004). Begin by jotting down the major skills required for the position you are seeking. Include five or six major skills such as:

- Administration/management.
- Teamwork/problem solving.
- Patient relations.
- Specialty proficiency.
- Technical skills.

Other

Academic honors, publications, research, and membership in professional organizations may be included. You are probably saying, "Wait a minute. I did not even take the NCLEX yet!" Were you active in your school's student nurses association? A church or community organization? Were you on the dean's list? What if you were "just a housewife" for many years? First, let's do an attitude adjustment: you were not "just a housewife" but a family manager. Explore your role in work-related terms such as *community volunteerism, personal relations, fund raising, counseling,* and *teaching.* A college career office, women's center, or professional résumé service can offer you assistance with analyzing the skills and talents you shared with your family and community. A student who lacks work experience has options as well. Examples of nonwork experience that show marketable skills include (Eubanks, 1991; Parker, 1989):

◆ Working on school paper or yearbook.

◆ Serving in student government.

◆ Leadership positions in clubs, bands, church activities.

◆ Community volunteerism.

◆ Coaching sports or tutoring children in academic areas.

Now that you have jotted down everything relevant about yourself, it is time to develop the highlights of your qualifications. This area could also be called the summary of qualifications or just summary. These are immodest one-liners designed to let your prospective employer know that you are qualified and talented and absolutely the best choice for the position. A typical group of highlights might include (Parker, 1989):

◆ Relevant experience.

◆ Formal training and credentials, if relevant.

◆ Significant accomplishments, very briefly stated.

◆ One or two outstanding skills or abilities.

◆ A reference to your values, commitment, or philosophy, if appropriate.

A new graduate's highlights could read:

◆ 5 years of experience as a licensed practical nurse in a large nursing home.

◆ Excellent client/family relationship skills.

◆ Experience with chronic psychiatric patients.

◆ Strong teamwork and communication skills.

◆ Special certification in rehabilitation and reambulation strategies.

Tailor the résumé to the job you are seeking. Include only relevant information, such as internships, summer jobs, inter-semester experiences, and volunteer work. Even if your previous experience is not directly related to nursing, your previous work experience can show transferable skills, motivation, and your potential to be a great employee.

Regardless of how wonderful you sound on paper, if the résumé itself is not high quality, it may end up in a trash can. As well, let your perspective employer know whether you have an answering machine or fax for leaving messages.

JOB SEARCH LETTERS

The most common job search letters are the cover letter, thank-you letter, and acceptance letter. Job search letters should be linked to the SWOT analysis you prepared earlier. Regardless of their specific purpose, letters should follow basic writing principles (Banis, 1994):

◆ State the purpose of your letter.

◆ State the most important items first and support them with facts.

◆ Keep the letter organized.

◆ Group similar items together in a paragraph, and then organize the paragraphs to flow logically.

◆ Business letters are formal, but they can also be personal and warm but professional.

◆ Avoid sending an identical form letter to everyone. Instead, personalize each letter to fit each individual situation.

◆ As you write the letter, keep it work-centered and employment-centered, not self-centered.

◆ Be direct and brief. Keep your letter to one page.

◆ Use the active voice and action verbs with a positive, optimistic tone.

◆ If possible, address your letters to a specific individual, using the correct title and business address. Letters addressed to "To Whom It May Concern" do not indicate much research or interest in your prospective employer.

◆ A timely (rapid) response demonstrates your knowledge of how to do business.

◆ Be honest. Use specific examples and evidence from your experience to support your claims.

Cover Letter

You have spent time carefully preparing the résumé that best sells you to your prospective employer. The cover letter will be your introduction. If it is true that first impressions are lasting ones, the cover letter will have a significant impact on your prospective employer. The purposes of the cover letter include (Beatty, 1989):

◆ Acting as a transmittal letter for your résumé.

◆ Presenting you and your credentials to the prospective employer.

◆ Generating interest in interviewing you.

Regardless of whether your cover letter will be read first by human resources personnel or by the individual nurse manager, the effectiveness of your cover letter cannot be overemphasized. A poor cover letter can eliminate you from the selection process before you even have an opportunity to compete. A sloppy, unorganized cover letter and résumé may suggest that you are sloppy and unorganized at work. A lengthy, wordy cover letter may suggest a verbose, unfocused individual (Beatty, 1991). The cover letter should include the following (Anderson, 1992):

◆ **State your purpose in applying and your interest in a specific position.** Identify how you learned about the position.

◆ **Emphasize your strongest qualifications that match the requirements for the position.** Provide evidence of experience and accomplishments that relate to the available position, and refer to your enclosed résumé.

◆ **Sell yourself!** Convince this employer that you have the qualifications and motivation to perform in this position.

◆ **Express appreciation to the reader for consideration.**

If possible, address your cover letter to a specific person. If you do not have a name, call the health-care facility, and obtain the name of the human resources supervisor. If you do not have a name, create a greeting by adding the word "manager" so that your greeting reads: Dear Human Resources Manager or Dear Personnel Manager (Zedlitz, 2003, p. 19). Figure 14-2 is an example of a cover letter.

Thank-You Letter

Thank-you letters are important but seldom used tools in a job search. You should send a thank-you letter to everyone who has helped in any way in your job search. As stated earlier, promptness is important. Thank-you letters should be sent out within 24 hours to anyone who has interviewed you. The thank-you letter (Banis, 1994, p. 4) should be used to:

◆ Express appreciation.

◆ Reemphasize your qualifications and the match between your qualifications and the available position.

◆ Restate your interest in the position.

◆ Provide any supplemental information not previously stated.

Figure 14-3 is a sample thank-you letter.

Acceptance Letter

Write an acceptance letter to accept an offered position; confirm the terms of employment, such as salary and starting date; and reiterate the employer's decision to hire you. The acceptance letter often follows a telephone conversation in which the terms of employment are discussed. Figure 14-4 is a sample acceptance letter.

Rejection Letter

Although not as common as the first three job search letters, you should send a rejection letter if you are declining an employment offer. When rejecting an employment offer, indicate that you have given the offer careful consideration but have decided that the position does

5734 Foster Road
Middleton, Indiana 46204

April 15, 2006

Ms. Joan Smith
Human Resources Manager
All Care Nursing Center
4431 Lakeside Drive
Middleton, Indiana 46204

Dear Ms. Smith:

I am applying for the registered nurse position that was advertised in the *Fort Lauderdale News* on April 14. The position seems to fit very well with my education, experience, and career interests.

Your position requires interest and experience in caring for the elderly and in IV certification. In addition to my clinical experience in the nursing program at Howard Community College (HCC), I worked as a certified nursing assistant at St. Mary's Nursing Home 25 hours/week during the 2 years I was enrolled in the HCC nursing program. My responsibilities included assisting the elderly clients with activities of daily living, including special range-of-motion and reambulation exercises. The experience of serving as a team member under the supervision of the registered nurse and physical therapist has been invaluable. I am currently enrolled in several continuing education courses at HCC. My enclosed résumé provides more details about my qualifications and education.

My background and career goals seem to match your job requirements. I am confident that I can perform the duties of a registered nurse at All Care Nursing Center. I am genuinely interested in pursuing a nursing career in care of the aging. Your agency has an excellent reputation in the community, and your parent company is likewise highly respected.

I am requesting a personal interview to discuss the possibilities of employment. I will call you during the week of April 21 to request an appointment. Should you need to reach me, please call 907-123-4567 or e-mail me at dwheatley@bellspot.com. My telephone has an answering machine. I will return your call or e-mail promptly.

Thank you for your consideration. I look forward to talking with you.

Sincerely yours,

Delores Wheatley

Delores Wheatley

FIGURE 14-2 ◆ Sample cover letter.

not fit your career objectives and interests at this time. As with your other letters, thank the employer for his or her consideration and offer. Figure 14-5 is a sample rejection letter.

Using the Internet

It is not uncommon to search the Internet for positions. Numerous sites either post positions or assist potential employees in matching their skills with available employment. More and more corporations are using the Internet to reach wider audiences. If you use the Internet in your search, it is always wise to follow up with a hard copy of your résumé if an address is listed. Mention in your cover letter that you sent your résumé via the Internet and the date you did so. If you are using an Internet-based service, follow up with an e-mail to ensure that your résumé was received.

THE INTERVIEW PROCESS

Initial Interview

Your first interview may be with the nurse manager, someone in the human resources office,

5734 Foster Road
Middleton, Indiana 46204

April 27, 2006

Ms. Martha Berrero
Human Resources Manager
All Care Nursing Center
4431 Lakeside Drive
Middleton, Indiana 46204

Dear Ms. Berrero:

Thank you very much for interviewing me yesterday for the registered nurse position at All Care Nursing Center. I enjoyed meeting you and learning more about the role of the registered nurse in long-term care with Jefferson Corporation.

My enthusiasm for the position and my interest in working with the elderly have increased as a result of the interview. I believe that my education and experience in long-term care fit with the job requirements. I know that currently I can make a contribution to the care of the residents and over time I hope to qualify as a nursing team leader.

I wish to reiterate my strong interest in working with you and your staff. I know that All Care Nursing Center can provide the kind of opportunities I am seeking. Please call me at 907-123-4567 if I can provide you with any additional information.

Again, thank you for the interview and for considering me for the registered nurse position.

Sincerely yours,

Delores Wheatley

Delores Wheatley

FIGURE 14-3 ◆ Sample thank-you letter.

or an interviewer at a job fair or even over the telephone. Regardless of with whom or where you interview, preparation is the key to success.

You began the first step in the preparation process with your SWOT analysis. If you did not obtain any of the following information regarding your prospective employer at that time, it is imperative that you do it now (Impollonia, 2004):

◆ Key people in the organization.

◆ Number of clients and employees.

◆ Types of services provided.

◆ Reputation in the community.

◆ Recent mergers and acquisitions.

◆ Review the prospective employer's Web site for current news releases.

You also need to review your qualifications for the position. What does your interviewer want to know about you? Consider the following:

◆ Why should I hire you?

◆ What kind of employee will you be?

◆ Will you get things done?

5734 Foster Road
Middleton, Indiana 46204

May 2, 2006

Ms. Martha Berrero
Human Resources Manager
All Care Nursing Center
4431 Lakeside Drive
Middleton, Indiana 46204

Dear Ms. Berrero:

I am writing to confirm my acceptance of your employment offer of May 1. I am delighted to be joining All Care Nursing Center. I feel confident that I can make a significant contribution to your team, and I appreciate the opportunity you have offered me.

As we discussed, I will report to the Personnel Office at 8 a.m. on May 15 for new employee orientation. I will have the medical examination, employee, and insurance forms completed when I arrive. I understand that the starting salary will be $33.10/hour with full benefits beginning May 15. Overtime salary in excess of 40 hours/week will be paid if you request overtime hours.

I appreciate your confidence in me and look forward to joining your team.

Sincerely yours,

Delores Wheatley

Delores Wheatley

FIGURE 14-4 ◆ Sample acceptance letter.

◆ How much will you cost the company?

◆ How long will you stay?

◆ What haven't you told us about your weaknesses?

Answering Questions

The interviewer may ask background questions, professional questions, and personal questions. If you are especially nervous about interviewing, role-play your interview with a friend or family member acting as the interviewer. Have this person help you evaluate not just what you say but how you say it. Voice inflection, eye contact, and friendliness are demonstrations of your enthusiasm for the position (Costlow, 1999).

Whatever the questions, know your key points and be able to explain in the interview why the company will be glad they hired you, say, 4 years from now. Never criticize your current employer before you leave. Personal and professional integrity will follow you from position to position. Many companies count on personal references when hiring, including those of faculty and administrators from your

5734 Foster Road
Middleton, Indiana 46204

May 2, 2006

Ms. Martha Berrero
Human Resources Manager
All Care Nursing Center
4431 Lakeside Drive
Middleton, Indiana 46204

Dear Ms. Berrero:

Thank you for offering me the position of staff nurse with All Care Nursing Center. I appreciate your taking the time to give me such extensive information about the position.

There are many aspects of the position that appeal to me. Jefferson Corporation is an excellent provider of health care services throughout this area and nationwide. However, after giving it much thought, I have decided to accept another position and must therefore decline your offer.

Again, thank you for your consideration and the courtesy extended to me. I enjoyed meeting you and your staff.

Sincerely yours,

Delores Wheatley

Delores Wheatley

FIGURE 14-5 ◆ Sample rejection letter.

nursing program. When leaving positions you held during school or on graduating from your program, it is wise not to take parting shots at someone. Doing a professional program evaluation is fine, but taking cheap shots at faculty or other employees is unacceptable (Costlow, 1999).

Background Questions

Background questions usually relate to information on your résumé. If you have no nursing experience, relate your prior school and work experience and other accomplishments in relevant ways to the position you are seeking without going through your entire autobiography with the interviewer. You may be asked to expand on the information in your résumé about your formal nursing education. Here is your opportunity to relate specific courses or clinical experiences you enjoyed, academic honors you received, and extracurricular activities or research projects you pursued. The background questions are an invitation for employers to get to know you. Be careful not to appear inconsistent with this information and what you say later.

Professional Questions

Many recruiters are looking for specifics, especially those related to skills and knowledge needed in the position available. They may start with questions related to your education, career goals, strengths, weaknesses, nursing philosophy, style, and abilities. Interviewers often open their questioning with words such as "review," "tell me," "explain," and "describe," followed by such phrases as "How did you do it?" or "Why did you do it that way?" (Mascolini & Supnick, 1993). How successful will you be with these types of questions?

When answering "how would you describe" questions, it is especially important that you remain specific. Cite your own experiences, and relate these behaviors to a demonstrated skill or strength. Examples of questions in this area include the following (Bischof, 1993):

◆ **What is your philosophy of nursing?** This question is asked frequently, so think about how you would answer it. Your response should relate to the position you are seeking.

◆ **What is your greatest weakness?** Your greatest strength? Do not be afraid to present a weakness, but present it to your best advantage, making it sound like a desirable characteristic. Even better, discuss a weakness that is already apparent such as lack of nursing experience, stating that you recognize your lack of nursing experience but that your own work or management experience has taught you skills that will assist you in this position. These skills might include organization, time management, team spirit, and communication. If you are asked for both strengths and weaknesses, start with your weakness, and end on a positive note with your strengths. Do not be too modest, but do not exaggerate. Relate your strengths to the prospective position. Skills such as interpersonal relationships, organization, and leadership are usually broad enough to fit most positions.

◆ **Where do you see yourself in 5 years?** Most interviewers want to gain insight into your long-term goals as well as some idea whether you are likely to use this position as a brief stop on the path to

another job. It is helpful for you to know some of the history regarding the position. For example, how long have others usually remained in that job? Your career planning should be consistent with the organization's needs.

◆ **What are your educational goals?** Be honest and specific. Include both professional education, such as RN or bachelor of science in nursing, and continuing education courses. If you want to pursue further education in related areas, such as a foreign language or computers, include this as a goal. Indicate schools to which you have applied or in which you are already enrolled.

◆ **Describe your leadership style.** Be prepared to discuss your style in terms of how effectively you work with others, and give examples of how you have implemented your leadership in the past.

◆ **What can you contribute to this position? What unique skill set do you offer?** Review your SWOT analysis as well as the job description for the position before the interview. Be specific in relating your contributions to the position. Emphasize your accomplishments. Be specific, and convey that, even as a new graduate, you are unique.

◆ **What are your salary requirements?** You may be asked about minimum salary range. Try to find out the prospective employer's salary range before this question comes up. Be honest about your expectations, but make it clear that you are willing to negotiate.

◆ **"What if" questions.** Prospective employers are increasingly using competency-based interview questions to determine people's preparation for a job. There is often no single correct answer to these questions. The interviewer may be assessing your clinical decision-making and leadership skills. Again, be concise and specific, focusing your answer in line with the organizational philosophy and goals. If you do not know the answer, tell the interviewer how you would go about finding the answer. You cannot be expected to have all the answers before you begin a job, but you can be expected to know how to obtain answers once you are in the position.

Personal Questions

Personal questions deal with your personality and motivation. Common questions include the following:

◆ **How would you describe yourself?** This is a standard question. Most people find it helpful to think about an answer in advance. You can repeat some of what you said in your résumé and cover letter, but do not provide an in-depth analysis of your personality.

◆ **How would your peers describe you?** Ask them! Again, be brief, describing several strengths. Forget about your weaknesses unless you are asked about them.

◆ **What would make you happy with this position?** Be prepared to discuss your needs related to your work environment. Do you enjoy self-direction, flexible hours, and strong leadership support? Now is the time to cite specifics related to your ideal work environment.

◆ **Describe your ideal work environment.** Give this question some thought before the interview. Be specific but realistic. If the norm in your community is two RNs to a floor with licensed practical nurses and other ancillary support, do not say that you believe a staff consisting only of RNs is needed for good client care.

◆ **Describe hobbies, community activities, and recreation.** Again, brevity is important. Many times this question is used to further observe the interviewee's communication and interpersonal skills.

Never pretend to be someone or something other than who or what you are. If pretending is necessary to obtain the position, then the position is not right for you.

Additional Points About the Interview

Federal, state, and local laws govern employment-related questions. Questions asked on the job application and in the interview must be related to the position advertised. Questions or statements that may lead to discrimination on the basis of age, gender, race, color, religion, or ethnicity are illegal. If you are asked a question that appears to be illegal, you may wish to take one of several approaches:

◆ You may answer the question, realizing that it is not a job-related question. Make it clear to the interviewer that you will answer the question even though you know it is not job-related.

◆ You may refuse to answer. You are within your rights but may be seen as uncooperative or confrontational.

◆ Examine the intent of the question and relate it to the job.

Just as important as the verbal exchanges of the interview are the nonverbal aspects. These include appearance, handshake, eye contact, posture, and listening skills.

Appearance

Dress in business attire. For women, a skirted suit or tailored jacket dress is appropriate. Men should wear a classic suit, light-colored shirt, and conservative tie. For both men and women, gray or navy blue is rarely wrong. Shoes should be polished, with appropriate heels. Nails and hair for both men and women should reflect cleanliness, good grooming, and willingness to work. The 2-inch red dagger nails worn on prom night will not support an image of the professional nurse. In many institutions, even clear, acrylic nails are not allowed. Paint stains on the hands from a weekend of house maintenance are equally unsuitable for presenting a professional image.

Handshake

Arrive at the interview 10 minutes before your scheduled time (allow yourself extra time to find the place if you have not previously been there). Introduce yourself courteously to the receptionist. Stand when your name is called, smile, and shake hands firmly. If you perspire easily, wipe your palms just before handshake time.

Eye Contact

During the interview, use the interviewer's title and last name as you speak. Never use the interviewer's first name unless specifically requested to do so. Use good listening skills (all those leadership skills you have learned). Smile and nod occasionally, making frequent eye contact. Do not fold your arms across your chest, but keep your hands at your sides or in your lap. Pay attention, and sound sure of yourself.

Posture and Listening Skills

Phrase your questions appropriately, and relate them to yourself as a candidate: "What would be my responsibility?" instead of "What are the responsibilities of the job?" Use appropriate grammar and diction. Words or phrases such as "yeah," "uh-huh," "uh," "you know," or "like" are too casual for an interview.

Do not say "I guess" or "I feel" about anything. These words make you sound indecisive and wishy-washy. Remember your action verbs—I analyzed, I organized, I developed. Do not evaluate your achievements as mediocre or unimpressive. (Of course, that walkathon you organized was a huge success!)

Asking Questions

At some point in the interview, you will be asked if you have any questions. Knowing what questions you want to ask is just as important as having prepared answers for the interviewer's questions. The interview is as much a time for you to learn the details of the job as it is for your potential employer to find out about you. You will need to obtain specific information about the job itself, including the type of clients you would be caring for, the people with whom you would be working, the salary and benefits, and your potential employer's expectations of you. Be prepared for the interviewer to say, "Is there anything else I can tell you about the job?" Jot down a few questions on an index card before going for the interview. You may want to ask a few questions based on your research, demonstrating knowledge about and interest in the company. In addition, you may want to ask questions similar to the ones listed next. Above all, be honest and sincere (Bhasin, 1998; Bischof, 1993; Johnson, 1999):

◆ What is this position's key responsibility?

◆ What kind of person are you looking for?

◆ What are the challenges of the position?

◆ Why is this position open?

◆ To whom would I report directly?

◆ Why did the previous person leave this position?

◆ What is the salary for this position?

◆ What are the opportunities for advancement?

◆ What kind of opportunities are there for continuing education?

◆ What are your expectations of me as an employee?

◆ How, when, and by whom are evaluations done?

◆ What other opportunities for professional growth are available here?

◆ How are promotion and advancement handled within the organization?

The following are a few additional tips about asking questions during a job interview:

◆ *Do not* begin with questions about vacations, benefits, or sick time. This gives the impression that these are the most important part of the job to you, not the work itself.

◆ *Do* begin with questions about the employer's expectations of you. This gives the impression that you want to know how you can contribute to the organization.

◆ *Do* be sure you know enough about the position to make a reasonable decision about accepting an offer if one is made.

◆ *Do* ask questions about the organization as a whole. The information is useful to you and demonstrates that you are able to see the big picture.

◆ *Do* bring a list of important points to discuss as an aid to you if you are nervous.

During the interview process, there are a few "red flags" to be alert for (Tyler, 1990):

◆ Lots of turnover in the position.

◆ A newly created position without a clear purpose.

◆ An organization in transition.

◆ A position that is not feasible for a new graduate.

◆ A "gut feeling" that things are not what they seem.

The exchange of information between you and the interviewer will go more smoothly if you review Box 14-2 before the interview.

After the Interview

If the interviewer does not offer the information, ask about the next step in the process. Thank the interviewer, shake hands, and exit. If the receptionist is still there, you may quickly smile and say thank you and good-bye. Do not linger and chat, and do not forget your thank-you letter.

The Second Interview

Being invited back for a second interview means that the first interview went well and that you made a favorable impression. Second visits may include a tour of the facility and meetings with a higher-level executive or a supervisor in the department in which the job opening exists and perhaps several colleagues.

In preparation for the second interview, review the information about the organization and your own strengths. It does not hurt to have a few résumés and potential references available. Pointers to make your second visit successful include the following (Muha & Orgiefsky, 1994; Knight, 2005):

◆ Dress professionally. Do not wear sandals or open-toed shoes, even with a great pedicure! Minimize jewelry and makeup.

◆ Be professional and pleasant with everyone, including secretaries and housekeeping and maintenance personnel.

◆ Do not smoke.

◆ Remember your manners.

◆ Avoid controversial topics for small talk.

◆ Obtain answers to questions you might have thought of since your first visit.

In most instances, the personnel director or nurse manager will let you know how long it will be before you are contacted again. It is appropriate to get this information before you leave the second interview. If you do receive an offer during this visit, graciously say "thank you," and ask for a little time to consider the offer (even if this is the offer you have anxiously been awaiting).

If the organization does not contact you by the expected date, do not panic. It is appropri-

---

BOX 14-2

Do's and Don'ts for Interviewing

Do:

◆ Shake the interviewer's hand firmly, and introduce yourself.
◆ Know the interviewer's name in advance, and use it in conversation.
◆ Remain standing until invited to sit.
◆ Use eye contact.
◆ Let the interviewer take the lead in the conversation.
◆ Talk in specific terms, relating everything to the position.
◆ Responses should be supported by personal experience and specific examples.
◆ Make connections for the interviewer. Relate your responses to the needs of the individual organization.
◆ Show interest in the facility.
◆ Ask questions about the position and the facility.

◆ Come across as sincere in your goals and committed to the profession.
◆ Indicate a willingness to start at the bottom.
◆ Take any examinations requested.
◆ Express your appreciation for the time.

Do Not:

◆ Place your purse, briefcase, papers, etc., on the interviewer's desk. Keep them in your lap or on the floor.
◆ Slouch in the chair.
◆ Play with your clothing, jewelry, or hair.
◆ Chew gum or smoke, even if the interviewer does.
◆ Be evasive, interrupt, brag, or mumble.
◆ Gossip about or criticize former agencies, schools, or employees.

Adapted from Bischof (1993), Mascolini & Supnick (1993), Krannich & Krannich (1993), Zedlitz (2003).

ate to call your contact person, state your continued interest, and tactfully express the need to know the status of your application so that you can respond to other deadlines.

MAKING THE RIGHT CHOICE

You have interviewed well, and now you have to decide among several job offers. Your choice not only will affect your immediate work but will also influence your future career opportunities. The nursing shortage of the early 1990s has led to greatly enhanced workplace enrichment programs as a recruitment and retention strategy. Career ladders, shared governance, particpatory management, staff nurse presence on major hospital committees, decentralization of operations, and a focus on quality interpersonal relationships are among some of these features. Be sure and inquire about the components of the professional practice environment (Joel, 2003). There are several additional factors to consider.

Job Content

The immediate work you will be doing should be a good match with your skills and interests. Although your work may be personally challenging and satisfying this year, what are the opportunities for growth? How will your desire for continued growth and challenge be satisfied?

Development

You should have learned from your interviews whether the initial training and orientation seem sufficient and well organized. Inquire about continuing education to keep you current in your field. Is tuition reimbursement available for further education? Is management training provided, or are supervisory skills learned on the job?

Direction

Good supervision and mentors are especially important in your first position. You may be able to judge prospective supervisors throughout the interview process, but you should also try to get a broader view of the overall philoso-phy of supervision. You may not be working for the same supervisor in a year, but the overall management philosophy is likely to remain consistent.

Work Climate

The day-to-day work climate must make you feel comfortable. Your preference may be formal or casual, structured or unstructured, complex or simple. It is easy to observe the way people dress, the layout of the unit, and lines of communication. It is more difficult to observe company values, factors that will affect your work comfort and satisfaction over the long term. Try to look beyond the work environment to get an idea of values. What is the unwritten message? Is there an open-door policy sending a message that "everyone is equal and important," or does the nurse manager appear too busy to be concerned with the needs of the employees? Is your supervisor the kind of person for whom you could work easily?

Compensation

In evaluating the compensation package, starting salary should be less important than the organization's philosophy on future compensation. What is the potential for salary growth? How are individual increases? Can you live on the wages being offered?

I CAN NOT FIND A JOB (OR I MOVED)

It is often said that finding the first job is the hardest. Many employers prefer to hire seasoned nurses who do not require a long orientation and mentoring. Some require new graduates to do postgraduate internships. Changes in skill mix with the implementation of various types of care delivery influence the market for the professional nurse. The new graduate may need to be armed with a variety of skills, such as intravenous certification, home assessment, advanced rehabilitation skills, and various respiratory modalities, to even warrant an initial interview. Keep informed about the demands of the market in your area, and be prepared to be flexible in seeking your first position. Even with the continuing nursing shortage, hiring you as a new graduate will depend on you selling yourself!

Even after all this searching and hard work, you still may not have found the position you want. You may be focusing on work arrangements or benefits rather than on the job description. Your lack of direction may come through in your résumé, cover letter, and personal presentation. You may also have unrealistic expectations for a new graduate or be trying to cut corners, ignoring the basic rules of marketing yourself discussed in this chapter. Go back to your SWOT analysis. Take another look at your résumé and cover letter. Become more assertive as you start again (Culp, 1999).

THE CRITICAL FIRST YEAR

Why a section on the "first year"? Don't you just get a nursing license and go to work? Aren't nurses always in demand? You have worked hard to succeed in college—won't those lessons help you to succeed in your new position? Of course they will, but some of the behaviors that were rewarded in school are not rewarded on the job. There are no syllabi, study questions, or extra credit points. Only "A's" are acceptable, and there do not appear to be many completely correct answers. Discovering this has been called "reality shock" (Kramer, 1974), which is discussed elsewhere in this book. Voluminous care plans and meticulous medication cards are out; multiple responsibilities and thinking on your feet are in. What is the new graduate to do?

Your first year will be a transition year. You are no longer a college student, but you are not yet a full-fledged professional. You are "the new kid on the block," and people will respond to you differently and judge you differently than when you were a student. To be successful, you have to respond differently. You may be thinking, "Oh, they always need nurses—it doesn't matter." Yes, it does matter. Many of your career opportunities will be influenced by the early impressions you make. The following section addresses what you can do to help ensure first-year success.

Attitude and Expectations

Adopt the right attitudes, and adjust your expectations. Now is the time to learn the art of being new. You felt like the most important, special person during the recruitment process. Now, in the real world, neither you nor the position may be as glamorous as you once thought. In addition, although you thought you learned a lot in school, your decisions and daily performance do not always warrant an "A." Above all, people shed the company manners that they displayed when you were interviewing, and organizational politics eventually surface. Your leadership skills and commitment to teamwork will get you through this transition period.

Impressions and Relationships

Manage a good impression, and build effective relationships. Remember, you are being watched: by peers, subordinates, and superiors. Because you as yet have no track record, first impressions are magnified. Although every organization is different, most are looking for someone with good judgment, a willingness to learn, a readiness to adapt, and a respect for the expertise of more experienced employees. Most people expect you to "pay your dues" to earn respect from them.

Organizational Savvy

Develop organizational savvy. An important person in this first year is your immediate supervisor. Support this person. Find out what is important to your supervisor and what he or she needs and expects from the team. Become a team player. Present solutions, not problems, as often as you can. You want to be a good leader someday; learn first to be a good follower. Finding a mentor is another important goal of your first year. Mentors are role models and guides who encourage, counsel, teach, and advocate for their mentee. In these relationships, both the mentor and mentee receive support and encouragement (Klein & Dickenson-Hazard, 2000). Mentoring was discussed in Chapter 13.

The spark that ignites a mentoring relationship may come from either the protégé or the mentor. Protégés often view mentors as founts of success, a bastion of life skills they wish to learn and emulate. Mentors often see the future that is hidden in another's personality and abilities (Klein & Dickenson-Hazard, pp. 20–21).

Skills and Knowledge

Master the skills and knowledge of the position. Technology is constantly changing, and contrary to popular belief, you did not learn everything in school. Be prepared to seek out new knowledge and skills on your own. This may entail extra hours of preparation and study, but who said that learning stopped after graduation (Holton, 1994; Johnson, 1994)?

◆ ADVANCING YOUR CAREER

Many of the ideas presented in this chapter will continue to be helpful as you advance in your nursing career. Continuing to develop your leadership and client care skills through practice and further education will be the key to your professional growth. The RN will be expected to develop and provide leadership to other members of the health-care team while providing competent care to clients. Getting your first job within the nursing shortage may not be so difficult, but advancing in your career will be your own responsibility.

◆ CONCLUSION

Finding your first position is more than being in the right place at the right time. It is a complex combination of learning about yourself and the organizations you are interested in and presenting your strengths and weaknesses in the most positive manner possible. Keeping the first position and using the position to grow and learn are also a planning process. Recognize that the independence and the ability to "do your own thing" that you enjoyed through college may not be the skills you need to keep you in your first position. There is an important lesson to be learned: becoming a team player and being savvy about organizational politics are as important as becoming proficient in nursing skills. Take the first step toward finding a mentor—before you know it, you will be one yourself!

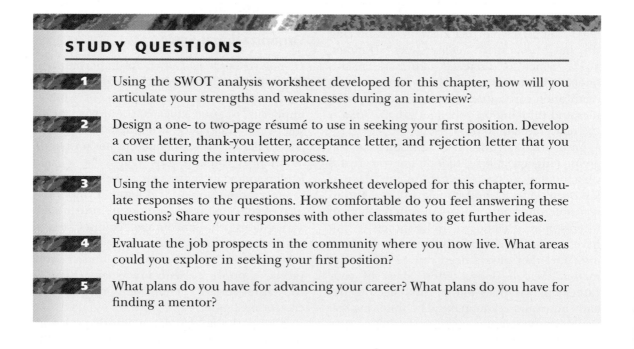

STUDY QUESTIONS

1 Using the SWOT analysis worksheet developed for this chapter, how will you articulate your strengths and weaknesses during an interview?

2 Design a one- to two-page résumé to use in seeking your first position. Develop a cover letter, thank-you letter, acceptance letter, and rejection letter that you can use during the interview process.

3 Using the interview preparation worksheet developed for this chapter, formulate responses to the questions. How comfortable do you feel answering these questions? Share your responses with other classmates to get further ideas.

4 Evaluate the job prospects in the community where you now live. What areas could you explore in seeking your first position?

5 What plans do you have for advancing your career? What plans do you have for finding a mentor?

SWOT Analysis Worksheet

Complete the following SWOT analysis

STRENGTHS	WEAKNESSES	OPPORTUNITIES	THREATS

CRITICAL THINKING EXERCISE

Paul Delane is interviewing for his first nursing position after obtaining his RN license. He has been interviewed by the nurse recruiter and is now being interviewed by the nurse manager on the pediatric floor. After a few minutes of social conversation, the nurse manager begins to ask some specific nursing-oriented questions: How would you respond if a mother of a seriously ill child asks you if her child will die? What attempts do you make to understand different cultural beliefs and their importance in health care when planning nursing care? How does your philosophy of nursing affect your ability to deliver care to children whose mothers are HIV-positive?

Paul is very flustered by these questions and responds with "it depends on the situation," "it depends on the culture," and "I don't ever discriminate."

1. What responses would have been more appropriate in this interview?

2. How could Paul have used these questions to demonstrate his strengths, experiences, and skills?

CHAPTER 14 SELF-ASSESSMENT
Interview Preparation Worksheet

Based upon the information presented in this chapter, formulate your responses to the following questions. Compare your responses with those of two peers. What suggestions did they make that would help you in the interview?

- How would you describe yourself?

- How would your peers describe you?

- What would make you happy with this position?

- Describe your ideal work environment.

- Describe your hobbies, community activities, and recreation.

- Your husband is a physician—do you really have to work?

REFERENCES

Anderson, J. (1992). Tips on résumé writing. *Imprint*, 39(1), 30–31.

Banis, W. (1994). The art of writing job-search letters. In College Placement Council, Inc. (ed.). *Planning Job Choices*. Philadelphia: College Placement Council, 44–51.

Beatty, R. (1989). *The Perfect Cover Letter.* New York: John Wiley & Sons.

Beatty, R. (1991). *Get the Right Job in 60 Days or Less.* New York: John Wiley & Sons.

Bhasin, R. (1998). Do's and don'ts of job interviews. *Pulp & Paper*, 72(2), 37.

Bischof, J. (1993). Preparing for job interview questions. *Critical Care Nurse*, 13(4), 97–100.

Chestnut, T. (1999). Some tips on taking the fear out of résumé writing. *Phoenix Business Journal*, 19(47), 28.

Costlow, T. (1999). How not to create a good first impression. *Fairfield County Business Journal*, 38(32), 17.

Crowther, K. (1994). How to research companies. In College Placement Council, Inc. (ed.). *Planning Job Choices*. Philadelphia: College Placement Council, 27–32.

Culp, M. (1999). Now's the time to turn the corner on your job search. *San Diego Business Journal,* 20(50), 35.

Ellis, M. (1999). Self-assessment: Discovering yourself and making the best choices for you! *Black Collegian,* 30(1), 30, 3p, 1c.

Eubanks, P. (1991). Experts: Making your résumé an asset. *Hospitals,* 5(20), 74.

Holton, E. (1994). The critical first year on the job. In College Placement Council, Inc. (ed.). *Planning Job Choices.* Philadelphia: College Placement Council, 68–71.

Hunsaker, P. (2001). *Training in Management Skills.* New Jersey: Prentice-Hall.

Impollonia, M. (2004), How to impress nursing recruiters to get the job you want. *Imprint,* March.

James, L. (2003). Vitae statistics. *Travel Weekly,* 1695, 70.

Joel, L. (2003). The role of the workplace in your transition from student to nurse. *Imprint,* April.

Johnson, K. (1994). Choose your first job with your whole future in mind. In College Placement Council, Inc. (ed.). *Planning Job Choices.* Philadelphia: College Placement Council, 65–67.

Johnson, K. (1999). Interview success demands research, practice, preparation. *Houston Business Journal,* 30(23), 38.

Klein, E., & Dickenson-Hazard, N. (2000). The spirit of mentoring. *Reflections on Nursing Leadership,* 26(3), 18–22.

Knight, K. (2005). New grad? Be prepared to look great. *Imprint,* January.

Kramer, M. (1974). *Reality Shock: Why Nurses Leave Nursing.* St. Louis: C.V. Mosby.

Krannich, C., & Krannich, R. (1993). *Interview for Success.* New York: Impact Publications.

Marino, K. (2000). *Resumes for the Health Care Professional.* New York: John Wiley & Sons.

Mascolini, M., & Supnick, R. (1993). Preparing students for the behavioral job interview. *Journal of Business and Technical Communication,* 7(4), 482–488.

Muha, D., & Orgiefsky, R. (1994). The 2nd interview: The plant or office visit. In College Placement Council, Inc. (ed.). *Planning Job Choices.* Philadelphia: College Placement Council, 58–60.

Parker, Y. (1989). *The Damn Good Résumé Guide.* Berkeley, CA: Ten Speed Press.

Pratt, C. (1994). Successful job-search strategies for the 90's. In College Placement Council, Inc. (ed.). *Planning Job Choices.* Philadelphia: College Placement Council, 15–18.

Rodriguez, K., & Robertson, D. (1992). Selling your talents with a résumé. *American Nurse,* 24(10), 27.

Shingleton, J. (1994). The job market for '94 grads. In College Placement Council, Inc. (ed.). *Planning Job Choices.* Philadelphia: College Placement Council, 19–26.

Tyler, L. (1990). Watch out for "red flags" on a job interview. *Hospitals,* 64(14), 46.

Unknown. (2005). The devil is in the resume details. *Fairfield County Business Journal,* 44(18), 17.

Waymon, L., & Baber, A. (1999). Surviving career. *Balance,* 3(2), 10–13.

Zedlitz, R. (2003). *How to Get a Job in Health Care.* New York: Delmar Learning.

chapter 15

Nursing Yesterday and Today

OBJECTIVES

After reading this chapter, the student should be able to:

- Compare and contrast historical and current definitions of nursing.
- Discuss Florence Nightingale's contribution to the development of modern nursing.
- Describe the effect Lillian Wald and the Henry Street Settlement had on community health care.
- Describe the contributions that Margaret Sanger made to women's health and social reform.
- Discuss Mary Mahoney's contributions to the advancement of black nurses.
- Describe Adelaide Nutting's contributions to nursing education.
- Discuss the role of Mildred Montag and the development of associate degree nursing programs.
- Discuss the contributions made by Virginia Henderson to modern nursing.
- Discuss the common characteristics of these historic leaders in nursing.
- Discuss the history of men in nursing.
- Analyze how men have changed modern nursing.
- Explain how nursing theory contributes to the advancement of nursing practice.
- Differentiate the roles of the American Nurses Association, the National League for Nursing, and the National Organization for Associate Degree Nursing.
- Differentiate between the various programs that offer nursing education.
- Identify methods nurses can use to project a positive image.
- Describe the characteristics considered indicative of a true profession.
- Evaluate nursing based on the criteria established for the profession.
- Evaluate strengths and weaknesses of self related to professional behaviors.
- Discuss some of the issues faced by the nursing profession over the past century.
- Identify the changes that will affect nursing's future

OUTLINE

■ INTRODUCTION

It is often said, "You don't know where you are going until you know where you have been." More than 30 years ago, Beletz (1974) wrote that society perceived nurses in gender-linked, task-oriented terms: "a female who performs unpleasant technical jobs and functions as an assistant to the physician" (p. 432). Although television programs and advertisements featuring nurses are more realistic than they were a decade ago, nurses are still often depicted as handmaidens who carry out physician orders.

In its history, the nursing profession has had many great leaders. From these, we have chosen seven who not only demonstrated the strengths of nursing's historic leaders but also reflect some of the most important issues that the profession has had to face over the past 100 years or so. Each of these leaders initiated change within the social environment of her time, using the theories of change and conflict resolution discussed earlier in the text.

Nursing Defined

The changes that have occurred in nursing are reflected in the definitions of nursing that have been developed since the time of Florence Nightingale. In 1859, Florence Nightingale defined the goal of nursing as putting the client "in the best possible condition for nature to act upon him" (Nightingale, 1859, p. 79). Virginia Henderson focused her definition on the uniqueness of nursing: "The unique function of the nurse is to assist the individual, sick or well, in the performance of those activities contributing to health or its recovery (or to peaceful death) that he would perform unaided if he had the necessary strength, will or knowledge. And to do this in such a way as to help him gain independence as rapidly as possible" (Henderson, 1966, p. 21). Martha Rogers defined nursing practice as "the process by which this body of knowledge, nursing science, is used for the purpose of assisting human beings to achieve maximum health within the potential of each person" (Rogers, 1988, p. 100). Rogers emphasized that nursing is concerned with *all* people, only a segment of whom is ill.

Florence Nightingale is probably the best known of the seven. She is considered the founder of modern nursing. Nightingale changed the care of soldiers, the keeping of hospital records, the status of nurses, and even the profession itself. Her concepts of nursing care became the basis of modern theory development in nursing.

Lillian Wald, founder of the Henry Street Settlement, is a role model for contemporary community health nursing. Ms. Wald developed a model for bringing health care to people. Her social conscience and determination to make changes in health care are a model for the modern health-care revolution.

Margaret Sanger, a political activist like the others, is best known for her courageous fight to make birth control information available to everyone who needed or wanted it. Her fight to make Congress aware of the plight of children in the labor force is less well known but led to important changes in the child labor laws. Sanger was perhaps the first nurse lobbyist.

Mary Eliza Mahoney became the first black graduate nurse in the United States. Her professional attitude helped to change the status of black nurses in this country.

Adelaide Nutting is probably best known of the early leaders in nursing education in the United States.

Mildred Montag proposed two levels of nursing, and she developed an associate's degree nursing program at Adelphi University.

Virginia Henderson, the final nursing leader discussed in this chapter, was a 20th century Florence Nightingale. Henderson wrote the nursing textbook used by nurse educators throughout the country for most of the preceding century.

The next part of the chapter discusses nursing organizations and their role in assisting the profession develop professionally and politically.

The final section of this chapter introduces you to nursing theory: what it is and why it is important to nursing as a profession. Nursing theory has helped nursing evolve into the scientifically based profession it is today.

As you read this chapter, you will see how each of these famous women exemplifies leadership in the nursing profession. Many of their characteristics—intelligence, courage, and foresight—are the same ones needed in today's nursing leaders.

FLORENCE NIGHTINGALE

Background

Florence Nightingale, an English noblewoman, was born in the city for which she was named, Florence, Italy, on May 12, 1820. She was the second daughter of William and Frances Nightingale. Her father was a well-educated, wealthy man who put considerable effort into the education of his two daughters (Donahue, 1985). Florence Nightingale learned French, German, and Italian. Mr. Nightingale personally instructed her in mathematics, classical art, and literature. The family made extended visits to London every year, which provided opportunities for contact with people in the highest social circles. These contacts were very valuable to Ms. Nightingale in later years.

Despite her family's ability to shelter her from the meaner side of life, Nightingale had always shown an interest in the welfare of those less fortunate than herself. It seems that she was never quite content with herself, as she was described as a "sensitive, introspective, and somewhat morbid child" (Schuyler, 1992). She was driven to improve herself and the world around her. When she expressed an interest in becoming a nurse, her parents objected strenuously. They wanted her to assume the traditional role of a well-to-do woman of the time: marry, have children, and take her "rightful" place in society.

Becoming a Nurse

In the fall of 1847, Nightingale left England for a tour of Europe with family friends. In Italy, she entered a convent for a retreat. This strengthened her religious beliefs, although she never converted from the Church of England to Catholicism. After this retreat, she believed that she had been called by God to help others. This experience made her more determined than ever to pursue nursing.

In 1851, Nightingale insisted on going to Kaiserswerth, Germany, to obtain training in nursing. Her family gave her their permission on the condition that no one would know where she was. When she returned from Kaiserswerth, she began to work on her plan to influence the health-care field.

Nightingale soon left for France to work with several Catholic nursing sisters. While in France, she received an offer from the committee that regulated the Establishment for Gentlewomen During Illness, a nursing home in London for governesses who became ill. She was appointed superintendent of the home and soon had it well organized, although she did have some difficulties with the committee.

Because of her knowledge of hospitals, Nightingale was often consulted by social reformers and by physicians who also recognized the need for this new type of nurse. Nightingale was offered a position as superintendent of nurses at King's College Hospital, but her family objected so strongly that she remained at home instead, until she went to the Crimea.

The Need for Reform

Fortunately for Nightingale, it was fashionable in the middle of the 19th century to become involved in the reform of medical and social institutions. After completing the reorganization of the nursing home, she began visiting hospitals and collecting information about nurses' working conditions. In the course of doing this, she realized that to improve nurses' working conditions, she would first have to improve the nurses.

Up to this time, the guiding principle of nursing had revolved around charity. Nursing services in Europe were provided primarily by the family or by members of religious orders. The Catholic organizations experienced a decline during the Reformation, when the government closed churches and monasteries. Hospitals were no longer run for charitable reasons but because of social necessity. Nursing lost its social standing when the religious orders declined. Nurses were no longer recruited from the respectable classes but from the lower classes of society. Women who needed to earn their keep entered domestic service, and nursing was considered a form of domestic service. Other women who could no longer earn a living by gambling or selling themselves also turned to nursing. Many came from criminal classes. They lacked the spirit of self-sacrifice found in the religious orders, and they often abused clients. Many consoled themselves with alcohol and snuff.

The duties of a nurse in those days were to take care of the physical needs of clients and to make sure they were reasonably clean. The conditions in which they had to accomplish these tasks were far less than ideal. Hospitals were dirty and unventilated. They were contaminated with infection and actually spread diseases instead of preventing them. The same bedsheets were used for several clients. The nurses dealt with people suffering from unrelenting pain, hemorrhage, infections, and gangrene (Kalisch & Kalisch, 2004).

To accomplish the needed reforms, Nightingale realized that she had to recruit her nurses from higher strata of society, as had been done in the past, and then educate them well. She concluded that this could be accomplished only by organizing a school to prepare reliable, qualified nurses.

The Crimean War

A letter written by war correspondent W.H. Russell comparing the nursing care in the British army unfavorably with that given to the French army created a tremendous stir in England. There was demand for change. In response, the Secretary of War, Sir Sidney Herbert, commissioned Nightingale to go to the Crimea (a peninsula in southeastern Ukraine) to investigate conditions there and make improvements.

On October 21, 1854, Nightingale left for the Crimea with a group of nurses on the steamer *Vectis* (Griffith & Griffith, 1965). They found a disaster when they arrived. The hospital that had been built to accommodate 1700 soldiers was filled with more than 3000 wounded and critically ill men. There were no plumbing or sewage disposal facilities. The mattresses, walls, and floors were wet with human waste. Rats, lice, and maggots thrived in this filthy environment (Kalisch & Kalisch, 2004).

The nurses went to work. They set up a kitchen, rented a house and converted it into a laundry, and hired soldiers' wives to do the laundry. Money was difficult to obtain, so Nightingale used the *Times* relief fund and her own personal funds to purchase medical supplies, food, and equipment. After the hospital had been cleaned and organized, she began to set up social services for the soldiers.

Nightingale rarely slept. She spent hours giving nursing care, wrote letters to families, prepared requests for more supplies, and reported to London on the conditions she had found and improved. At night, she made rounds accompanied by an 11-year-old boy who held her lamp when she sat by a dying soldier or assisted during emergency surgery. This is how she earned the title "The Lady with the Lamp" from the poet Longfellow (1868).

Despite their strenuous efforts and enormous accomplishments, the physicians and army officers resented the nurses. They regarded these nurses as intruders who interfered with their work and undermined their authority. There was also some conflict between Nightingale and Dr. John Hall, the chief of the medical staff. At one time, after Dr. Hall had been awarded the Knight Commander of the Order of the Bath, Nightingale sarcastically referred to him as "Dr. Hall, K.C.B., Knight of the Crimean Burial Grounds." When Nightingale contracted Crimean fever, Hall used this as an excuse to send her back to England. However, Nightingale thwarted his resistance and eventually won over the medical staff by creating an operating room and supplying the instruments with her own resources. Although she returned to duty, she never fully recovered from the fever. She returned to England in 1865 a national heroine but remained a semi-invalid for the rest of her life.

A School for Nurses

After her return from the Crimea, Nightingale pursued two goals: reform of military health care and establishment of an official training school for nurses. The British public contributed more than $220,000 to the Nightingale Fund for the purpose of establishing the school.

Although opposed by most of the physicians in Britain, Nightingale continued her efforts, and the Nightingale Training School for Nurses opened in 1860. The school was an independent educational institution financed by the Nightingale Fund. Fifteen probationers were admitted to the first class. Their training lasted a year. Although Nightingale was not an instructor at the school, she was consulted about all of the details of student selection, instruction, and organization. Her book, *Notes on Nursing: What It Is and What It Is Not,* established the fundamental principles of nursing.

The following is an example of her writing:

On What Nursing Ought To Do
I use the word nursing for want of a better. It has been limited to signify little more than the administration of medicines and the application of poultices. It ought to signify the proper use of air, light, warmth, cleanliness, quiet and the proper selection and administration of diet—all at the least expense of vital power to the patient. (Nightingale, 1859)

This book was one of the first nursing textbooks and is still widely quoted today. Many nursing theorists have used Nightingale's thoughts as a basis for constructing their view of nursing. The basic principles on which the Nightingale school was founded are the following:

1. Nurses should be technically trained in schools organized for that purpose.
2. Nurses should come from homes that are of good moral standing.

Nightingale believed that schools of nursing must be independent institutions and that women who were selected to attend the schools should be from the higher levels of society. Many of Nightingale's beliefs about nursing education are still applicable, particularly those involved with the progress of students, the use of diaries kept by students, and the need for integrating theory into clinical practice (Roberts, 1937).

The Nightingale school served as a model for nursing education. Its graduates were sought worldwide. Many established other schools and became matrons (superintendents) in hospitals in other parts of England, the Commonwealth, and the United States. However, very few schools were able to remain financially independent of the hospitals, and therefore they lost much of their autonomy. This was in contradiction to Nightingale's philosophy that the training schools were educational institutions, not part of any service agency.

Health-Care Reform

Nightingale's other goal was the improvement of military health care. As a result of her documentation of the conditions in the Crimea and the nurses' efforts to improve them, reforms were undertaken. Her work marked the beginning of modern military nursing. Nurses are still active in health-care reform efforts.

Nightingale's statistics were so accurate and clearly reported that she was elected a member of the British Statistical Society, the first woman to hold this position. At their conference in 1860, she presented a paper entitled, "Miss Nightingale's Scheme for Uniform Hospital Statistics." Before this paper was written, each hospital had used its own names and classification systems for diseases.

Nightingale's continuous efforts to study and improve health care made her an expert in her day. Her opinions on these subjects were constantly solicited. This led to another publication, *Notes on Hospitals.*

For more than 40 years, Nightingale played an influential part in most of the important health-care reforms of her time. At the turn of the 20th century, however, her energies had waned, and she spent most of the next 10 years confined to her home on South Street in London. She died in her sleep on August 13, 1910.

Nightingale's Contributions

Nightingale is believed to have been in error in only two areas. First, she did not believe in or appreciate the significance of the germ theory of infection, although her insistence on fresh air, physical hygiene, and environmental cleanliness certainly did a great deal to decrease the transmission of infectious diseases. Second, she did not support a central registry or testing for nurses similar to what was in place for physicians. She was convinced that this would undermine the profession and that a letter of recommendation from the school matron was sufficient to attest to the skill and character of the nurse.

Florence Nightingale was a woman of vision and determination. Her strong belief in herself and her abilities allowed her to pursue and achieve her goals. She was a political activist and a revolutionary in her time. Her accomplishments went beyond the scope of nursing and nursing education, penetrating into all aspects of health care and social reform.

Many memorials have been established in honor of Florence Nightingale, and it is the legacy she has left to all of us who follow in her footsteps that perpetuates her name. Through today's nurses, Nightingale's spirit and determination remain alive. She has handed her lamp to each of us, and we have become the keepers of the lamp.

LILLIAN WALD

Background

Born in Cincinnati, Ohio, in 1867, Lillian Wald moved to Rochester, New York, where she spent most of her childhood. She received her education at Miss Crittenden's English and French Boarding and Day School for Young Ladies and Little Girls. Her relatives were physicians and had a tremendous influence on her. They encouraged her to choose nursing as a career.

Wald attended the New York Hospital School of Nursing. After graduation, she worked as a nurse in the New York Juvenile Asylum. She felt a need for more medically oriented knowledge, so she entered Women's Medical College in New York.

Turning Point

During this time, Wald and a colleague, Mary Brewster, were asked to go to New York's Lower East Side to give a lecture to immigrant mothers on caring for the sick. Wald and Brewster were shocked by what they discovered there.

While showing a group of mothers how to make a bed, a child came up to Wald and asked for help. The boy took her to a squalid tene-ment apartment where nine poorly nourished people were living in two rooms. A woman lay on a bed. Although she was seriously ill, it was apparent that no one had attended to her needs for several days (Kalisch & Kalisch, 2004). Miss Crittenden's School had not prepared Wald for this, but she went right to work anyway. She bathed the woman, washed and changed the bedclothes, sent for a physician, and cleaned the room.

This incident was a turning point in her life. Wald left medical school and began a career as an advocate and helper of the poor and sick, joined by her friend Mary Brewster. They soon found that there were thousands of cases similar to the first in just one small neighborhood.

The Visiting Nurses

Wald and Brewster established a settlement house in 1893 in a rented tenement apartment in a poor section of New York's Lower East Side. To be closer to their clients, they gave up their comfortable living quarters and moved into a smaller, upper-floor apartment there.

It did not take long for the women to build up a nursing practice. At first, they had to seek out the sick, but within weeks calls came to them by the hundreds. The people of the neighborhood trusted them and relied on them for help. Gradually, they also developed a reputation among the physicians and hospitals in the area, and requests to see clients came from these sources as well.

Lillian Wald and her nursing colleagues brought basic nursing care to the people in their home environment. These nurses were independent practitioners who made their own decisions and followed up on their own assessments of families' needs. Like Nightingale, they were very aware of the effect of the environment on the health of their clients and worked hard to improve their clients' surroundings.

Wald was convinced that many illnesses resulted from causes outside individual control and that treatment needed to be holistic. She claimed she chose the title *public health nurse* to emphasize the value of the nurse whose work was built on an understanding of the social and economic problems that inevitably accompanied the clients' ills (Bueheler-Wilkerson, 1993).

Because she had the freedom to explore alternatives for care during numerous births, illnesses, and deaths, Wald began to organize an impressive group of offerings, ranging from private relief to services from the medical establishment. She developed cooperative relationships with various organizations, which allowed her access to goods and jobs for her clients. News of her successes spread. Private physicians sought her out and referred their clients to her for service.

The Henry Street Settlement House

Within 2 years, the nurses had outgrown their original quarters. They needed larger facilities and more nurses. With the help of Jacob Schiff, a banker and philanthropist, they moved to a larger building at 265 Henry Street. This became known as the Henry Street Settlement House (Mayer, 1994). Nine graduate nurses moved in soon after.

By 1909, the Henry Street Settlement House had grown into a well-organized social services system with many departments. The staff included 37 nurses, 5 of whom were managers, and other men and women performed the many activities of the settlement house.

Other Accomplishments

Wald is credited with the development of school health nursing. Health conditions were so bad in the New York City schools that 15–20 children per school were sent home every day. These ill children were returned to school by their parents in the same condition. As a result, illnesses spread from child to child. Ringworm, scabies, and pediculosis were common.

To prove her point about the value of community health nurses, Wald set up an experiment using one nurse for 1 month in one school. During that time, the number of children dismissed from classes dropped from more than 10,000 to 1100. The New York Board of Health was so impressed that they hired nurses to continue the original nurse's work. Wald's nurses treated illnesses, explained the modes of transmission, and explained the

reasons that some children had to be excluded from class and why others did not. The nurses also followed up on the children at home to prevent the recurrence of illnesses.

Wald was also responsible for organizing the Children's Bureau, the Nursing Service Division of the Metropolitan Life Insurance Company, and the Town and Country Nursing Service of the American Red Cross. Her dreams of expanding public health nursing, obtaining insurance coverage for home-based preventive care, and developing a national health nursing service have not become a reality. However, in view of today's health-care demands, she was a visionary who believed that health care belongs in the community and that nurses have a vital role to play in community-based care. She died in 1940 and is remembered as one of the foremost leaders in public health nursing.

▨ MARGARET SANGER

Background

Margaret Higgins was born in Corning, New York, on September 14, 1879. After recovering from tuberculosis, which she contracted while caring for her mother, she attended nursing school at the White Plains Hospital School of Nursing. In her autobiography, she described the school as rigid and at times inhuman; perhaps this provides an indication of where her future interests would take her (Sanger, 1938). During her affiliation at the Manhattan Eye and Ear Hospital, she met William Sanger. They married and moved to a suburb of New York, where she stayed at home to raise their three children.

Labor Reformer

Sanger was very concerned about the working conditions faced by people living in poverty. Many workers were paid barely enough to buy food for themselves and their families. At that time, the income for a family with two working parents was about $12–$14 a week. If only the father worked, earnings dropped to $8 a week. Obviously, when only the mother worked, the family income was even lower. A portion of this income was paid back to the company as rent for company housing. Food was often purchased through a company store, and very little was left for other expenses, including health care.

A major strike of industrial workers in Lawrence, Massachusetts, marked the beginning of Sanger's career as an advocate and social reformer. The workers had previously attempted a strike for better conditions but conceded because of threatening starvation. If the workers went on strike, there was no money for food. Strike sympathizers in New York offered to help the workers and to take the children from Lawrence into their homes. Because of her interest in the situation of the underpaid workers and her involvement with New York laborers, Sanger was asked to assist in the evacuation of children from the unsettled and sometimes violent conditions in Lawrence.

Following an outbreak of serious rioting, she was called to Washington to testify before the House Committee on Rules about the condition of the children. She testified that the children were poorly nourished, ill, ragged, and living in conditions worse than those in impoverished city slums.

Two months later, the owners of the mills sat down to talk with the workers and gave in to their demands. Sanger's interventions on behalf of the children had brought the workers' plight to the attention of the general public and to the people in Washington.

A New Concern for Sanger

In the spring of 1912, Sanger returned to work as a public health nurse. She was assigned to maternity cases in New York City's Lower East Side. One case became a turning point in her life. Sanger was caring for a 28-year-old mother of three children who had attempted to self-abort. This woman and her husband were already struggling to feed and clothe the children they had and could not afford any more. After 3 weeks, the woman had regained her health. However, during the physician's final visit to her home, he told the young woman that she had been lucky to survive this time but

that if she tried to self-abort again, she would not need his services but those of a funeral director. The young woman pleaded with him for a way to prevent another pregnancy. The doctor replied, "Tell your husband to sleep on the roof" (Sanger, 1938). The young woman then turned to Sanger, who remained silent.

Three months later, Sanger was called to the same home. This time, the woman was in a coma and died within minutes of Sanger's arrival. At that moment, Sanger dedicated herself to learning about and disseminating information about birth control.

Contraception Reform

This task turned out to be far more difficult than Sanger had expected. The Comstock Act of 1873 classified birth control information as obscene. Unrewarding research at the Boston Public Library, the Library of Congress, and the New York Academy of Medicine only increased her frustration. Very little information about birth control was available anywhere in the United States at that time.

But contraception was widely practiced in many European countries, so Sanger went to Europe. She studied methods of birth control in France, and when she returned to the United States, she began to publish a journal called *The Woman Rebel*. This journal carried articles about contraception, family planning, and other matters related to women's rights.

The first birth control clinic in the United States opened at 46 Amboy Street in Brooklyn, New York, in 1916. Sanger operated the clinic with her sister, Ethel Byrne, and another nurse, Fania Mindell. On the first day, more than 150 women asked them for help. Everything went smoothly until a policewoman masquerading as a client arrested the three women and recorded the names of all the by-now frightened clients. To bring attention to their plight and to the closing of the clinic, Sanger refused to ride in the police wagon. Instead, she walked the mile to the courthouse.

Several weeks later, Sanger returned to a courthouse overflowing with friends and supporters to face the charges that had been filed against her. The public found it difficult to believe that this attractive mother, flanked by her two sons, was either "demented" or "over-sexed," as her adversaries had claimed. She did not deny the charges of disseminating birth control information, but she did challenge the law that made this information illegal. Because she refused to abide by that law, the judge sentenced her to 30 days in the workhouse.

After completing her 30 days, Sanger continued her work for many years. She solicited the support of wealthy women and used their help to gain financial backing to continue her fight. She gave talks and organized meetings. In 1921, she organized the Birth Control Conference in New York (Kalisch & Kalisch, 2004). In 1928, she established the National Committee on Federal Legislation for Birth Control, which eventually became the Planned Parenthood Foundation. Sanger was also an accomplished author, writing *What Every Girl Should Know, What Every Mother Should Know,* and *Motherhood in Bondage.*

Conservative religious and political groups were the most vocal in their opposition to Sanger's work. In the end, however, Sanger won. Planned Parenthood is a thriving organization, and birth control information is available to anyone who seeks it, although some groups oppose its availability on religious or political grounds.

Sanger could fairly be labeled an early example of the liberated woman. She was independent and assertive during a time when it was considered politically incorrect for a woman to behave in such a manner. Perhaps her most important contributions to the community were her tenacity and her ability to bring the needs of the poor to society's attention and not just the needs of the favored few who had sufficient money. As a nurse, she represented that part of caring that operates in the political arena to bring about change to improve people's health and save lives.

MARY ELIZA MAHONEY

Background

Mary Eliza Mahoney was the first African American registered nurse (RN) in the United States. She was born free on May 7, 1845, in Dorchester, Massachusetts; however, an unverified paper reports the official date as April 16 of the same year. She grew up in Roxbury with her parents and showed an interest in nursing during her adolescence. She worked for 15 years at the New England Hospital for Women and Children (now Dimock Community Health Center). She was a cook, a janitor, a washerwoman, and an unofficial nurse's assistant.

Nursing Education

In 1878, at the age of 33, she applied to the hospital's nursing program and was accepted as a student. She spent her training days washing, ironing, and cleaning and scrubbing, expected competencies of that time. Sixteen months later, of the 43 students who began the rigorous course, Mary and 4 white students were the only ones who completed it. After graduation she worked mostly as a private duty nurse. She ended her nursing career as director of an orphanage in Long Island, New York, a position she had held for a decade. She never married.

Contribution to Nursing

Mahoney recognized the need for nurses to work together to advance the status of black nurses within the profession. In 1896, Mahoney became one of the original members of the predominately white Nurses Associated Alumnae of the United States and Canada (later known as the American Nurses Association [ANA]). She cofounded the National Association of Colored Graduate Nurses (NACGN). Mahoney delivered the welcoming speech at the first convention of the NACGN and served as its national chaplain. Mahoney died on January 4, 1926, and was buried in the Woodlawn Cemetery in Everett, Massachusetts.

In 1936, the NACGN created an award in her honor for women who contributed to racial integration in nursing. After the NACGN was dissolved in 1951, the ANA continued to offer this award to deserving black women. In 1976, 50 years after her death, Mary Eliza Mahoney was inducted into the Nursing Hall of Fame.

When she entered nurse's training, Mahoney never envisioned how her simple act of becoming a nurse would change the status of black nurses and help them to attain leadership positions within the profession. Her dedication and untiring will to inspire future generations has been an inspiration to many men and women of color who remain dedicated members of the nursing profession.

ADELAIDE NUTTING

Background

Adelaide Nutting was born on November 1, 1858, in Frost Village, Quebec, Canada. She was the first graduate of the Johns Hopkins School of Nursing in Baltimore, Maryland. During her student days, the journal *Trained Nurse* offered a $10 prize for an essay on a typhoid fever case. Nutting submitted her essay and won the prize. Her essay was printed in the March 1910 issue, but that was just the beginning for this dynamic nurse leader.

Nutting was a close friend of Isabel Hampton, the director of the Johns Hopkins School of Nursing. When Hampton resigned her position in 1894, Nutting became the superintendent of nurses and the principal.

Nursing Education

Nutting established the 3-year, 8-hour-per-day program that became the prototype for diploma school education in nursing. She later came to believe that more background in the basic sciences was a necessity, and she developed a 6-month course that also became a model for other schools. Although associated with a hospital school of nursing, Nutting was convinced that nursing education would advance only if the profession developed more autonomy. Like Nightingale, Nutting believed that schools of nursing should be independent of hospital control or ownership.

Higher Education

Nutting is probably best known for her work in the creation of the Department of Nursing and Health at Teachers College of Columbia University. After leaving Johns Hopkins in 1907 to take the first chair in nursing at Columbia University, she became the first professor of nursing in the world. She held this position until 1925, when she was succeeded by Isabel Stewart, a former student and colleague.

Other Interests

Nutting was interested in many aspects of nursing. In 1918, she approached the Rockefeller Foundation to request funds for her alma mater, Johns Hopkins. During the interview, she stressed the need for improvement in the education of public health nurses. This meeting led to the formation of a blue-ribbon committee that studied the situation and released a report that emphasized the need for university education of nurses.

Nutting also recognized the importance of cultivating benefactors for nursing. For example, she became very close to Frances Payne Bolton, a wealthy and influential citizen of Cleveland, Ohio. She convinced Bolton to fund an Army Nurse Training School at a time when women were being trained as aides rather than as professional nurses. Nutting opposed their training as aides because she believed that soldiers with war wounds needed professionals to care for them.

The three major nursing organizations of the time supported the establishment of the school, but the U.S. War Department rejected the idea. In response, Bolton went to Washington to persuade the War Department to prepare the women as nurses. The Frances Payne Bolton School of Nursing at Case Western Reserve University in Cleveland, Ohio, is named after this supporter of nursing.

Nutting was committed to the promotion of nursing and nursing education. She was in the forefront of educational reform, first by establishing standards of diploma education and later by supporting the move to the university setting. One of her best achievements was improving the preparation of teachers of nursing. She realized early that the quality of nurses is greatly influenced by the quality of the teachers of nursing students.

MILDRED MONTAG

Background

During World War II, a nursing shortage became evident. To meet the demands for nurses, Congress enacted the Bolton Act of 1943. This created the United States Cadet Nurse Corps. According to the Bolton Act, nurses could be educated in fewer than 3 years and perform nursing duties and responsibilities like their counterparts from the traditional 3-year diploma schools (Applegate, 1988). Mildred Montag developed this program at Adelphi University.

After the war, the federal funds were withdrawn, and the numbers of nursing graduates declined. The acute nursing shortage continued. In 1952, however, a project aimed at developing nursing education programs in junior and community colleges was discussed. Montag, now an assistant professor of nursing at Columbia Teacher's College, was appointed the project coordinator.

The time for a change in nursing education had come. The postwar era created other job opportunities for women, and hospital-based diploma school was not a popular career choice. The health-care delivery system was disease-oriented and patient-centered. New technologies had entered the field of health care, requiring nurses to have a stronger background in the sciences and be able to use these technologies at the bedside.

Montag proposed two levels of nursing. She described a curriculum that would educate what she referred to as the *technical nurse*. This nurse would provide direct, safe nursing care under the supervision of the professional nurse in an acute care setting (Haase, 1990). Today, associate degree programs provide more graduate nurses than any other nursing programs, providing the majority of the nurse workforce.

Associate degree nursing education has had a profound effect on nursing education. The associate degree is the primary model for basic registered nurse education. Montag's major achievement with this innovation was to shift nursing education from the hospital, service-based institutions to the institutions of higher learning. The curriculum included general education courses to prepare the nurse for social and personal competency as well as skill competency.

VIRGINIA HENDERSON

Background

Virginia Henderson was born November 30, 1897, in Kansas City, Missouri. She attended the U.S. Army School of Nursing during World War I. Her mentor was Annie Goodrich, head of the Army School. Goodrich later became the first dean of the Yale School of Nursing. After the war, Henderson continued her nursing career in public health in New York City and Washington, D.C.

Henderson decided to enter nursing education and took her first faculty position at the Norfolk Virginia Protestant Hospital School of Nursing. In 1929, she returned to New York and enrolled in Columbia Teacher's College to further her nursing education. Here she earned her bachelor's and master's degrees. In 1934, she joined the faculty of Columbia Teacher's College. She taught nursing at Columbia from 1934 to 1948.

In 1953, she joined the faculty of the Yale School of Nursing in New Haven, Connecticut, as a research associate and spent the last four decades of her life at Yale. She began a 19-year project to review nursing literature and published the four-volume *Nursing Studies Index*, which indexed the English-language nursing literature from 1900 through 1960.

Contributions to 20th-Century Nursing

Virginia Henderson pioneered the work that is the essence of modern nursing. Her most important writing, *Principles and Practice of Nursing*, is considered the 20th century's equivalent to Nightingale's *Notes on Nursing*. Nightingale emphasized nature as the primary healer. With the advent of antibiotic therapy and other technological advances, Nightingale's work became dated (Henderson, 1955).

In her textbook revision in 1955, Henderson first offered her description of nursing: "I say that the nurse does for others what they would do for themselves if they had the strength, the will and the knowledge. But I go on to say that the nurse makes the patient independent of him or her as soon as possible" (Henderson, 1955). Henderson wrote three editions of this textbook. Unlike other nursing textbooks, this one emphasized the importance of nursing research, not just routine nursing techniques. Nurse educators continued using the book throughout the remainder of the century.

As a nursing professional, Henderson actively participated in nursing organizations. She founded the Interagency Council on Information Resources for Nursing. She was a member of the ANA and acted as a consultant to the National Library of Medicine and the American Journal of Nursing Company. Henderson received many awards for her work and efforts to increase the status of the nursing profession. The Sigma Theta Tau International Nurses Honor Society named its library in honor of her outstanding contributions to nursing.

Henderson believed that nursing complemented the patient by giving him or her what was needed in "will or strength" to perform the daily activities and carry out the physician's treatment. She believed strongly in "getting inside the skin" of her patients as a way of knowing what he or she needed. As she said, "The nurse is temporarily the consciousness of the unconscious, the love of life for the suicidal, the leg of the amputee, the eyes of the newly blind, a means of locomotion for the infant and the knowledge and confidence of the new mother" (Henderson, 1955).

Henderson's beginnings were in public health, and this contributed to her definition of nursing. Because of this background, Henderson was a proponent of publicly financed, universally accessible health-care services. She understood that nurses maintained roots in the communities where they lived, and she believed that nursing belonged in the forefront of health-care reform. She also believed that nurses should take this opportunity to advance the profession by becoming leaders in developing plans for implementing accessible health care.

Henderson is recognized as the "First Lady of Nursing" and is thought by many to be the most important nursing figure in the 20th century. Her colleagues refer to her as the 20th century Florence Nightingale (ualberta.ca/~jmorris/nt/henderson.htm, 2000). She represents the essence and the spirit of nursing in the 20th century to all of us.

MEN IN NURSING

Men's participation in nursing did not begin in the latter part of the 20th century. Early Egyptian priests practiced nursing. The priests who served the goddess Sekhmet held high social rank. The first nursing school in the world started in India in about 250 B.C., and only men were considered "pure" enough for admission.

During the Byzantine Empire, nursing was practiced primarily by men and was a separate profession (Kalisch & Kalisch, 2004). In every plague that swept through Europe, men risked their lives to provide nursing care. In 300 A.D. the Parabolani, a group of men, started a hospital to care for victims of the Black Plague. Two hundred years later, St. Benedict founded the Benedictine Nursing Order (Kalisch & Kalisch, 2004). Throughout the Middle Ages military, religious, and lay orders of men continued to provide nursing care.

Before the Civil War, male and female slaves were identified as "nurses." During the Civil War, the Union used mainly female nurse volunteers, although some men also filled this responsibility. Walt Whitman, for example, served as a volunteer nurse in the Union Army. The Confederate Army took a more formal stand and identified 30 men in each regiment to serve as military nurses. Charged with this responsibility, these men tended to the ill on the battlefields (Clay, 1928). During this war, more men died than in any other war in U.S. history.

The Alexian Brothers, named after St. Alexis, a 5th century nurse, were first organized in the 1300s to provide nursing care to those afflicted with the Black Death. In 1863, the Alexian Brothers opened their first hospital in the United States to educate men as nurses. The Mills School for Nursing and St. Vincent's School for men were organized in New York in 1888. At that time, men did not attend female nursing schools.

Nursing continued to develop as a predominantly female profession, excluding men from entering into schools of nursing and its professional organization. The Nurses Associated Alumnae of the United States and Canada held its first annual meeting in Baltimore in 1897. This organization developed into the ANA in 1911 and continued to exclude men until 1930. One of the early acts of the organization was to prevent men from practicing as nurses in the military.

The Army Nurse Corps, created in 1901, barred men from serving as nurses (Kalisch & Kalisch, 2004). The U.S. military changed from predominantly male nurses to female. At the conclusion of the Korean War, the armed services permitted men to serve as military nurses (Brown, 1942).

Once men entered the military as nurses, their numbers increased in civilian nursing as well. Nursing schools admitted men into the classroom. The numbers of men in nursing gradually increased. Today, although still a comparatively small group, the number of men pursing nursing careers continues to increase. Men are attaining graduate degrees and specialty certifications; men continue to enhance nursing by resuming their historical role as caring, nurturing professionals.

◼ PROFESSIONAL ORGANIZATIONS

American Nurses Association

In 1896, delegates from 10 nursing schools' alumnae associations met to organize a national professional association for nurses. The constitution and bylaws were completed in 1907, and the Nurses Associated Alumnae of the United States and Canada was created. The name was changed in 1911 to the American Nurses Association (ANA), which in 1982 became a federation of constituent state nurses associations.

The purposes of the ANA are to (nursingworld.org/about/index.htm):

1. Work for the improvement of health standards and the availability of health-care services for all people.
2. Foster high standards for nursing.
3. Stimulate and promote the professional development of nurses.
4. Promote the economic and general welfare of nurses in the workplace.
5. Project a positive and realistic view of nursing.
6. Lobby Congress and regulatory agencies about health-care issues affecting nursing and the public.

These purposes, reviewed in each biennial meeting by the House of Delegates, are unrestricted by consideration of age, color, creed, disability, gender, health status, lifestyle, nationality, religion, race, or sexual orientation (ANA, 2005). The core issues identified by the ANA in 2005 were (ana.org):

◆ Nursing shortage.
◆ Workplace rights.
◆ Workplace health and safety.
◆ Appropriate staffing.
◆ Patient safety and advocacy.

Although more than 2 million people are members of the nursing profession in the United States, only about 10% of the nation's RNs are members of their professional organization. The many different subgroups and numerous specialty nursing organizations contribute to this fragmentation, which makes presenting a united front from which to bargain for nursing difficult. As the ANA works on the goal of preparing nurses during the 21st century, nurses must work together in their efforts to identify and promote their unique, autonomous role within the health-care system.

Many advantages are available to nurses who join the ANA. Membership offers benefits such as informative publications, group life and health insurance, malpractice insurance, and continuing education courses. The ANA also helps state nurses associations to support their members regarding workplace and client care issues such as salaries, working conditions, and staffing.

As the major voice of nursing, the ANA lobbies the government to influence laws that affect the practice of nursing and the safety of consumers. The power of the ANA was apparent when nurses lobbied against the American Medical Association's (AMA) proposal to create a new category of health-care worker, the registered care technician, as an answer to the nursing shortage of the 1980s. The registered care technician category was never established, despite the AMA's vigorous support. The ANA frequently publishes position statements outlining the organization's position on particular topics important to the health and welfare of the public and/or the nurse. Table 15-1 summarizes some of the current position statements available from the ANA, which can be accessed on the ANA website (nursingworld. org/readroom/position/index.htm) or are available by mail on request.

Finally, the ANA offers certification in various specialty areas. Certification is a formal, voluntary process by which the professional demonstrates knowledge of and expertise in a specific area of practice. It is a way to establish the nurse's expertise beyond the basic requirements for licensure and is an important part of peer recognition for nurses. In many areas, certification entitles the nurse to salary increases and position advancement. Some specialty nursing organizations also have certification programs.

National League for Nursing

Another large nursing organization is the National League for Nursing (NLN). Unlike ANA membership, NLN membership is open to other health professionals and interested consumers. Over 1500 nursing schools and health-care agencies and more than 5000 nurses, educators, administrators, consumers, and students are members of the NLN (nln.org/aboutnln/info-history.htm).

The NLN participates in test services, research, and publication. It also lobbies actively for nursing issues and is currently working cooperatively with the ANA and other nursing organizations on health-care reform. To do such things more effectively, the ANA, NLN, American Association of Colleges of Nursing, and American Organization of Nurse Executives have formed a coalition called the TriCouncil for the purpose of dealing with issues that are important to all nurses.

The NLN formed a separate accrediting agency, the National League for Nursing Accrediting Agency (NLNAC). The NLNAC is responsible for the specialized accreditation of nursing education schools and programs, both postsecondary and higher degree (master's degree, baccalaureate degree, associate degree, diploma, and practical nursing program).

National Organization for Associate Degree Nursing

Associate degree nursing programs prepare the largest number of new graduates for RN licensure. Many of these individuals would never have had the opportunity to become RNs without the access afforded by the community college system. The move to begin a national organization that would only address associate degree nursing began in 1986. The organization identified two major goals: (1) to maintain eligibility for licensure for associate degree graduates; and (2) to interact with other nursing organizations. Today, the mission of the National Organization for Associate Degree Nursing (NOADN) includes supporting the associate degree graduate through (noadn.org conventionstate.htm):

◆ Strong educational programs.
◆ Dynamic curricula education of students in a variety of settings.
◆ Emphasis on lifelong learning.
◆ Continued articulation with colleges and universities.

Specialty Organizations

In addition to the national nursing organizations, nurses may join specialty practice organizations such as the American Association of Critical Care Nurses; the Academy of Medical Surgical Nurses; American Assembly for Men in Nursing; American Association of Neuroscience Nurses; and the Association of Women's Health, Obstetric and Neonatal Nurses. These organizations provide nurses with information regarding evidence-based practice, trends in the field. and approved stan-

TABLE 15–1
Position Statements

American Nurses Association

Bloodborne and Airborne Diseases

- Education and Barrier Use for Sexually Transmitted Diseases and HIV Infection
- The Health Care Service System and Linkage of Primary Care, Substance Abuse, Mental Health, and HIV/AIDS-Related Services
- AIDS/HIV Disease and Socio-Culturally Diverse Populations
- Availability of Equipment and Safety Procedures to Prevent Transmission of Bloodborne Diseases
- Guidelines for Disclosure to a Known Third Party About Possible HIV Infection
- HIV Infected Nurse, Ethical Obligations and Disclosure
- Tuberculosis and HIV
- HIV Disease and Correctional Inmates
- Needle Exchange and HIV
- Support for Confidential Notification Services and a Limited Privilege to Disclose
- Personnel Policies and HIV in the Workplace
- Post-Exposure Programs in the Event of Occupational Exposure to HIV/HBV
- HIV Exposure from Rape/Sexual Assault
- HIV Infection and Nursing Students
- Tuberculosis and Public Health Nursing
- HIV Infection and U.S. Teenagers
- HIV Testing
- Travel Restrictions for Persons with HIV/AIDS
- HIV Disease and Women

Ethics and Human Rights

- Human Cloning by Means of Blastomere Splitting and Nuclear Transplantation
- Privacy and Confidentiality
- Assisted Suicide
- Nurses' Participation in Capital Punishment
- The Non-Negotiable Nature of the Code for Nurses (**Note:** This is **not** the Code for Nurses; to order the Code for Nurses, go the Publications Catalog.)
- Promotion of Comfort and Relief of Pain in Dying Patients
- Cultural Diversity in Nursing Practice
- Discrimination and Racism in Health Care
- Nursing Care and Do-Not-Resuscitate Decisions
- Ethics and Human Rights
- Active Euthanasia
- Foregoing Nutrition and Hydration
- Mechanisms Through Which SNAs Consider Ethical/Human Rights Issues
- Nursing and the Patient Self-Determination Acts
- Risk Versus Responsibility in Providing Nursing Care
- Reduction of Patient Restraint and Seclusion in Health-care Settings

Social Causes and Health-care

- Adult Immunization
- Cessation of Tobacco Use
- Childhood Immunizations
- Environmental Tobacco Smoke
- Home Care for Mother, Infant, and Family Following Birth
- Informal Caregiving
- Lead Poisoning and Screening
- Long-Term Care
- Nutrition Screening for the Elderly
- Physical Violence Against Women

(Continued on following page)

TABLE 15–1 *(Continued)*
Position Statements

American Nurses Association

- Prevention of Tobacco Use in Youth
- Health Promotion and Disease Prevention
- Reproductive Health
- Use of Placebos for Pain Management in Patients with Cancer

Drug and Alcohol Abuse

- Abuse of Prescription Drugs
- Polypharmacy and the Older Adult
- Opposition to Criminal Prosecution of Women for Use of Drugs While Pregnant
- Support for Treatment Services for Alcohol and Drug Dependent Women of Childbearing Age
- Drug Testing for Health-care Workers

Nursing Education

- Guideline for Commercial Support for Continuing Nursing Education

Nursing Practice

- A National Nursing Database to Support Clinical Nursing Practice
- Nurse-Midwifery
- Privatization and For-profit Conversion
- Psychiatric Mental Health Nursing and Managed Care

Nursing Research

- Education for Participation in Nursing Research

Consumer Advocacy

- Referrals to the Most Appropriate Provider

Workplace Advocacy

- Latex Allergy
- The Right to Accept or Reject an Assignment
- -Restructuring, Work Redesign, and the Job and Career Security of Registered Nurses
- Sexual Harassment
- Polygraph Testing of Health-care Workers
- Opposition to Mandatory Overtime

Unlicensed Assistive Personnel (Note: ANA work on the UAP issue is ongoing.)

- Registered Nurse Utilization of Unlicensed Assistive Personnel
- Registered Nurse Education Relating to the Utilization of Unlicensed Assistive Personnel

Joint Statements

- AORN Official Statement on RN First Assistants
- Role of the Registered Nurse (RN) in the Management of Analgesia by Catheter Techniques
- Paper on Computer-based Patient Record Standards
- Paper on Authentication in a Computer-based Patient Record
- On Access to Patient Data
- Role of the Registered Nurse (RN) in the Management of Patients Receiving IV Conscious Sedation
- Maintaining Professional and Legal Standards During a Shortage of Nursing Personnel
- Services to Families Following a SIDS (Sudden Infant Death Syndrome)

nursingworld.org/readroom/position/index.htm

dards of specialty practice. Links to nursing organizations may be found at nursingsociety.org/career/nursing_orgs.html.

NURSING THEORY

The word *theory* comes from the Greek word *theoria*, which means to contemplate (Johnson & Webber, 2001) or think about. A theory provides an explanation of why something happens the way it does. Because individuals may have different thoughts as to why some things happen, often several theories about the same phenomenon may exist.

Throughout your nursing education you have come in contact with several theories, particularly those of human development. Maslow's Theory of Human Motivation is one such theory. His theory suggests that basic needs must be met before higher level needs become important. Nursing education often uses this theory to teach students about priority setting in patient care.

Nurses integrate many theories into their care models. These include psychological theories, developmental theories, sociocultural theories, family theories, and systems theory. Two other theories familiar to most nursing students are Freud's Theory of Psychosexual Development and Erickson's Psychosocial Stages of Development. Both these theories look at the same phenomenon, human development, but explain it differently.

Nurses use theory to help them think critically and make decisions supported by scientific principles. Nursing theory provides a knowledge base for nurses to use in decision making. Throughout history, most of nursing care has been built on tradition and intuition, not necessarily on scientific principles (Upton, 1999). For this reason, many consumers do not understand what nursing really is and what nurses really do. To establish a strong scientific nursing foundation, nurses need to conduct research to validate nursing actions. Many nursing programs have changed their curricula by incorporating a theoretical framework.

Over the years, many nurse theorists have attempted to explain the relationship nursing has to individuals and to the environment in which they live and to the concept of health. Some of these theories are based on how individuals adapt to changes, and others are based on a systems perspective. No one theory seems to be able to include the entirety of nursing. More information on nurse theorists and nursing theory can be found at sandiego.edu/nursing/theory/

Nursing Theory as a Basis for Practice

Does nursing have its own unique, systematic body of knowledge? Those who say "no" to this question argue that nursing has borrowed from other disciplines, such as the social sciences, biological sciences, and medicine. These same critics believe that knowledge from these other disciplines, technical skills, intuition, and experience have been combined into what is called nursing knowledge. Many disciplines use knowledge from other professions. Physicists use knowledge from mathematics, and pharmacists rely on their background in chemistry.

Those who say "yes" argue that nursing theorists and nursing researchers have identified and described a unique body of knowledge. As the results of their work are used in practice, the unique body of knowledge becomes more widely recognized.

Contrary to the critics and taking into consideration that other disciplines incorporate and utilize knowledge from other professions, nurses in the middle of the 20th century believed that theories from other disciplines could enhance nursing practice but could not effectively describe nursing practice. During this time, an interest in defining nursing knowledge increased, and with more nurses receiving graduate degrees, nurse theorists evolved. These nurses started creating philosophies, or systems of basic principles, and conceptual models, picture representations of ideas and their relationships to one another, to explain nursing. As more nurses obtained doctoral degrees, research methods and data collection increased. This research supported the theoretical propositions in the nursing theories.

Defining nursing as a profession requires nurses to conduct research to increase the existing knowledge base, create new knowledge, and validate nursing theories. Originally, nursing research was based on the scientific method and modeled after the natural and physical sciences. Nursing theories have allowed nurses to examine human experiences and behavior responses more closely.

Although nursing research may be conducted by advanced practice nurses, practicing nurses play a major part in identifying researchable patient problems. They also help in gathering data for ongoing research. It is important for practicing nurses to understand the necessity for nursing research and what part they may play in the research process.

Managed Care

In a managed care system, consumers select a primary care physician provider from an approved list generated by their plan. Each provider is paid a predetermined (capitation) rate for each client, usually on a monthly basis. The primary care provider is the "gatekeeper" because the client must obtain a referral from the primary care physician before seeing a specialist. Those who want to see an out-of-plan provider usually have to pay for new services out-of-pocket.

The original idea behind managed care was that emphasizing preventive health care, including yearly physicals, immunizations, and health education, was an effective way to avoid illness and future hospitalizations, thereby reducing costs (Richards, 1996). Managed care was based on evidence that eight of the nine leading causes of death in the United States could be reduced by attention to lifestyle changes: smoking, lack of exercise, unsafe sex, unsafe driving, and poor diets (Hayes, 2000). If clients did become ill, the physicians in the plan were often given powerful incentives to control costs (Buerhaus, 1996) by limiting the number of diagnostic tests done, for example, or by avoiding a hospital stay altogether, if possible.

Among the industrialized countries around the world, the United States is the only one that does not provide basic health-care coverage to every citizen (Lieberman, 2003). In fact, one in seven people in the United States does not have health insurance (Pear, 2002). The United States does have technologically advanced, highly sophisticated health care and spends more per capita (per person) than most countries. This amount is increasing. Yet, the U.S. health-care system has been described as a "shipwreck" (O'Connor, 2002), a system with "growing cracks" in it that are serious enough to raise high levels of concern (McGinley & Lueck, 2002). One study of medical errors estimated that 36% of all patients admitted to a teaching hospital can expect to encounter some iatrogenic event during their stay (Yourstone & Smith, 2002). An Institute of Medicine report estimated that somewhere between 44,000 and 98,000 hospital patients a year die as a consequence of medical error (Mechanic, 2002). This is equivalent to having a jumbo jet crash every day (Yourstone & Smith, 2002).

If the United states has the most advanced knowledge and equipment and spends a great deal of money on health care, why the cause for alarm? What is wrong? Why doesn't everyone have health-care insurance? Why are people so worried about the quality of care? The answer is complex.

◆ For most people, health insurance comes through their place of employment. One problem with this is that many employers are motivated to keep the cost as low as possible or transfer much of the cost to the employee. Another problem is that if you lose your job, you also lose your health insurance.

◆ Managed care is designed to limit the amount spent on health care. Some have said that it has become a way to limit choices and ration care (Mechanic, 2002) rather than prevent illness.

◆ As managed care plans grow and spread across the country, these companies become powerful enough to be able to negotiate reduced rates (discounts) from local hospitals (Trinh & O'Connor, 2002). They can, in effect, say, "We can get an appendectomy for $2300 at hospital A; why should we pay you $2700?" If hospital B does not agree, the hospital may lose all the patients enrolled in that managed care plan. This pressures hospital B to reduce costs and spread staff even thinner than before.

◆ Similar price pressures come from Medicare, Medicaid, and other health insurance companies. To keep costs under control, some states have cut benefits for people receiving Medicaid (state-supported health benefits for low-income people) (Pear, 2002).

◆ Although always an important issue, health care took a back seat to national security after the September 11, 2001, attacks and the conflict in the Middle East (Pear, 2002). The national debate on how to fix the U.S. health-care system needs to be renewed.

◆ With the upsurge in for-profit health plans and the purchase of not-for-profit hospitals by for-profit companies, U.S. health care has become increasingly "corporatized." It had been thought that this would yield a highly efficient, responsive system ("the customer is always right"), but that has not happened because the "customer" who pays for insurance coverage is actually the employer, not the individual patient. The care provided by the for-profits appears to be of lesser quality than the old not-for-profit or fee-for-service plans (Mechanic, 2002).

◆ There is a limit to the extent to which cost cutting can increase efficiency without endangering patients. A series of important research studies has shown that increasing the number of RNs providing care in a hospital has a direct effect on improving the outcomes of patient care. The opposite is also true: each additional patient assigned to a nurse increases the odds of the patient dying within 30 days of admission by 7% (Aiken, et al., 2002).

For many years, the United States has been trying to fix its health-care system by applying patches over its worst cracks, but this has apparently not worked very well. Does the system need a major overhaul? Probably, but first, groups need to agree on a vision of what it should be and what it should do (O'Connor, 2002). Whatever way that vision develops, it is certain that nurses will have an important role in a future health-care system. As Aiken and colleagues (2002) wrote, "nurses contribute importantly to surveillance, early detection and timely interventions that save lives" (p. 18).

Community-Based Care

Another alternative to the acute care setting is to provide care in ambulatory settings and in the home. Many types of surgery can be done on an outpatient basis, and many therapies once considered too complex to do at home (intravenous therapies and dialysis, for example) are now being done safely and effectively in clients' homes. The specialization common in acute facilities is entering home care: wound care, dialysis care, perinatal care, and congestive heart failure management are a few examples (McClure, 2000). Buerhaus (1996) listed characteristics of the past and future health-care delivery systems (Table 15-2).

EFFECT ON NURSING

The past decade has seen pronounced changes in the organization and delivery of health-care services. Several related to nursing were identified in both North America and Europe:

1. Decentralization of allied health services, such as physical and respiratory therapy. In some cases, much of the responsibility

---

TABLE 15-2
Comparison of the Past and Future Health-Care Delivery Systems

Past/Traditional	Future Managed Health-Care System
Episodic illness-focused	Wellness- and prevention-oriented
Insurance-based payment	Managed care
Inpatient care	Ambulatory and community-based
Hospitals as profit centers	Hospitals as cost centers
Specialist providers	Primary care providers
Independent solo physicians	Multispecialty group practices
Fee-for-service payments	Predetermined capitated fee
Heavily regulated environment	Highly competitive environment
Provider-driven system	Cost-driven system
Presumption of high quality	Systematic evaluation of quality indicators

Adapted from Buerhaus, P.I. (1996). A heads up on capitation. Nursing Policy Forum, 2(3), 21.

was moved back to nursing; in others, the therapists were asked to supervise ancillary personnel (technicians, aides) so that more patients could be treated at a lower cost.

2. Cross-training of workers with varying education and expertise levels to assume tasks traditionally outside their scope of work so that workers can do interchangeable tasks and therefore be substituted for each other.

3. Assignment of ancillary personnel, such as housekeeping, to patient units.

4. Skill mix reductions, with a decreasing percentage of RNs on patient units (Aiken, Clarke, & Sloan, 2000).

As predicted, nurses have moved into other settings, causing major concerns about the severe nuring shortage (Bleich, Santos, & Cox, 2003). As more opportunities open outside of the traditional hospital settings, nurses will continue to explore other career options.

Communicating Nursing's Role

The TriCouncil (ANA, NLN, American Association of Colleges of Nursing, and American Organization of Nurse Executives) organized a campaign in 1993 designed specifically to communicate the significant contributions of nurses. Three areas were emphasized (Swirsky, 1993):

1. Nurses as resource people available to interpret technical health information for consumers.

2. Nurses as health-care coordinators who assist consumers in identifying and using appropriate health-care services.

3. Nurses as expert practitioners in the provision of health care.

Collectively, nurses have more potential power and influence than they currently exhibit. To be able to use this power, nurses need to become more aware of it and more skilled in its use. To improve their confidence, Hess (1993) suggested that nurses think of themselves as "special agents" who have the following responsibilities:

1. *Carry your license.* The strongest legitimate power that nurses have is the exclusive license to provide the kind of care that the public sees as vitally important. This license provides nurses with intimate access to those entrusted to their care. Your license should also be advertised in the professional appearance that you maintain. Although you may believe that people should not be judged by their appearance, they often are. Think, for example, of how you would feel at a restaurant if the person serving you had dirty hair or fingernails.

2. *Use your special training and experience.* Only nurses know what they know. No one else in health care has their broad, specialized education and skills. Be both self-confident and respectful of others when sharing your knowledge and skills with them.

3. *Become a double agent.* Use your personal knowledge and experience to form professional and personal coalitions, both at work and elsewhere.

4. *Network and empower your colleagues.* Extend your knowledge of caring to other nurses. Nurses can help each other increase their skills and advance their careers. Empowerment is defined as "the enabling of people and groups of people to act and make decisions where an equitable distribution of power exists" (Mason, Backer, & Georges, 1993). Focusing on consensus building and group decision making will help empower nurses.

5. *Eliminate the enemy within.* The greatest enemy is self-defeating thoughts and behaviors. Mobilize yourself and others to plan for change positively. Destructive attitudes, criticism, and manipulation of others do not foster a spirit of group collectivity and equality.

6. *Focus on operations.* No matter what level you are, participate. Instead of focusing on the problem, become part of the solution. For example, be a positive infiltrator of relevant hospital committees and professional associations.

7. RNs comprise the largest segment of the health-care workforce. There are more than 2.5 million licensed RNs, and approximately 2 million are employed in the profession (ANA, 2002). The future of nursing depends on nurses' ability to organize as a group, recognize and accept their differences, and develop the skills necessary to negotiate and manage within the changing health-care system.

CONCLUSION

As nursing moves forward in the 21st century, the need for courageous and innovative nurse leaders is greater than ever. Society's demand for high-quality health care at an affordable cost is a contemporary force for change. Nursing has become as diversified as the populations it serves.

Nurses began in hospitals, moved to the community, moved back into the hospitals, and are now seeing a move back to the community. Men were the earliest nurses, then left the profession and have now returned, bringing with them new ideas and leadership abilities. The development and integration of nursing theory into nursing practice and nursing research has laid new foundations for nursing knowledge and nursing practice. We will be the Nightingales, Walds, Sangers, Mahoneys, Nuttings, Montags, and Hendersons of the future; the creativity and dedication of these nurses are part of all of us.

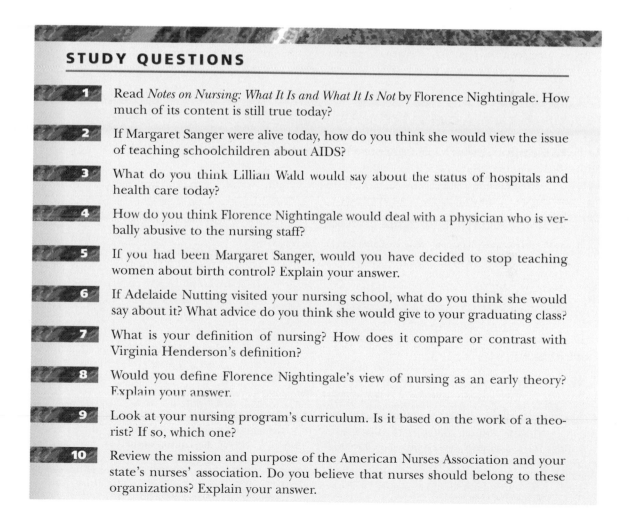

STUDY QUESTIONS

1 Read *Notes on Nursing: What It Is and What It Is Not* by Florence Nightingale. How much of its content is still true today?

2 If Margaret Sanger were alive today, how do you think she would view the issue of teaching schoolchildren about AIDS?

3 What do you think Lillian Wald would say about the status of hospitals and health care today?

4 How do you think Florence Nightingale would deal with a physician who is verbally abusive to the nursing staff?

5 If you had been Margaret Sanger, would you have decided to stop teaching women about birth control? Explain your answer.

6 If Adelaide Nutting visited your nursing school, what do you think she would say about it? What advice do you think she would give to your graduating class?

7 What is your definition of nursing? How does it compare or contrast with Virginia Henderson's definition?

8 Would you define Florence Nightingale's view of nursing as an early theory? Explain your answer.

9 Look at your nursing program's curriculum. Is it based on the work of a theorist? If so, which one?

10 Review the mission and purpose of the American Nurses Association and your state's nurses' association. Do you believe that nurses should belong to these organizations? Explain your answer.

CRITICAL THINKING EXERCISE

Alina went to nursing school on an Air Force scholarship. She has received her assignment, which is to establish a comprehensive primary care and health promotion program clinic on board NASA's newest international space station. The crew is to remain on board the station for 6 months at a time. The crew will consist of professional military men and women.

1. What medical and nursing equipment should Alina plan to have in this center?

2. What would the physical environment on board need to have to satisfy Florence Nightingale and Lillian Wald?

3. How do you believe Virginia Henderson would describe the role of the nurse in this environment?

4. How would a background in a nursing theory help her to plan for the possible interactions that may occur among the concepts of health, person, environment, and nursing?

5. Develop a possible nursing research topic for study in this situation.

STUDENT ACTIVITIES

1. Identify a researchable issue on your clinical unit. Describe the problem.

2. How would you research this problem?

REFERENCES

Aiken, L., Clarke, S.P., Sloane, D., Sochalski, J., & Silber, J.H. (2002). Hospital nurse staffing and patient mortality, nurse burnout and job dissatisfaction. *JAMA,* 288(16), 1987–1993.

Aiken, L., Clarke, S., & Sloane, D. (2000). Hospital restructuring: Does it adversely affect care and outcomes? *Journal of Nursing Administration,* 30(10), 457–465.

American Nurses Association (2005). Retrieved on May 3, 2006 from nursingworld.org/readroom/position/index.htm

Applegate, M. (1988). Associate degree nursing and health care. In *Perspectives of Nursing 1987–1989,* pp. 207–219.

Beletz, E. (1974). Is nursing's public image up-to-date? *Nursing Outlook,* 22, 432–435.

Bleich, M.R., Santos, S.R., & Cox, K.S. (2003). Analysis of the nursing workforce crisis: A call to action. *American Journal of Nursing,* 103(4), 66–74.

Brown, D. (1942). Men nurses in the U.S. Navy. *American Journal of Nursing,* 42, 499–501.

Bueheler-Wilkerson, K. (1993). Bring care to the people: Lillian Wald's legacy to public health nursing. *American Journal of Public Health,* 83, 1778–1785.

Buerhaus, P.I. (1996). A heads up on capitation. *Nursing Policy Forum*, 2(3), 21.

Clay, V. (1928). Home life of a Southern lady. In Albert B. Hart (ed.). *American History Told by Contemporaries*, vol. 4, p. 244. New York: Macmillan.

Donahue, H.P. (1985). *Nursing, the Oldest Art*. St. Louis: C.V. Mosby.

Griffith, G.J., & Griffith, H.J. (1965). *Jensen's History and Trends in Professional Nursing*, 5th ed. St. Louis: C.V. Mosby.

Haase, P. (1990). The origins and rise of associate degree nursing education. Durham, NC: Duke University Press.

Hayes, P.G. (2000). Observations on apparent paradoxes: Health care markets in the new millennium. *The Forum*, 79–84.

Henderson, V. (1966). *The Nature of Nursing*. New York: Macmillan.

Henderson, V. (1955). ualberta.ca/~jmorris/nt/henderson.htm retrieved on May 9, 2000, unc.edu/ehallora/henderson.htm

Hess, R. (1993). In nursing as in life—No risks, no rewards. *Revolution: The Journal of Nurse Empowerment*, 3(1), 84–86, 111–112.

Johnson, B.M. & Webber, P.B. (2001). *An Introduction to Theory and Reasoning in Nursing*. Philadelphia: Lippincott.

Kalisch, P.A. & Kalisch, B.J. (2004). *American Nursing: A History*. Philadelphia: Lippincott, Williams & Wilkins.

Lieberman, T. (2003). Bruised and broken: The US health system. *AARP Bulletin*, 44(3), 3–5.

Longfellow, H.W. (1868). The lady with the lamp. In Williams, M. (1975). *How Does a Poem Mean?* Boston: Houghton Mifflin.

Mason, D., Backer, B., & Georges, A. (1993). Toward a feminist model for the political empowerment of nurses. *Revolution: Journal of Nurse Empowerment*, 3(1), 63–71, 106–108.

Mayer, S. (1994). Amelia Greenwald: Pioneer in international public health nursing. *Nursing and Health Care*, 15(2), 74–78.

McGinley, L. & Lueck, S. (November 14, 2002). Gore's position on health care signals a sharp shift in mood. *Wall Street Journal*, A8.

Mechanic, D. (2002). Sociocultural implications of changing organizational technologies in the provision of care. *Social Science and Medicine*, 54, 459–467.

National League for Nursing. Retrieved on May 4, 2006, from nln.org/aboutnln/info-history.htm

National Organization of Associate Degree Nursing. Retrieved on May 3, 2006, from noadn.org convention-state .htm

Nightingale, F. (1859). *Notes on Nursing: What It Is and What It Is Not*. Reprinted 1992. Philadelphia: J.B. Lippincott.

O'Connor, K. (April 8, 2002). Healthcare in need of a fix. *Modern Healthcare*, 27.

Pear, R. (November 20, 2002). Report: Health system in crisis. *Sun Sentinel*, 3A.

Richards, S. (1996). The pulse of managed care: Managed care 101. *Nursing Policy Forum*, 2(3), 13.

Roberts, M. (1937). Florence Nightingale as a nurse educator. *American Journal of Nursing*, 37, 775.

Rogers, M.E. (1988). Nursing science and art: A prospective. *Nursing Science Quarterly*, 1, 99–102.

Sanger, M. (1938). *Margaret Sanger: An Autobiography*. New York: W.W. Norton.

Schuyler, C.B. (1992). Florence Nightingale. In *Notes on Nursing: What It Is and What It Is Not*. Philadelphia: J.B. Lippincott.

Sigma Theta Tau International Nursing Honor Society. (2006). Retrieved on May 3, 2006, from nursingsociety.org/career/nursing_orgs.html

Swirsky, J. (1993). Exclusive interview with Virginia Trotter Betts, President of the American Nurses Association. *Revolution: The Journal of Nurse Empowerment*, 3(1), 41–48.

Trinh, H.Q. & O'Connor, S.J. (2002). Helpful or harmful? The impact of strategic change on the performance of U.S. urban hospitals. *Health Services Research*, 37(1), 145–171.

Upton, D. (1999). How can we achieve evidence-based practice if we have a theory-practice gap in nursing today? *Journal of Advanced Nursing*, 29(3), 549–555.

Yourstone, S.A. & Smith, H.L. (2002). Managing system errors and failures in health care organizations: Suggestions for practice and research. *Health Care Management Review*, 27(1), 50–61.

Nursing Today

*E*_{*pilogue:*} "A short addition or concluding section at the end of a literary work, often dealing with the future of its characters" (dictionary.com). In the Third Edition of this book, the final chapter was titled "Looking to the Future." However, what were then trends has become reality. Nurses must play a key role in this implementation. What are the functions of nurses? Where are they going to fit in the big picture of local, national, and international health care?

It is impossible to get an accurate idea of the current and future status of health care without considering some of the key players.

INSTITUTE OF MEDICINE

The Institute of Medicine (IOM) (iom.edu) was cited in the discussions of quality and safety initiatives. The IOM is a private, nongovernmental organization that serves as an advisor to policy makers, health-care leaders, and the public. The majority of the work done by the IOM is at the request of government agencies. Its focus currently is on child obesity, health communication, quality issues, and combating cancer.

Child Obesity

"Since the 1970s, the prevalence (or percentage) of obesity has more than doubled for preschool children aged 2–5 years and adolescents aged 12–19 years, and it has more than tripled for children aged 6–11 years. At present, approximately nine million children over

six years of age are obese" (iom.edu/CMS/22593.aspx).

Health Communication

Currently, almost half of all deaths in the United States are linked to smoking, diet, alcohol use, sedentary lifestyle, and accidents. However, less than five percent of $1 trillion spent annually on healthcare addresses reducing risks posed by these conditions (iom.edu/CMS/6095.aspx).

Quality Issues

The IOM has been addressing quality issues since 1996. However, the IOM quality initiative is broader than just safety. The IOM defines quality as "the degree to which health services for individuals and populations increase the likelihood of desired health outcomes and are consistent with current professional knowledge" (iom.edu/CMS/8089.aspx).

2001–2002. The IOM focused on a vision of the role of the federal government in health-care services and quality.

2003. The IOM quality issues explored included:
◆ Priority areas for national action (Box E-1).
◆ A report related to the education of current and future health professionals recommending that students and working professionals develop and maintain proficiency in five core areas: delivering patient-centered care, working as part of interdiscipli-

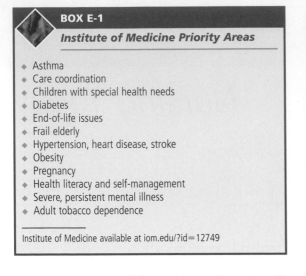

BOX E-1

Institute of Medicine Priority Areas

- Asthma
- Care coordination
- Children with special health needs
- Diabetes
- End-of-life issues
- Frail elderly
- Hypertension, heart disease, stroke
- Obesity
- Pregnancy
- Health literacy and self-management
- Severe, persistent mental illness
- Adult tobacco dependence

Institute of Medicine available at iom.edu/?id=12749

BOX E-3

Patient Safety Key Issues

- Safety is a system property.
- Transparency is necessary; secrecy is harmful.
- Needs are anticipated.
- Cooperation among clinicians is a priority.
- Waste is continuously decreased.
- Care is based on continuous healing relationship.
- Care provided according to patient needs and values.
- Patient is source of control of care.
- Knowledge is shared.
- Decisions are evidence-based.

nary teams, practicing evidence-based medicine, focusing on quality improvement, and using information technology (iom. edu/?id=12749)

◆ Identification of a set of eight core care delivery functions that electronic health records (EHR) systems should be capable of performing (Box E-2).

◆ A report addressing key areas related to patient safety (Box E-3).

2004. The quality report focused on work environments that threaten patient safety through their effect on nursing care. The publication, *Keeping Patients Safe: Transforming the Work Environment of Nurses*, presents evidence and recommendations from a multitude of research studies that address issues of staffing, work hours, and mandatory overtime. Also, the future of rural health care was addressed. For nurses who live in rural areas, the need to maintain health-care professions and access to services is an ongoing challenge. See Box E-4 for safety research results.

2005. The delivery of care for mental and substance use conditions differs from overall health-care delivery. These issues were addressed to develop a comprehensive framework that meets the needs of these clients.

BOX E-2

Functions of an EHR System

- Health information and data
- Result management
- Order management
- Decision support
- Electronic communication and connectivity
- Patient support
- Administrative processes and reporting
- Reporting and population health

Institute of Medicine available at iom.edu/?id=12749

BOX E-4

IOM Current Safety Reports

- Between 44,000 and 98,000 Americans die from medical errors annually.
- Only 55% of patients in a recent random sample of adults received recommended care, with little difference found between care recommended for prevention, to address acute episodes or to treat chronic conditions.
- Medication-related errors for hospitalized patients cost roughly $2 billion annually.
- 41 million uninsured Americans exhibit consistently worse clinical outcomes than the insured and are at increased risk for dying prematurely.
- The lag between the discovery of more effective forms of treatment and their incorporation into routine patient care averages 17 years.
- 18,000 Americans die each year from heart attacks because they did not receive preventive medications, although they were eligible for them.
- Medical errors kill more people per year than breast cancer, AIDS, or motor vehicle accidents.
- More than 50% of patients with diabetes, hypertension, tobacco addiction, hyperlipidemia, congestive heart failure, asthma, depression, and chronic atrial fibrillation are currently managed inadequately.

Institute of Medicine available at iom.edu/CMS/8089/14980.aspx

JOINT COMMISSION ON ACCREDITATION OF HEALTHCARE ORGANIZATIONS

Established more than 50 years ago, the Joint Commission on Accreditation of Healthcare Organizations (JCAHO) (jcaho.org) evaluates the quality and safety of care for more than 15,000 health-care organizations. In order to be accredited, an agency must be reviewed by JCAHO at least once every 3 years. The patient safety initiatives, including monitoring of patient safety goals and sentinel events, are the responsibility of the JCAHO. It is the agency that publishes the official "do not use" list of abbreviations. This list is part of the JCAHO national patient safety initiative. Health-care facilities and providers must keep abreast of changes in the updated list (jcaho.org/accred-ited+organizations/patient+safety/dnu.htm).

HUMAN GENOME PROJECT

The Human Genome Project (HGP) (doegenomes.org)was a 13-year project coordinated by the U.S. Department of Energy and the National Institutes of Health. Project goals included (ornl.gov/sci/techresources/Human_Genome/home.shtml):

◆ *Identifying* all the approximately 20,000 25,000 genes in human DNA.

◆ *Determining* the sequences of the 3 billion chemical base pairs that make up human DNA.

◆ *Storing* this information in databases.

◆ *Improving* tools for data analysis.

◆ *Transferring* related technologies to the private sector.

◆ *Addressing* the ethical, legal, and social issues that may arise from the project.

CENTERS FOR DISEASE CONTROL

The Centers for Disease Control and Prevention (CDC) (cdc.gov)is part of the Department of Health and Human Services (HHS) of the United States government. The current health and safety goals of the CDC include:

◆ Emerging infectious diseases (SARS, monkeypox, pandemic influenza).

◆ Terrorism.

◆ Environmental threats (hurricanes, wildfires, toxic chemical spills).

◆ Aging population.

◆ Lifestyle choices (tobacco use, poor nutrition, lack of physical fitness).

AGENCY FOR HEALTHCARE QUALITY AND RESEARCH

Another arm of the U.S. Department of HHS, the Agency for Healthcare Quality and Research (AHRQ) (ahrq.gov) works in conjunction with the biomedical research mission of its sister agency, the National Institutes of Health. The AHRQ supports research centers that specialize in major areas of health-care research:

◆ Quality improvement and patient safety.

◆ Outcomes and effectiveness of care.

◆ Clinical practice and technology assessment.

◆ Health-care organization and delivery systems.

◆ Primary care (including preventive services).

◆ Health-care costs and sources of payment (ahcpr.gov/about/whatis.htm).

Evidence-Based Practice

The AHRQ also supports a center for evidence-based practice. Instrumental in the development of clinical practice guidelines and research into evidence-based practice, the AHRQ is a clearinghouse for promoting the practice of medicine using evidence.

A new paradigm for medical practice is emerging. Evidence-based medicine deemphasizes intuition, unsystematic clinical experience, and pathophysiological rationales as sufficient grounds for clinical decision making; instead, it stresses the examination of evidence from clinical research. Evidence-based medicine requires new skills of the physician, including efficient literature searching and applying formal rules of evidence in evaluating the clinical literature (cche.net/usersguides/ebm.asp)

Nursing has also begun focusing on practicing using evidence. The Academic Center for Evidence-Based Nursing at the University of Texas (acestar.uthscsa.edu/about.htm) is one example of nursing striving to bridge research into practice.

CONCLUSION

The above are only a few of the players in the quest for health-care change and quality that are focusing on the present as well as the future.

The question is what is *not* nursing's role? Indeed, nursing's role is part of every agency, every goal, and every outcome. The issues are not limited to healthy aging, genetics, and prevention of chronic diseases, technology, infectious diseases and bioterrorism—the list goes on and on. Nursing must be at the forefront in this century, coupled with the timeless nursing values of advocacy, caring, compassion, quality, commitment, and trust. Evidence continues to grow that nursing is vital to building and maintaining safe, patient-centered, and affordable health care (Aiken, 2002).

To claim—as *nursing* does—that each person has an uncontested and undeniable right to be valued and treated with dignity; and to strive—as *nurses* do—to fashion their work in the service of that belief is the proud tradition of this profession and its practitioners. (Manthey, et al., 2000, p. 5.)

REFERENCES

Academic Center for Evidence Based Nursing (ACE) available at acestar.uthscsa.edu/About.htm

Agency for Healthcare Quality available at ahcpr.gov/

Aiken L.H., Clarke S.P., & Sloane D.M., (2002). Hospital nurse staffing and patient mortality, nurse burnout, and job dissatisfaction. *JAMA,* 288, 1987–1993.

Center for Health Evidence available at cche.net/usersguides/ebm.asp

Centers for Disease Control (CDC) available at cdc.gov/about/goals/default.htm

Dictionary.com available at http://dictionary.reference.com/search?q=epilogue

Human Genome Project available at ornl.gov/sci techresources/Human_Genome/home.shtml

Institute of Medicine available at iom.edu

Institute of Medicine available at iom.edu/CMS/22593.aspx

Institute of Medicine available at iom.edu/CMS/6095.aspx

Institute of Medicine available at iom.edu/?id=12749

Institute of Medicine available at iom.edu/CMS/8089/14980.aspx

Joint Commission on Accreditation of Healthcare Organizations available at jcaho.org/accredited+organizations/patient+safety/dnu.htm

Manthey, M.W., Zane, R., Carlson, K., Salmon, M.E., & Moccia, P. (2000). *Creative Nursing,* 6(1), 5–11.

Code of Ethics for Nurses

AMERICAN NURSES ASSOCIATION CODE OF ETHICS FOR NURSES

1 The nurse, in all professional relationships, practices with compassion and respect for the inherent dignity, worth, and uniqueness of every individual, unrestricted by considerations of social or economic status, personal attributes, or the nature of health problems.

2 The nurse's primary commitment is to the patient, whether an individual, family, group, or community.

3 The nurse promotes, advocates for, and strives to protect the health, safety, and rights of the patient.

4 The nurse is responsible and accountable for individual nursing practice and determines the appropriate delegation of tasks consistent with the nurse's obligation to provide optimum patient care.

5 The nurse owes the same duties to self as to others, including the responsibility to preserve integrity and safety, to maintain competence, and to continue personal and professional growth.

6 The nurse participates in establishing, maintaining, and improving health care environments and conditions of employment conducive to the provision of quality health care and consistent with the values of the profession through individual and collective action.

7 The nurse participates in the advancement of the profession through contributions to practice, education, administration, and knowledge development.

8 The nurse collaborates with other health professionals and the public in promoting community, national, and international efforts to meet health needs.

9 The profession of nursing, as represented by associations and their members, is responsible for articulating nursing values, for maintaining the integrity of the profession and its practice, and for shaping social policy.[1]

Approved July 2001.

Web site: nursingworld.org/ethics/chcode.htm

CANADIAN NURSE ASSOCIATION CODE OF ETHICS FOR REGISTERED NURSES

Values

A value is something that is prized or held dear; something that is deeply cared about. This code is organized around eight primary values that are central to ethical nursing practice:

Safe, Competent and Ethical Care
Nurses value the ability to provide safe, competent, and ethical care that allows them to fulfill their ethical and professional obligations to the people they serve.

Health and Well-Being

Nurses value health promotion and well-being and assisting persons to achieve their optimum level of health in situations of normal health, illness, injury, disability, or at the end of life.

Choice

Nurses respect and promote the autonomy of persons and help them to express their health needs and values, and also to obtain desired information and services so they can make informed decisions.

Dignity

Nurses recognize and respect the inherent worth of each person and advocate for respectful treatment of all persons.

Confidentiality

Nurses safeguard information learned in the context of a professional relationship, and ensure it is shared outside the health care team only with the person's informed consent, or as may be legally required, or where the failure to disclose would cause significant harm.

Justice

Nurses uphold principles of equity and fairness to assist persons in receiving a share of health services and resources proportionate to their needs and in promoting social justice.

Accountability

Nurses are answerable for their practice, and they act in a manner consistent with their professional responsibilities and standards of practice.

Quality Practice Environments

Nurses value and advocate for practice environments that have the organizational structures and resources necessary to ensure safety, support, and respect for all persons in the work setting.[2]

Approved September 2002.

Web site: cna-nurses.ca/pages/ethics/ethics-frame.htm

---

[2]Reprinted with permission from the Canadian Nurses Association.

THE INTERNATIONAL COUNCIL OF NURSES CODE OF ETHICS FOR NURSES

Nurses and People

The nurse's primary professional responsibility is to people requiring nursing care.

In providing nursing care, the nurse promotes an environment in which the human rights, values, customs, and spiritual beliefs of the individual, family, and community are respected.

The nurse ensures that the individual receives sufficient information on which to base consent for care and related treatment.

The nurse holds in confidence personal information and uses judgment in sharing this information.

The nurse shares with society the responsibility for initiating and supporting action to meet the health and social needs of the public, in particular those of vulnerable populations.

The nurse also shares responsibility to sustain and protect the natural environment from depletion, pollution, degradation, and destruction.

Nurses and Practice

The nurse carries personal responsibility and accountability for nursing practice, and for maintaining competence by continual learning.

The nurse maintains a standard personal health such that the ability to provide care is not compromised.

The nurse uses judgment regarding individual competence when accepting and delegating responsibility.

The nurse at all times maintains standards of personal conduct which reflect well on the profession and enhance public confidence.

The nurse, in providing care, ensures that use of technology and scientific advances are compatible with safety, dignity, and rights of people.

Nurses and the Profession

The nurse assumes the major role in determining and implementing acceptable standards of clinical nursing practice, management, research, and education.

The nurse is active in developing a core research-based professional knowledge.

The nurse, acting through professional organization, participates in creating and maintaining equitable social and economic working conditions in nursing.

Nurses and Co-Workers

The nurse sustains a co-operative relationship with co-workers in nursing and other fields.

The nurse takes appropriate action to safeguard individuals when their care is endangered by a co-worker or any other person.[3]
Approved 2000.
Web site: cn.ch/ethics.htm

---

[3]Used with permission International Council of Nurses, Geneva, Switzerland, copyright 2000.

Standards Published by the American Nurses Association

Faith Community Nursing: Scope and Standards of Practice

Intellectual and Developmental Disabilities Nursing: Scope and Standards of Practice

Neonatal Nursing: Scope and Standards of Practice

Pain Management Nursing: Scope and Standards of Practice

Plastic Surgery Nursing: Scope and Standards of Practice

School Nursing: Scope and Standards of Practice

Scope and Standards for Nurse Administrators

Scope and Standards of Addictions Nursing Practice

Scope and Standards of College Health Nursing Practice

Scope and Standards of Diabetes Nursing Practice

Scope and Standards of Gerontological Nursing Practice

Scope and Standards of Home Health Nursing Practice

Scope and Standards of Hospice and Palliative Nursing Practice

Scope and Standards of Neuroscience Nursing Practice

Scope and Standards of Nursing Informatics Practice

Scope and Standards of Pediatric Nursing Practice

Scope and Standards of Pediatric Oncology Nursing

Scope and Standards of Practice for Nursing Professional Development

Scope and Standards of Psychiatric-Mental Health Nursing Practice

Scope and Standards of Public Health Nursing Practice

Scope and Standards of Vascular Nursing Practice

Standards of Addictions Nursing Practice with Selected Diagnoses and Criteria

nursingworld.org/books/

National Organization for Associate Degree Nursing (N-OADN) Resolution: Differentiated Nursing Practice

Whereas differentiated nursing practice is an approach to assuring quality nursing care through the appropriate utilization of nursing resources; and

Whereas the approach may include a variety of models for the roles and functions of registered nurses defined by criteria which include, but are not limited to, experience, competence, and life-long learning; and

Whereas differentiated nursing practice is a response to an environment challenged by changing health care trends as well as cost containment; and

Whereas the model for differentiated nursing practice is developed by the registered nurse employed within a practice environment and requires the identification of nursing competencies needed to provide quality nursing care; therefore

Be It Resolved that N-OADN strongly support those practice models affording the registered nurse the opportunity to participate in the development of competencies for roles in varied practice environments; and

Be It Further Resolved that N-OADN advocates registered nurses to have the opportunity to assume roles appropriate to their capabilities and experience; and

Be It Further Resolved that N-OADN strongly supports differentiated practice models that value the registered nurse and his/her practice; and

Be It Further Resolved that this resolution be widely distributed to nursing and health care organizations.

(Adopted: N-OADN Convention, November 1997)

National Organization for Associate Degree Nursing noadn.org

Guidelines for the Registered Nurse in Giving, Accepting, or Rejecting a Work Assignment

Registered Nurses, as licensed professionals, share the responsibility and accountability along with their employer to ensure that safe, quality nursing care is provided. The scope of professional nurses' accountability involves legal, ethical, and professional guidelines for assuring safe, quality patient care. Legal responsibility for the provisions, delegation and supervision of patient care is specified in the Nurse Practice Act 464.001, and the Administrative Rules Chapter 59S. The American Nurses Association (ANA) Code for Nurses with Interpretive Statements (1985) guides ethical conduct and decision making of professional nurses. The ANA Standards and Scope of Practice (1997) provides a systematic application of nursing process for patient care management across patient care settings. In addition, the ANA Restructuring Survival Kit (1996) suggests common strategies to assist the professional nurse facing assignment and delegation issues during reassignment and reorganization, temporary or permanent. Lastly, the employer requirements for safe, competent staffing are outlined in facility policies and guidelines.

Within ethical and legal parameters the nurse exercises informed judgment and uses individual competence and qualifications as criteria in seeking consultation, accepting responsibilities and delegating nursing activities to others. The nurse's decision regarding accepting or making work assignments is based on the legal, ethical and professional obligation to assume responsibility for nursing judgment and action.

The document offers strategies for problem solving as the staff nurse, nurse manager, chief nurse executive and administrator practice within the complex environment of the health care system.

NURSING CARE DELIVERY

Only a Registered Nurse (RN) will assess, plan and evaluate a patient's or client's nursing care needs. No nurse shall be required or directed to delegate nursing activities to other personnel in a manner inconsistent with the Nurse Practice Act, the standards of the Joint Commission on Accreditation of Health Organizations, the ANA Standards of Practice or Hospital Policy. Consistent with the preceding sentence, the individual RN has the autonomy to delegate (or not delegate) those aspects of nursing care the nurse determines appropriate based on the patient assessment.

When a nurse is floated to a unit or area where the nurse receives an assignment that is considered unsafe to perform independently, the RN has the right and obligation to request and receive a modified assignment, which reflects the RN's level of competence.

*Reproduced with permission of Florida Nurses Association, 1999, Orlando, Florida.

The Florida Nurses Association (FNA), the Florida Organization of Nurse Executives (FONE), and the FNA Labor Employee Relations Commission (LERC) recognize that changes in the health care delivery system have occurred and will continue to occur, while emphasizing the common goal to provide safe quality patient care. The parties also recognize that RNs have a right and responsibility to participate in decisions affecting delivery of nursing care and related terms and conditions of employment. All parties have a mutual interest in developing systems, which will provide quality care on a cost efficient basis without jeopardizing patient outcomes. Thus, commitment to measuring the impact of staffing and assignments to patient outcomes is a shared commitment of all professional nurses irrespective of organizational structure.

ASSIGNMENT DESPITE OBJECTION (ADO)/DOCUMENTATION OF PRACTICE SITUATION (DOPS)

Staff nurses today face often untenable assignments that need to be documented as such. Critical, clinical judgment should be utilized when evaluating the appropriateness of an assignment. Refusal to accept an assignment without appropriate discussion within the chain of command can be defined as insubordinate behavior. Each Registered Nurse should become familiar with organizational policies, procedures and documentation regarding refusal to accept an unsafe assignment. ANA has recently adopted a position statement and model ADO form available for use by SNA members. (Please contact Florida Nurses Association for further information.)

Staffing

In the event a Registered Nurse determines in his/her professional opinion that he/she has been given an assignment that does not allow for appropriate patient care, he/she shall notify the Supervisor or designee who shall review the concerns of the nurse. If the nurse's concerns cannot be resolved by telephone, the Supervisor or designee, except in instances of compelling business reasons that preclude him/her from doing so, will then come to the unit within four (4) hours of being contacted by the nurse to assess the staffing. Such assessment shall be documented with a copy given to the nurse. Nothing herein shall prohibit a Registered Nurse from completing and submitting a protest of assignment form.

NURSE PRACTICE ACT, 1994, ADMINISTRATIVE RULES CHAPT. 59S, 14.001 DEFINITIONS (4/29/96)

"Assignments" - are the normal daily functions of the UAPs based on institutional or agency job duties to which do not involve delegation of nursing functions or nursing judgment.

"Competency" - is the demonstrated ability to carry out specified tasks or activities with reasonable skill and safety that adheres to the prevailing standard of practice in the nursing community.

"Delegation" - is the transference to a competent individual the authority to perform a selected nursing task or activity in a selected situation by a nurse qualified by licensure and experience to perform the task or activity.

"Supervision" - is the provision of guidance by a qualified nurse and periodic inspection by the nurse for the accomplishment of a nursing task or activity, provided the nurse is qualified and legally entitled to perform such task or activity. The supervisor may be the delegator or a person of equal or greater licensure to the delegator.

SCENARIO

◆ Suppose you are asked to care for an unfamiliar patient population or to go to a unit for which you feel unqualified—what do you do?

◆ Suppose you are approached by your supervisor and asked to work an additional shift. Your immediate response is that you don't want to work another shift—what do you do?

Such situations are familiar and emphasize the rights and responsibilities of the RN to make informed decisions. Yet all members of the health care team, from staff nurses to administrator, share a joint responsibility to ensure that quality patient care is provided. At times, though, difference in interpretation of legal or ethical principles may lead to conflict.

Guidelines for decision making are offered to assist RN problem-solve work assignment issues. Applications of these guidelines are presented in the form of scenarios, examples of unsafe assignments experienced by RNs.

 ## GUIDELINES FOR DECISION MAKING

The complexity of the delivery of nursing care is such that only professional nurses with appropriate education and experience can provide nursing care. Upon employment with a health care facility, the nurse contracts or enters into an agreement with that facility to provide nursing services in a collaborative practice environment.

It is the Registered Nurse's Responsibility to:

◆ provide competent nursing care to the patient

◆ exercise informed judgment and use individual competence and qualifications as criteria in seeking consultation, accepting responsibilities and delegating nursing activities to others

◆ clarify assignments, assess personal capabilities, jointly identify options for patient care assignments when he/she does not feel personally competent or adequately prepared to carry out a specific function

◆ refuse an assignment that he/she does not feel prepared to assume after appropriate consultation with supervisor

It is Nursing Management's Responsibility to:

◆ ensure competent nursing care is provided to the patient

◆ evaluate the nurse's ability to provide specialized patient care

◆ organize resources to ensure that patients receive appropriate nursing care

◆ collaborate with the staff nurse to clarify assignments, assess personal capabilities, jointly identify options for patient care assignments when the nurse does not feel personally competent or adequately prepared to carry out a specific function.

◆ take appropriate disciplinary action according to facility policies

◆ communicate in written policies to the staff the process to make assignment and reassignment decisions

◆ provide education to staff and supervisory personnel in the decision making process regarding patient care assignments and reassignments, including patient placement and allocation of resources

◆ plan and budget for staffing patterns based upon patient's requirements and priorities for care

◆ provide a clearly defined written mechanism for immediate internal review of proposed assignments, which includes the participation of the staff involved, to help avoid conflict

Issues Central to Potential Dilemmas Are:

◆ the right of the patient to receive safe professional nursing care at an acceptable level of quality

◆ the responsibility for an appropriate utilization and distribution of nursing care services when nursing becomes a scare resource

◆ the responsibility for providing a practice environment that assures adequate nursing resources for the facility, while meeting the current socioeconomic and political realities of shrinking health care dollars

░ LEGAL ISSUES

Behaviors and activities relevant to giving, accepting, or rejecting a work assignment that could lead to disciplinary action include:

◆ practicing or offering to practice beyond the scope permitted by law, or accepting and performing professional responsibilities which the licensee knows or has reason to know that he or she is not competent to perform

◆ performing, without adequate supervision, professional services which the licensee is authorized to perform only under the supervision of a licensed professional, except in an emergency situation where a person's life or health is in danger

◆ abandoning or neglecting a patient or client who is in need of nursing care without making reasonable arrangements for the continuation of such care

◆ failure to exercise supervision over persons who are authorized to practice only under the supervision of the licensed professional

Of the above, the issue of abandonment or neglect has thus far proven the most legally devastating. Abandonment or neglect has been legally defined to include such actions as insufficient observation (frequency of contact), failure to assure competent intervention when the patient's condition changes (qualified physician not in attendance), and withdrawal of services without provision for qualified coverage. Since nurses at all levels most frequently act as agents of the employing facility, the facility shares the risk of liability with the nurse.

░ APPLICATION OF GUIDELINES FOR DECISION MAKING

Two clinical scenarios are presented for the RN to demonstrate appropriate decision making when faced with an unsafe assignment. Sometimes an example or two can help the RN objectively examine legal, ethical and professional issues prior to making a final decision. Additional resources are listed following the scenarios.

Scenario—A Question of Competence

An example of a potential dilemma is when an evening supervisor pulls a psychiatric nurse to the coronary care unit because of a lack of nursing staff. The CCU census has risen and there is not additional qualified staff available.

Suppose you are asked to care for an unfamiliar patient population or to go to a unit for which you feel unqualified—what do you do?

1 CLARIFY what it is you are being asked to do.

◆ How many patients will you be expected to care for?
◆ Does the care of these patients require you to have specialty knowledge and skills in order to deliver safe nursing care?
◆ Will there be qualified and experienced RNs on the unit?
◆ What procedures and/or medications will you be expected to administer?
◆ What kind of orientation do you need to function safely in the unfamiliar setting?

2 ASSESS yourself. Do you have the knowledge and skill to meet the expectations that have been outlined for you? Have you had experience with similar patient populations? Have you been oriented to this unit or a similar unit? Would the perceived discrepancies between your abilities and the expectations lead to an unsafe patient care situation?

3 IDENTIFY OPTIONS and implications of your decision.

a) If you perceive that you can provide safe patient care, you should accept the assignment. You would now be ethically and legally responsible for the nursing care of these patients.

b) If you perceive there is a discrepancy between abilities and the expectations of the assignment, further dialogue with the nurse supervisor is needed before you reach a decision. At this point it may be appropriate to consult the next level of management, such as the house supervisor or the chief nurse executive.

In further dialogue, continue to assess whether you are qualified to accept either a portion or the whole of the requested assignment. Also point out options which might be mutually beneficial. For example, obviously it would be unsafe for you to administer chemotherapy without prior training. However, if someone else administered the chemotherapy, perhaps you could provide the remainder of the required nursing care for that patient. If you feel unqualified for the assignment in its entirety, the dilemma becomes more complex.

At this point the RN must be aware of the legal rights of the facility. Even though the RN may have legitimate concern for patient safety and one's own legal accountability in providing safe care, the facility has legal precedent to initiate disciplinary action, including termination, if you refuse to accept an assignment. Therefore, it is important to continue to explore options in a positive manner, recognizing that both the RN and the facility have a responsibility for safe patient care.

4 POINT OF DECISION/IMPLICATIONS
If none of the options are acceptable, you are at your final decision point.

a) Accept the assignment, documenting carefully your concern for patient safety and the process you used to inform the facility (manager) of your concerns. Keep a personal copy of this documentation and send a copy to the manager(s) involved. Once you have reached this decision it is unwise to discuss the situation or your feelings with other staff or patients. Now you are legally accountable for these patients. From this point, withdrawal from the agreed upon assignment may constitute abandonment.

b) Refuse the assignment, being prepared for disciplinary action. Document your concern for patient safety and the process you used to inform the facility (manager) of your concerns. Keep a personal copy of this documentation and send a copy to the Nurse Executive. Courtesy suggests that you also send a copy to the manager(s) involved.

c) Document the steps taken in making your decision. It may be necessary for you to use the facility's grievance procedure.

Scenario—A Question of an Additional Shift

An example of another potential dilemma is when a nurse who recognizes his/her fatigue and its potential for patient harm is required to work an additional shift.

Suppose you are approached by your supervisor and asked to work an additional shift. Your immediate response is that you don't want to work another shift—what do you do?

1 CLARIFY what it is you are expected to do.
◆ For example, would the additional shift be with the same patients you are currently caring for, or would it involve a new patient assignment?
◆ Is your reluctance to work another shift because of a new patient assignment you do not feel competent to accept? (If the answer is yes, then refer to the previous example, "A Question of Competence.")
◆ Is your reluctance due to work fatigue, or do you have other plans?
◆ Is this a chronic request due to poor scheduling, inadequate staffing, or chronic absenteeism?
◆ Are you being asked to work because there is no relief nurse coming for your present patient assignment? Because your unit will be short of professional staff on the next shift? Because another unit will be short of professional staff on the next shift?
◆ How long are you being asked to work—the entire shift or a portion of the shift?

2 ASSESS yourself.
◆ Are you really tired, or do you just not feel like working? Is your fatigue level such that your care may be unsafe? Remember, you are legally responsible for the care of your current patient assignment if relief is not available.

3 IDENTIFY OPTIONS and implications of your decision.
a) If you perceive that you can provide safe patient care and are willing to work the additional shift, accept the assignment.
b) If you perceive that you can provide safe patient care but are unwilling to stay due to other plans or the chronic nature of the request, inform the manager of

your reasons for not wishing to accept the assignment.

c) If you perceive that your fatigue will interfere with your ability to safely care for patients, indicate this fact to the manager.

If you do not accept the assignment and the manager continues to attempt to persuade you it may be appropriate to consult the next level of management, such as the house supervisor or the nurse executive.

In further dialogue, continue to weigh your reasons for refusal versus the facility's need for an RN. If you have a strong alternate commitment, such as no child care, or if you seriously feel your fatigue will interfere with safe patient care, restate your reasons for refusal.

At this point, it is important for you to be aware of the legal rights of the facility. Even though you may have legitimate concern for patient safety and your own legal accountability in providing safe care, or legitimate concern for the safety of your children or other commitments, the facility has legal precedent to initiate disciplinary action, including termination, if you refuse to accept an assignment. Therefore, it is important to continue to explore options in a positive manner, recognizing both you and the facility have a responsibility for safe patient care.

4 POINT OF DECISION/IMPLICATIONS

a) Accept the assignment, documenting your professional concern for patient safety and the process you used to inform the facility (manager) of your concerns. Keep a personal copy of this documentation and send a copy to the nurse executive. Courtesy suggests that you also send a copy to the manager(s) involved. Once you have reached this decision it is unwise to discuss the situation of your feelings with other staff and/or patients.

b) Accept the assignment, documenting your professional concerns for the chronic nature of the request and possible long-term consequences in reducing the quality of care. Documentation should follow the procedures outlined in (a).

c) Accept the assignment, documenting your personal concerns regarding working conditions in which management decides the legitimacy of employee personal commitments. This documentation should go to your manager. You may wish to request a meeting with your manager to discuss the incident and your concerns regarding future requests.

d) Refuse the assignment, being prepared for disciplinary action. If your reasons for refusal were patient safety or an imperative personal commitment, document this carefully, including the process you used to inform the facility (nurse manager) of your concerns. Keep a personal copy of this documentation and send a copy to the chief nurse executive. Courtesy suggests that you also send a copy to the manager(s) involved.

e) Document the rationale for your decision. It may be necessary to use the facility's grievance procedure.

SUMMARY

Two scenarios of how an RN may apply the guidelines for decision making in the actual work situation have been presented. Staffing dilemmas will always be present and mandate that active communication between staff nurses and all levels of nursing management be maintained to assure patient safety. The likelihood of a satisfactory solution will increase if there is prior consideration of the choices available. This consideration of available alternatives should include recognition that professional nurses are intelligent adults who should be involved in the decision making process. Professional nurses are accountable for nursing judgments and actions regardless of the personal consequences. Providing safe nursing care to the patient is the ultimate objective of the professional nurse and the health care facility.

The Florida Nurses Association Labor and Employment Relations Commission acknowledges:

◆ the Florida Organization of Nurse Executives for input and collaboration in this document and the development of the previous 1989 edition of this document.

◆ the **Florida Nurses Association Labor and Employment Relations Commission** for final preparation of the revised 1999 edition of this document:

Michael Nilsson, CRRN, RN,
     Chairman
Patricia Quigley, Ph.D.,ARNP, CRRN
   Nancy Hartley
   Mary Healy Smith, ARNP
Patricia Cox, R.N.
Dorothy Walsh, R.N.
O'dell Anderson, R.N.

RESOURCES

To maintain current and accurate information on accountability of registered nurses for giving, accepting, or rejecting a work assignment, the following resources are suggested:

◆ **Health Care Facility**: Nurses are encouraged to seek consultation with their nurse manager/executives to discuss the facility's missions and goals as well as policies and procedures.

◆ The **Florida Nurses Association,** the largest statewide organization for registered nurses, represents nursing in the governmental, policy making arena and maintains current information and publications relative to the nurse's practice environment. Contact FNA, P.O. Box 536985, Orlando, FL 32853-6985, (407) 896-3261 or check out our website *http://www.floridanurse.org* for the benefits and services of membership, as well as priorities and activities of the Association.

◆ The **American Nurses Association** serves as the national clearing-house of information and offers publications on contemporary issues, including standards of practice, nursing ethics, as well as legal and regulatory issues. Contact ANA for a complimentary copy of the Publications Catalogue: ANA, 600 Maryland Avenue, SW, Suite 100 West, Washington, DC 20024-2571 or phone (202) 651-7000.

◆ ANA Survival Kit (1996) available through the American Nurses Association.

◆ ANA Basic Guide to Safe Delegation available through the American Nurses Association.

◆ ANA Code of Ethics for Nurses (1998) available through the American Nurses Association.

◆ ANA Standards and Scope of Practice (1997) available through the American Nurses Association.

◆ Nurse Practice Act (Florida Statutes 464, January 1994) and Administrative Rules (59S).

◆ Board of Nursing: 4080 Woodcock Drive, Jacksonville, FL 32207, or phone (904) 858-6940. A complimentary copy of the Nurse Practice Act is available to each registered nurse upon request.

Revised 08/99

Index

Page numbers followed by b indicate boxes, those followed by f indicate figures, and those followed by t indicate tables.

Publicly supported health-care organizations
  defined, 65
Punishment
  in effective management, 19f, 20
  in management theory, 17, 18f

Q

Quality Chasm Series
  of Institute of Medicine, 153
Quality of care
  delegation and, 135
  evaluation of, 151–157
    American Nurses Association in, 152t, 152–153
    continuous quality improvement in, 151, 154, 155f
    Institute of Medicine in, 153–154, 307–308, 308b
    JCAHO in, 151–153, 153b
    outcome in, 156t, 156–157
    process in, 155–156, 156t
    structure in, 155, 156t
  improvement in, 157–162, 158b, 160t–162t
Quality practice environments
  in codes of ethics, 295–296
Quasi-intentional tort
  overview of, 26
  slander and libel as, 27
Quebec
  licensure of nurses in, 37
Questionable practices
  reporting of, 205b, 205–206
Questions
  in job interview, 254–259
Quid pro quo
  in sexual harassment, 195

R

Rawls
  on justice, 50
Reality shock
  work-related stress and, 220
Recognition
  in empowerment, 71
  feedback for, 88
Record-keeping
  time management and, 176
Reframing
  in stress management, 232
Refreezing
  in change process, 113, 113f
Refusal of assignment
  in limit setting, 175
Refusal of treatment
  battery and, 28–29
Registered nurses
  as care managers, 147
  in client-focused care delivery model, 149
  delegation and, 124–130
  in differentiated practice care delivery model, 149–151
  shortage of, 144
  time management and, 171
  work assignment guidelines for, 303–309

in assignment despite objection, 304–305
  decision-making in, 305–308
  documentation of practice situation and, 304–305
  legal issues in, 306
  Nurse Practice Act and, 304
  nursing care delivery and, 303–304
  resources for, 309
Rejection letters
  job search, 251–252, 255f
Relationship-oriented concerns
  in delegation, 133–134, 134b
Relaxation
  in stress management, 230b, 230–231
Repetitive stress injuries
  workplace, 201
Reports
  of client information, 83–87
  of questionable practices, 205b, 205–206
  of sexual harassment, 196
  time management and, 174
Representation
  in effective management, 19f, 20
Research
  expertise enhanced by, 73–74
  supported by Agency for Healthcare Quality and Research, 293–294
Research-based knowledge
  code of ethics and, 297
Resistance
  in stress response, 218
Resistance to change, 113–117
  lowering of, 115–117
  planning and, 118
  recognition of, 115, 115t
  sources of, 114f, 114–115
Resolution
  in response to conflict, 98b
Resource allocation
  in client care economics, 142
  distributive justice and, 50
  in effective management, 19f, 20
  as source of conflict, 100, 100b
Resources
  as power source, 72
Respect
  in advance directive procedure, 35
  in code of ethics, 291
  in cultural diversity, 209–210
  in effective leadership, 10
Respondeat superior
  in malpractice, 26
Response
  to conflict, 98b
  to stress, 218–220, 219t
Responsibility
  in guidelines for work assignments, 305
Rest
  in stress management, 230
Restraints
  as false imprisonment, 28
  standards of practice and, 28

Standards of practice (*Continued*)
    informed consent as, 30
    negligence malpractice suits and, 29
    nursing boards and, 29
    Patient's Bill of Rights as, 30
    restraining patients and, 28
State Board Test Pool Examination, 37
Status
    as organizational goal, 67
    resistance to change and, 114–115
Statutory law
    overview of, 24
Strategic planning
    in quality improvement, 157–159, 158b, 160t–162t
Streamlining of work
    in time management, 176–177
Stress
    benefits of, 219–220
    continuum of response to, 218–220, 219t
    defined, 218
    management of, 228b–233b, 228–233
      in effective leadership, 9
      self-assessment of, 234b–235b
    work-related, 217–238
      adaptation to, 220–224, 221t–222t, 224t
      burnout and, 26b, 224–228
      delegation and, 133
      in response to change, 118
      in response to conflict, 99
Stressors
    categories of, 218
Strong Interest Inventory, 243
Structure
    organizational, 67–69, 68b, 68f
    in quality evaluation, 155
Structured care methodologies
    in quality improvement, 158–159
Substance abuse
    workplace, 201–202
Supervision
    delegation and, 125
    delegation *versus,* 126
    in guidelines for work assignments, 306
    Nurse Practice Act definition of, 304
Supervisory support
    value of, 206–207
Support
    in adaptation to workplace, 223
    in effective followership, 5
    as power source, 72
    in sexual harassment, 196
    in stress management, 232
    value of peer and supervisory, 206–207
Survival
    as organizational goal, 67
SWOT analysis
    in job search, 242–243, 263b
    in quality improvement, 157

T

Task *versus* relationship theory
    of leadership, 7

Tasks
    conflict from assignment of, 100, 100b
    delegation of, 130, 132b, 132f, 132–133
    efficient organizing of, 172–175, 173b–174b
    elimination of unnecessary, 175–176
Taylorism
    defined, 17
Team approach
    in client information conferences, 84
    in quality improvement, 157–158
Team care delivery model, 145
Technology
    burnout and, 226–227
    in client care economics, 144
    code of ethics and, 296
    in ethical dilemmas, 57–59
    in time management, 174, 177, 179
Teleological ethical theories, 47–48
Terminal condition
    defined, 35
Territoriality
    as source of conflict, 99b–100b, 99–100
Terrorism
    readiness for, 187–188, 206
Thank-you letters
    job search, 251, 253f
Theories
    on human motivation, 283
    nursing, 283–285
    of psychosexual development, 283
    of psychosocial development stages, 283
    X and Y of management, 17–18, 18f
Threats
    to professional identity
      resistance to change and, 114–115
      as source of conflict, 100, 100b
    to safety and security, 187–192, 188t, 189b, 190t
      defined, 192
      resistance to change and, 114
      as sources of conflict, 100, 100b
      workplace violence as, 192t, 192–195, 193b–194b, 194t
    in SWOT analysis, 243
Time management, 169–181
    cultural diversity and, 209
    direct client care and, 171–172
    documentation and, 171
    fallacies in, 171
    limit-setting in, 175–176
    organization in, 172–175, 174b
    overview of, 170
    rhythm model in, 179, 180t
    schedule for, 84, 85f, 177, 178f
    staff makeup and, 170–171
    streamlining in, 176–177, 178f, 179, 180t
    time log in, 176, 178f
    time perception in, 170, 170b
Tort law. *See also* specific issues
    overview of, 25–26
Total care delivery model, 145
Total quality management
    defined, 151